Label-Free Biosensor Methods in Drug Discovery

Edited by

Ye Fang

*Biochemical Technologies, Science and Technology Division,
Corning Incorporated, Corning, NY, USA*

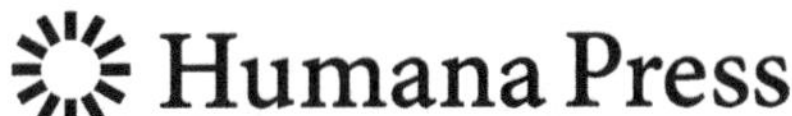

Humana Press

Editor
Ye Fang
Biochemical Technologies
Science and Technology Division
Corning Incorporated
Corning, NY, USA

ISSN 1557-2153   ISSN 1940-6053   (electronic)
Methods in Pharmacology and Toxicology
ISBN 978-1-4939-2616-9   ISBN 978-1-4939-2617-6   (eBook)
DOI 10.1007/978-1-4939-2617-6

Library of Congress Control Number: 2015936478

Springer New York Heidelberg Dordrecht London

Humana Press is a brand of Springer
Springer Science+Business Media LLC New York is part of Springer Science+Business Media (www.springer.com)

Preface

The past decade has witnessed a great expansion of label-free biosensor platforms and methods. Although surface plasmon resonance (SPR) still is a leading player in label-free biosensor market, data points generated by other newer techniques have quickly surpassed those obtained using SPR in the recent years. This is largely due to the development and implementation of high-throughput screening-compatible biosensor systems and innovative assay methods for drug screening and profiling. Nowadays, label-free techniques have been implemented in various stages of drug discovery process including hit identification, lead optimization, target engagement determination, drug safety assessment, and clinical diagnostics.

Label-free is advantageous in that it bypasses the need of labels, reporters, and cell engineering, all of which are common to labeled techniques but may introduce artifacts in assay results. Label-free is also advantageous in that it enables continuous monitoring of biomolecular interactions and cellular responses in real time, so the kinetics of drug-target binding or cell signaling can be characterized in detail. However, label-free generally suffers from relatively low sensitivity for biochemical assays or relatively poor molecular specificity for cell-based measurements due to the facts that these biosensors typically monitor an integrated cellular response upon drug stimulation and many drugs display polypharmacology. Therefore, assay design to improve sensitivity and specificity is essential to adopt label-free in many applications.

Aiming to assist academic and industrial researchers involved in drug and probe discovery to adopt label-free techniques for their research, this inaugural book, *Label-Free Biosensor Methods in Drug Discovery*, provides a new avenue for rapid access to a focused collection of highly regarded contributions in the field. This book addresses several fundamental and practical aspects as to how to implement label-free methods in drug discovery process. This book covers a wide range of topics, including binding kinetics determination, fragment screening, antibody epitope mapping, protein–protein interaction profiling and screening, receptor pathway deconvolution, drug pharmacology profiling and screening, target identification, drug toxicity assessment, and physical phenotype profiling and diagnostics based on various cellular processes such as cell adhesion, migration, invasion, infection, and inflammation.

Corning, NY, USA   *Ye Fang*

Contents

Contributors

BENJAMIN AROETI • *Department of Cell and Developmental Biology, The Alexander Silberman Institute of Life Sciences, The Hebrew University of Jerusalem, Jerusalem, Israel*

CARYN E. BACON • *Lilly Research Laboratories, Eli Lilly and Company, Indianapolis, IN, USA*

MELVYN BAEZ • *Lilly Research Laboratories, Eli Lilly and Company, Indianapolis, IN, USA*

AUDREY B. BERGERON • *Corning Life Sciences, Corning Incorporated, Kennebunk, ME, USA*

SZILVIA BŐSZE • *Research Group of Peptide Chemistry, Hungarian Academy of Sciences, Eötvös Loránd University, Budapest, Hungary*

PHILIPPE BOURASSA • *Département de pharmacologie et physiologie, Université de Sherbrooke, Sherbrooke, QC, Canada*

BILLY BRETON • *Biomolecular Screening Facility, School of Life Sciences, Ecole Polytechnique Fédérale de Lausanne (EPFL), Lausanne, Switzerland*

LISA M. BROAD • *Lilly Research Center, Eli Lilly and Company, Windlesham, Surrey, UK*

BENJAMIN D. BROOKS • *Wasatch Microfluidics, LLC, Salt Lake City, UT, USA*

AMANDA E. BROOKS • *Department of Pharmaceutics, North Dakota State Univerisity, Fargo, ND, UT, USA*

RUFUS W. BURLINGAME • *Genalyte, Inc., San Diego, CA, USA*

RHONDA L. CARTER • *Center for Translational Medicine, Temple University School of Medicine, Philadelphia, PA, USA*

PAUL G. CHARETTE • *Département de génie électrique et informatique, Université de Sherbrooke, Sherbrooke, QC, Canada*

JENNIFER Y. CHEN • *Department of Chemistry, Drexel University, Philadelphia, PA, USA*

MATTHEW COOPER • *Institute for Molecular Bioscience, Queensland Bioscience Precinct, The University of Queensland, St. Lucia, QLD, Australia*

S. NICOLE DAVIDOFF • *Wasatch Microfluidics, LLC, Salt Lake City, UT, USA*

NOAH T. DITTO • *Wasatch Microfluidics, LLC, Salt Lake City, UT, USA*

DARIO DOLLER • *Lundbeck Research USA, Paramus, NJ, USA*

JOSH ECKMAN • *Wasatch Microfluidics, LLC, Salt Lake City, UT, USA*

YE FANG • *Biochemical Technologies, Science and Technology Division, Corning Incorporated, Corning, NY, USA*

CHRISTIAN C. FELDER • *Lilly Research Laboratories, Eli Lilly and Company, Indianapolis, IN, USA*

ALICE GAO • *Corning Life Science, Corning Incorporated, Corning, NY, USA*

MARCELA P. GARCIA • *Department of Chemistry, Drexel University, Philadelphia, PA, USA*

LOUIS GENDRON • *Département de physiologie et biophysique, Centre de recherche du CHU de Sherbrooke, Institut de pharmacologie de Sherbrooke, Université de Sherbrooke, Sherbrooke, QC, Canada*

STEFAN GESCHWINDNER • *Discovery Sciences, AstraZeneca R&D, Mölndal, Sweden*

HANNAH J. GITSCHIER • *Corning Life Sciences, Corning Incorporated, Kennebunk, ME, USA*

MARTIN A. GLEESON • *Genalyte, Inc., San Diego, CA, USA*

PAUL J. GOLDSMITH • *Lilly Research Center, Eli Lilly and Company, Windlesham, Surrey, UK*

MICHEL GRANDBOIS • *Département de pharmacologie, Centre de recherche du CHU de Sherbrooke, Institut de pharmacologie de Sherbrooke, Université de Sherbrooke, Sherbrooke, QC, Canada*

TYLER GROVE • *Genalyte, Inc., San Diego, CA, USA*

REENA HALAI • *The University of Queensland, St. Lucia, QLD, Australia*

JÜRGEN HESCHELER • *Institute of Neurophysiology, University of Cologne, Cologne, Germany*

MICHIHIRO HIDE • *Department of Dermatology, Graduate School of Biomedical and Health Science, Hiroshima University, Hiroshima, Japan*

ROBERT HORVATH • *Nanobiosensorics Group, Research Centre for Natural Sciences, Institute for Technical Physics and Materials Science, Hungarian Academy of Sciences, Budapest, Hungary*

XINYAN HUANG • *Lundbeck Research USA, Paramus, NJ, USA*

MUZAMMIL IQBAL • *Genalyte, Inc., San Diego, CA, USA*

FABIEN KUTTLER • *Biomolecular Screening Facility, School of Life Sciences, Ecole Polytechnique Fédérale de Lausanne (EPFL),, Lausanne, Switzerland*

PAUL H. LEE • *Molecular Structure and Characterization, Amgen Inc., Thousand Oaks, CA, USA*

XINMIAO LIANG • *Key Laboratory of Separation Science for Analytical Chemistry, Dalian Institute of Chemical Physics, Chinese Academy of Sciences, Dalian, Liaoning, China*

RIDHA LIMAME • *Laboratory of Experimental Cancer Research, Department of Radiation Oncology and Experimental Cancer Research, Ghent University Hospital, Ghent, Belgium*

SHUANG LIU • *Department of Pharmacology and Molecular Science, Johns Hopkins University School of Medicine, Baltimore, MD, USA; Institute of Physics, Chinese Academy of Sciences, Beijing, China*

HUIBIN LU • *Institute of Physics, Chinese Academy of Sciences, Beijing, China*

JEAN-SÉBASTIEN MALTAIS • *Département de pharmacologie, Université de Sherbrooke, Sherbrooke, QC, Canada*

FILOMAIN NGUEMO • *Institute of Neurophysiology, University of Cologne, Cologne, Germany*

NORBERT ORGOVAN • *Department of Biological Physics, Eötvös Loránd University, Budapest, Hungary; Nanobiosensorics Group, Research Centre for Natural Sciences, Institute for Technical Physics and Materials Science, Hungarian Academy of Sciences, Budapest, Hungary*

LYNN S. PENN • *Department of Chemistry, Drexel University, Philadelphia, PA, USA*

BEATRIX PETER • *Nanobiosensorics Group, Research Centre for Natural Sciences, Institute for Technical Physics and Materials Science, Hungarian Academy of Sciences, Budapest, Hungary; Faculty of Information Technology, Doctoral School of Molecular- and Nanotechnologies University of Pannonia, Veszprém, Hungary*

XIANXIN QIU • *Biosensor National Special Laboratory, Department of Biomedical Engineering, Zhejiang University, Hangzhou, China*

JEREMY J. RAMSDEN • *Clore Laboratory, University of Buckingham, Buckingham, UK; Centre for Molecular Recognition, Collegium Basilea (Institute of Advanced Study), Basel, Switzerland*

DAVID H. RANDLE • *Corning Life Sciences, Corning Incorporated, Kennebunk, ME, USA*

BENJAMIN RAPPAZ • *Biomolecular Screening Facility, School of Life Sciences, Ecole Polytechnique Fédérale de Lausanne (EPFL), Lausanne, Switzerland*

ASHLEY A. REPAS • *Center for Translational Medicine, Temple University School of Medicine, Philadelphia, PA, USA*

RANDY ROMERO • *Genalyte, Inc., San Diego, CA, USA*

DOUGLAS A. SCHOBER • *Lilly Research Laboratories, Eli Lilly and Company, Indianapolis, IN, USA*

JUDITH SEMMLER • *Institute of Neurophysiology, University of Cologne, Cologne, Germany*

THOMAS SÖLLRADL • *Département de génie électrique et informatique, Université de Sherbrooke, Sherbrooke, QC, Canada*

BÁLINT SZABÓ • *Department of Biological Physics, Eötvös Loránd University, Budapest, Hungary*

INNA SZÉKÁCS • *Research Centre for Natural Sciences, Institute of Technical Physics and Materials Science, Hungarian Academy of Sciences, Budapest, Hungary*

DOUGLAS G. TILLEY • *Department of Pharmacology and Center for Translational Medicine, Temple University School of Medicine, Philadelphia, PA, USA*

GERARDO TURCATTI • *Biomolecular Screening Facility, School of Life Sciences, Ecole Polytechnique Fédérale de Lausanne (EPFL), Lausanne, Switzerland*

ANNABEL WANG • *Genalyte, Inc., San Diego, CA, USA*

JIXIA WANG • *Key Laboratory of Separation Science for Analytical Chemistry, Dalian Institute of Chemical Physics, Chinese Academy of Sciences, Dalian, Liaoning, China*

PING WANG • *Biosensor National Special Laboratory, Department of Biomedical Engineering, Zhejiang University, Hangzhou, China*

OLIVIER DE WEVER • *Laboratory of Experimental Cancer Research, Department of Radiation Oncology and Experimental Cancer Research, Ghent University Hospital, Ghent, Belgium*

SOO-HANG WONG • *Molecular Structure and Characterization, Amgen Inc., Thousand Oaks, CA, USA*

JUN XI • *Department of Chemistry, Drexel University, Philadelphia, PA, USA*

YUHKI YANASE • *Department of Dermatology, Graduate School of Biomedical and Health Science, Hiroshima University, Hiroshima, Japan*

GUOZHEN YANG • *Institute of Physics, Chinese Academy of Sciences, Beijing, China*

PEIYI YANG • *Lilly Research Laboratories, Eli Lilly and Company, Indianapolis, IN, USA*

VICTOR YASHUNSKY • *Robert H. Smith Faculty of Agriculture, Food and Environment, Institute of Biochemistry, Food Science and Nutrition, The Hebrew University of Jerusalem, Rehovot, Israel*

XIULI ZHANG • *Key Laboratory of Separation Science for Analytical Chemistry, Dalian Institute of Chemical Physics, Chinese Academy of Sciences, Dalian, Liaoning, China*

HUAILING ZHONG • *U-Pharm Laboratories LLC, Parsippany, NJ, USA*

JIE ZHOU • *Biosensor National Special Laboratory, Department of Biomedical Engineering, Zhejiang University, Hangzhou, China*

HENG ZHU • *Department of Pharmacology and Molecular Science, Johns Hopkins University School of Medicine, Baltimore, MD, USA*

Part I

Review

Chapter 1

Label-Free Technologies: Which Technique to Use and What to Watch Out for!

Reena Halai and Matthew Cooper

Abstract

The number of different label-free platforms available for drug discovery and life science research has exploded in the last decade. Until the late 1990s, the field was dominated by just four technologies: mass spectrometry (MS), nuclear magnetic resonance (NMR), calorimetry, and surface plasmon resonance (SPR). Commercial systems based on these technologies were marketed as "easy to use," with companies and review writers (including ourselves ☺) promoting the virtues of "label-free" assays, their inherent simplicity, and direct, easy-to-interpret results. However, label-free technologies often require carefully designed experimental controls and analytical rigor in the interpretation of what at first appears to be simplistic data. As with any assay technology, label-free platforms are also affected by physical and biological artifacts, which can be erroneously interpreted to be related to drug action. In this chapter we review the fundamentals of drug action in a biological system, the physical basis of different label-free systems, and then discuss the advantages and artifacts associated with each technique. We hope that this will help guide the reader towards a rational choice of technology for their particular project. Forearmed with an awareness of the pitfalls that can lead a beguiled label-free devotee astray, label-free assays can indeed illuminate the complex biology of drug action.

Key words Drug action, Design of experiment, Data quality, Robustness, Reproducibility, Experimental controls, Binding affinity, Binding specificity, Binding kinetics, Binding thermodynamics

1 Drug Action and Biosensors

A drug candidate that is designed to act against a particular target must first bind to the target to initiate the desired biological response. Drug efficacy can be associated with target-binding kinetics and thermodynamics, residence time, and type of target modulation that leads to a biological response. Compounds that exhibit the same binding potency may have completely different on and off rates and enthalpies and entropies of binding, and subsequently show very different functional therapeutic effects [1]. An in-depth review by Copeland et al. in 2006 [2] highlights the advantages of longer residence times for target selectivity and pharmacological effect, with the underlying take home message

Ye Fang (ed.), *Label-Free Biosensor Methods in Drug Discovery*, Methods in Pharmacology and Toxicology,
DOI 10.1007/978-1-4939-2617-6_1, © Springer Science+Business Media New York 2015

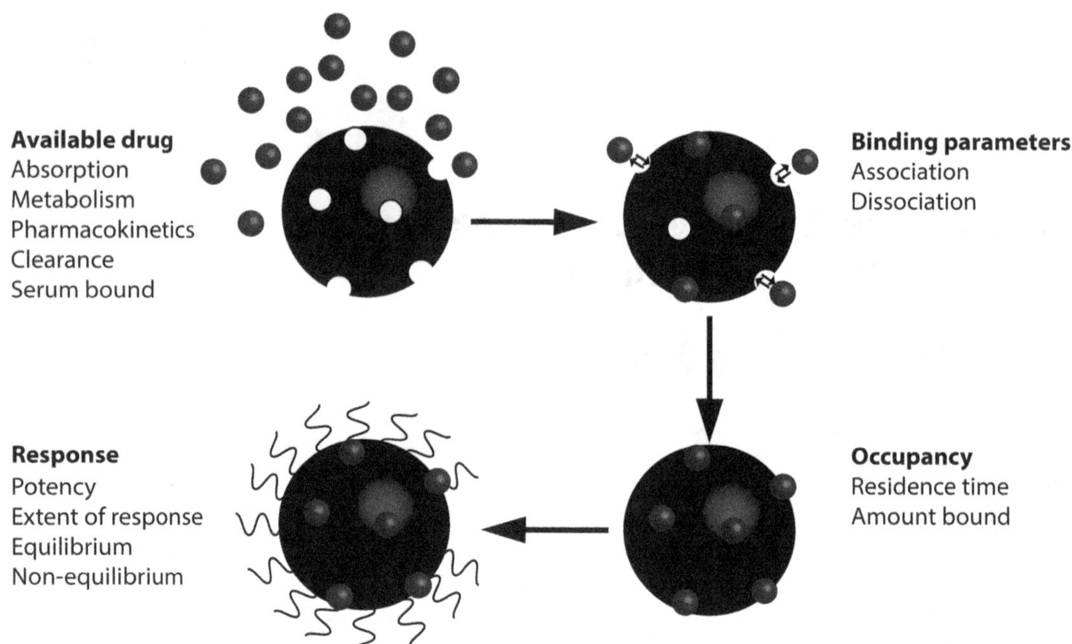

Fig. 1 A schematic of drug action and the key parameters that regulate this process. Before a drug can reach its target, it encounters and must overcome numerous obstacles, such as metabolism, clearance, serum binding, absorption, and membrane transport, the latter of which is critical for intracellular targets. When the drug eventually does reach the binding site on its cognate target, it is further governed by how quickly it can associate with and dissociate from the target, and how long it can occupy the receptor. Generally speaking a fast on-rate and a slow off-rate (with concomitant higher affinity) are ideal characteristics of a good drug; however if seeking fast-acting, short-lived drugs, slower off-rates can be disadvantageous

being simply the longer a receptor-ligand complex is maintained, the longer the drug can have an effect. The residence time for a drug binding to its receptor is a function of its dissociation rate, which is purely a function of the molecular recognition between receptor and drug, and the number of collisions per unit time with the receptor-binding site, often termed the observed on-rate, which is a function of drug concentration and association rate: ($k_{obs} = [\text{drug}].k_{ass}$). The latter value can thus be modified by changing drug dosing levels, bioavailability, and formulation, all of which affect pharmacokinetics and pharmacodynamics (PK-PD) (Fig. 1).

An understanding of binding kinetics, thermodynamics, along with a detailed nature of a molecular recognition event, is a fundamental pre-requisite to success in drug design and discovery. In order to gain such an understanding of binding dynamics, traditional assays utilized labels (such as particles, chemiluminescent, bioluminescent, and fluorescent tags). However, these reporter molecules have the potential to interfere with the binding interaction itself. Furthermore, such assays are generally restricted to end-point measurements, where a particular time for readout of the response is sometimes chosen arbitrarily. However, there are now numerous different methods that allow direct detection of such biochemical interactions without the use of labels, where data is produced in real time. These methods exploit various physical properties of the analyte and/or receptor, and use a biosensor to transduce changes in these properties into a quantifiable signal. The introduction of label-free biosensors to study drug-receptor interactions has provided a more in-depth understanding of receptor-ligand binding kinetics, without the hindrance of labels. Advancements in the field have seen the introduction of different instruments with new modes of detection, each with their own advantages and disadvantages, performance, and data quality (Table 1).

2   Solution-Based Measurements

Before the introduction of high-throughput optical biosensors, techniques such as isothermal titration calorimetry (ITC) and nuclear magnetic resonance (NMR) were the methods of choice to study ligand-receptor interactions. Mass spectrometry was then used extensively in the 1990s to screen for drug-receptor interactions. More recently, microscale thermophoresis (MST) combines a flow-based, low-volume format in free solution with label-free readout of drugs binding to receptors.

2.1   Mass Spectrometry

Mass spectrometry continues to be used for protein-ligand binding interactions with the use of electrospray ionization mass spectrometry (ESI-MS). Nanoelectrospray ionization mass spectrometry (nESI-MS) has been popular to study non-covalent interactions and their associated kinetics [3, 4]. Using ESI-MS, mass shift change indications from ligand titration quantify bound and unbound proteins, where using a ratio of the ion signal from these two states allows the dissociation constant to be calculated [4]. To be able to infer this from the experiment, it is assumed that the ligand-bound conformation has the same ionizing potential as the unbound form and that no ligand dissociates from the protein in the mass spectrometer [5]. However, despite the success of ESI-MS for detecting such interactions, whether or not the solution conformations are the same in the gas phase is a concern [6, 7]. Furthermore, sample quality is a key feature with mass spectrometry, where samples that may contain degraded protein and other nonnative structural proteins can severely hamper the success of this technique [8]. Another technical consideration with mass spectroscopy is its limitations in sensitivity [9], and compatibility of buffer solutions [10], making ITC and MST more favorable techniques in these cases.

Table 1
Label-free biosensor techniques, and their key applications, advantages, and disadvantages

Technology	Where used[a]	Major applications	Main advantages	Main disadvantages
Calorimetry (DSC, ITC)	H2L, LO	– Binding thermodynamics – Binding stoichiometry – Compound purity and stability	– Solution-based—true label free – Wide range of interactions and solvents – Relative ease of use – Development in automation and higher throughput in progress	– Solubility and dissolution artifacts – Currently low throughput – Large amounts of sample required – Buffer incompatibilities – Current lack of automation
Cell impedance	HTS, H2L, LO	– Whole-cell screening – Secondary screening – Cardiotoxicity screening	– Wide Mwt range – Pathway-independent readout – Ease of use	– Limited utility with non-adherent cells – Averaged cell response—including off-target effects – Matrix ionic strength artifacts
Mass spectrometry	HTS, H2L, LO, ADME/T Clinical	– Proteomics, metabolomics – Target de-orphaning – Fragment screening – Metabolite ID – Drug pharmacokinetics – Drug efficacy biomarkers	– High sensitivity – High specificity – Small sample volume required – Interface with multiple separation techniques and sample types	– Sample heterogeneity – Matrix effects – Limited dynamic range for some compounds

Nuclear magnetic resonance	H2L, LO	– Fragment screening – Structure determination – Purity determination – Mode of action/binding	– Solution-based—true label free – Sample recovery after screen – High information content – Minimal sample preparation	– Low throughput – Limited utility with many important targets (e.g., GPCRs, ion channels) – Sensitivity issues
Resonant waveguides	HTS, H2L	– Whole-cell screening – Binding affinity – Epitope mapping and immunoassays – Plasma protein binding	– Wide Mwt range – Pathway-independent readout – Ease of use	– Averaged cell response—includes off-target effects – Bulk refractive index artifacts
Surface plasmon resonance/bio-layer interferometry	H2L, LO	– Binding affinity and kinetics – Immunoassays – Epitope mapping – Plasma protein binding	– Sensitive with high Mwt compounds – Regeneration allows reuse of chips	– Limited sensitivity with low Mwt compounds – Bulk refractive index artifacts

[a]Key: *ADME/T* absorption digestion metabolism excretion toxicity, *DSC* Differential scanning calorimetry, *H2L* hit to lead, *HTS* high-throughput screening, *LO* lead optimization, *Clinical* phase I–III clinical trials and post-launch phase IV drug efficacy/toxicity monitoring, *Mwt* molecular weight

2.2 Isothermal Titration Calorimetry (ITC)

When a reaction takes place there is a change in heat (enthalpy); differences between the amount of heat given off and the amount of heat taken in is the enthalpy change of a reaction [11] and the basis of what is exploited for ITC. ITC works on maintaining the temperature of the cell during an experiment over several injections. By measuring any changes in heat either absorbed or released during bond formation, one can infer calculations of enthalpy, dissociation constant, and stoichiometry [12]. Unlike surface chemistry-based techniques, protein immobilization is not required, but the relatively low sensitivity of the ITC instruments means that high concentrations are needed for low-affinity binders [4]. Furthermore, a study by Baranauskiene et al. [13] highlighted that inconsistencies in validation and lack of attention to experimental parameters such as pH, temperature, and buffers can lead to reports of enthalpies that vary significantly from scientist to scientist for the same biological system under investigation. In particular, heats of dilution related to ligand addition can sometimes be misinterpreted as resulting from receptor binding.

2.3 Microscale Thermophoresis

MST is another solution-based method by which affinities, stoichiometry, competition, and dissociation constants can be measured. Changes in the movement of molecules along temperature gradients [14] related to solvation entropy, size, and charge are monitored to determine binding affinities and kinetics. Unlike some of the techniques highlighted above, MST appears far more resilient to the common problems of buffer incompatibilities, or crude samples; binding data has been reported with unprocessed blood samples, thus saving time on sample preparation and allowing measurements in a relevant clinical matrix [15].

3 Optical Biosensors

Although there are many different types of biosensors, optical biosensors are more readily used for understanding receptor-binding kinetics [16], and essentially all exploit some characteristic of light as a method of detection [17]. For example, since the introduction of the BIAcore from Pharmacia Biotechnology (now part of GE Healthcare), surface plasmon resonance (SPR) has by far become the most popular method for the measurement of binding kinetics. However, not all optical based biosensors are the same; differences in their sensitivity, cost, ease of use, resolution, and robustness must be considered in evaluating the instrument and the quality of the data generated bearing technical restrictions and configurations in mind.

The lack of a wider uptake of optical biosensors by big pharmaceutical companies can largely be attributed to one of the named factors: cost [18]. In the early stages of drug discovery, screening campaigns of half a million compounds or more are usually undertaken. It is therefore of utmost importance to consider the cost per data point. As optical based biosensors are manufactured with expensive components, the cost of the biosensors is high [18]. There is a small trade-off as the cost of labels to tag the protein/ligand is no longer needed, and an attempt to reduce cost by allowing consumers to reuse the senor is possible [18]. Improvements in manufacturing and new competitors entering the market have seen costs reduced over time, but there is still significant room for improvement. As well as large pharmaceutical companies, optical instruments such as the BIAcore have established themselves well in numerous academic laboratories. Academic laboratories are generally financially constrained and research scientists are obligated to get more "bang for their buck." In these instances, due to the high cost of the sensor chips, research scientists may attempt to regenerate the sensor chips a few times to many, and inadvertently compromise data quality, so it is absolutely essential to reduce costs to a point where data can be generated without compromising on quality and reliability.

4 Types of Optical Biosensors

4.1 BIAcore

The BIAcore utilizes SPR to detect changes close to the sensor surface by shifts in the refractive index [16]. Since the release of the first BIAcore instrument almost a quarter of a century ago in 1990, a number of new models have been released with increased sensitivity and throughput, such as the T200 and BIAcore 4000. The T200 system is able to run 384 samples unattended and quickly co-evaluate up to 5,000 samples in a single evaluation according to the manufacturer's product description, whilst the 4,000 can run 60 h of unattended operation with parallel analysis of up to 16 targets or 4,800 interactions in 24 h. This is a vast improvement on some of the earlier systems that were developed and underutilized by big pharmaceutical companies due to their lack of throughput. As well as the improved throughput, the second key component of the newer models is improved sensitivity, which is crucial for the detection of low-molecular-weight compounds. Since the refractive index change at the sensor surface in SPR is directly related to the mass of the ligand, small-molecular-weight compounds will generate a much smaller response relative to those with larger molecular weights. In this instance, small-molecular-weight ligands could compromise the quality of the data due to working at ranges close to the limits of detection. This is by no means to say that high-quality data cannot be generated if the correct controls are included in the experimental design [19, 20]. The general issues of the quality of data generated using the SPR can also be attributed to the quality of the compounds, the solubility of the compounds, their purity and selectivity, and the quality of the software that exists for their analysis [16]. Here it is important to include negative control compounds for screening, account and calibrate for the effects of differential solvent partitioning on different flow cells (e.g., dimethyl sulfoxide, DMSO, titration), and choose at least one or more surface controls (e.g., a non-related receptor *in addition* to a blank flow cell control).

4.2 Octet® Systems

The Octet® system by ForteBIO (now part of Pall Corp.) is another optical label-free biosensor that allows for the detection of biomolecular interactions. It utilizes a phenomenon known as bio-layer interferometry (BLI) to detect shifts in interference patterns of reflected white light. Biomolecular interactions between a target and an analyte cause a change at the biosensor tip, which results in real-time detection of the binding event displayed as a shift in the wavelength. BLI technology can be used to probe protein-binding interactions, affinity, and kinetics, similar to the abilities of the BIAcore, except that the direct interaction at the sensor surface means that lysate, media, and other complex biological samples can be used with little effect from interfering components of the sample matrix.

4.3 BIND®

The SRU biosystems BIND® is a high-throughput optical label-free biosensor based on a guided-mode resonant filter that is made from multiple plastic films embedded into a microplate [18]. Utilizing the properties of a photonic crystal, the microplates and sensor are compatible with multiple different assay formats, including protein-ligand interaction assays, cell-based assays, and screening style assays. The liquid-handling robotics and ease of automation using these instruments have seen them being used by large pharmaceutical companies [17].

4.4 EPIC®
and Enspire®

The benchtop PerkinElmer Enpire® and its predecessor the Corning® EPIC® system are two other high-throughput optical systems currently on the market. These two label-free plate readers exploit the properties of an evanescent wave to provide changes in "dynamic mass redistribution" [21] within the cells. The EPIC® system is a higher throughput version of the benchtop version introduced by PerkinElmer. There are slight changes in temperature control and plate-handling robotics between the two instruments, but fundamentally they use the same detection system as a readout of the biological interactions under investigation [22]. Much like the SRU Bind®, these instruments can detect protein-ligand interactions and cell-based phenomena such as receptor signalling, toxicity, and proliferation, amongst others.

5   Quality and Assessment Measures

Although label-free instruments have been around for some time now and can be used with relative ease, several key parameters need to be considered to ensure high-quality data. For SPR and other surface-based optical biosensors, target immobilization, analyte affinity, regenerations, signal corrections, wash procedures, and inclusion of the correct controls are required in order to obtain the most reliable and accurate data.

5.1   Immobilization

The protein (target) must be immobilized onto the sensor surface without any interference to its activity or blockade of its active site [23]. There are two ways to achieve this, by either direct immobilization or indirect immobilization. Direct immobilization involves covalent coupling whereas indirect immobilization utilizes a capture method that exploits reagents immobilized to the sensor surface that recognize specific parts of the target being exploited. Both methods have their advantages and disadvantages; for example direct coupling allows the immobilization of a broader range of proteins that are reasonably pure [24]. However, this comes at the cost of protein coupling heterogeneity and the inability to regenerate the senor surface for reuse. With respect to this, the indirect coupling method proves more beneficial as the sensor surface can be regenerated with the use of agents that specifically allow the covalent interaction between the target and analyte to be disrupted. Furthermore, there is a far reduced chance of any impact on the activity of the protein with indirect capture, and less heterogeneity in the protein orientation during capture as a tag is required to capture the target to the immobilized reagent on the sensor surface [23, 24]. Where possible, a tagged receptor for more controlled, oriented immobilization is preferred. In the case of random, carbodiimide-mediated coupling, the drug-binding site can be blocked with an endogenous ligand (if available) during the coupling procedure.

5.2   Affinity

The power of some optical biosensors to measure a range of interactions from as low as picomolar to millimolar has seen their use in early stages of drug discovery where the detection of weak interactions is required [25–27].

5.3   Solubility

The use of solvents such as DMSO is often needed when handling early-stage and library compounds with limited aqueous solubility. However, as is the case with many biological assays, solvents are not recommended at high concentrations in label-free assays. Although solubility of the analyte can affect the lower limit of the affinity, high concentrations of such solvents can be detrimental to the protein of interest and thus produce artifacts in the results. Stringent controls can help to identify and ameliorate the effect of these artifacts, but not completely eliminate them [23].

5.4 Regeneration

Sensor chip regeneration refers to the restoration of the sensor surface to its original state prior to the analysis of any analyte. Although a simplistic idea, the regeneration process has a few caveats one must bear in mind if the quality of the data after regeneration is not to be compromised. If the regeneration process is not carried out efficiently or to completion each time, this will directly impact the quality of the assay and furthermore reduce the number of times the sensor surface can be regenerated and reused. When direct target immobilization has been employed the regeneration process will remove the bound analyte. If a capture method has been employed for immobilization, then both target and analyte will be removed. The buffer needed for regeneration depends on the strength of the interaction, where ideally conditions that allow analyte to dissociate, but keep the activity of the immobilized receptor, are ideal [23]. If the analyte is able to dissociate fast and the baseline is reached with the normal washing procedure, there is no need to use regeneration buffers (GE Healthcare BIAcore sensor surface handbook). However, when needed, and considering regeneration buffers, the pH of the solution and the use of different detergents are necessary depending on the type of target that has been immobilized. For example the regeneration condition for small molecules is likely to be significantly different to antibodies. In such situations, it is recommended to undertake scouting experiments, where multiple combinations of compositions are tested to find the optimal condition overall [23].

To judge if the ideal regeneration condition has been met, one must see the same analyte response over multiple cycles of regeneration. If a creeping regeneration baseline is observed, there may be a problem in the regeneration condition. For example, a gradual incline in the baseline over multiple regenerations may suggest only partial regeneration. On the other hand a fairly large drop in the baseline is likely to indicate incompatibilities between the stability of the target and the regeneration conditions [23]. A small decline in the baseline is acceptable as long as the analyte response is normal. In an ideal world with complete regeneration, the baseline should return to normal and all analyte responses between cycles should be the same; however this is not always the case. One must make the judgement call that if the analyte response is consistent relative to baseline, increasing and decreasing trends in the baseline can be somewhat overlooked.

6   Controls

6.1 Verifying the Surface

The functional verification of the sensor chip is important when the sensor surface has been generated for the first experiment, but more importantly when the sensor has been stored over time. This can be done by simply testing multiple increasing concentrations of analyte or testing the maximum binding activity and comparing it to the theoretical calculation, to determine changes in the efficiency of the immobilized target.

6.2 Immobilization Levels

To ensure that the correct level of target immobilization is achieved, a number of different factors need to be considered. One would assume that saturating the surface with the target would be the best way and in some instances it is; for example if the analyte is small relative to the immobilized target, high immobilization levels may be necessary to observe a response. However, if the immobilized target is small, large amounts of target immobilized onto the surface can cause what is known as steric hindrance and surface crowding, particularly at high concentrations of analyte [28].

6.3 Bulk Refractive Index

Bulk refractive index artifacts arise as SPR or other optical detection systems fundamentally measure changes in the dielectric constant at the sensor surface, which are measured as changes in refractive index imparted by ligands binding to surface-associated receptors. As well as detecting changes in the refractive index that arise from the receptor-ligand interaction, changes in the refractive index that arise from incompatibilities between the running buffer and the analyte buffer are also detected, and referred to as bulk refractive index changes. There are ways to reduce this effect by avoiding large amounts of DMSO, salt, and other interfering components in the analyte buffer. The bulk refractive index is readily detectable if a reference surface is used and identifiable by a distinct square shape signal. This signal on the reference pad should be subtracted from the signal generated on the binding surface, to yield the signal from the analyte–target interaction [23]. With solvents or solutes that can impart a large refractive index change (e.g., DMSO), it is best to run a titration of this interferent in the running buffer to produce a calibration curve, which can be used to further normalize the bulk refractive index change [29].

6.4 Nonspecific Binding

Not only is the reference surface useful for detecting bulk refractive index changes, but also nonspecific binding. Providing that both the reference surface and binding surface have been subjected to the same conditions, nonspecific analyte binding, resulting from hydrophobic or electrostatic interactions, can be identified on the reference surface.

7 Conclusion

This chapter has highlighted some of the different label-free biosensors available to study ligand-receptor interactions, whether they are based on solution phase or surface-interface detection. Label-free biosensors can generate high-quality reliable data, if the methodology and experimental design are well thought out. A number of key issues that relate to individual instruments and types of detection have been touched upon in this chapter. If the experimenter is able to address these issues and include the relevant controls, these technologies have enormous potential. Indeed some of the issues are a common theme amongst all the technologies, such as levels of DMSO or compound solubility issues for example. With the real-time measurements and the increased sensitivity of label-free biosensors, these issues are of greater concern as this method of detection can be less forgiving than some of the traditional methods for probing biomolecular interactions. However, these are not insurmountable and thus still make label-free detection of ligand-receptor interaction a more representative method of detection to label-based methods.

References

1. Yin N, Pei J, Lai L (2013) A comprehensive analysis of the influence of drug binding kinetics on drug action at molecular and systems levels. Mol Biosyst 9:1381–1389

2. Copeland RA, Pompliano DL, Meek TD (2006) Drug-target residence time and its implications for lead optimization. Nat Rev Drug Discov 5:730–739

3. Jecklin MC, Touboul D, Bovet C, Wortmann A, Zenobi R (2008) Which electrospray-based ionization method best reflects protein-ligand interactions found in solution? a comparison of ESI, nanoESI, and ESSI for the determination of dissociation constants with mass spectrometry. J Am Soc Mass Spectrom 19:332–343

4. Jecklin MC, Schauer S, Dumelin CE, Zenobi R (2009) Label-free determination of protein-ligand binding constants using mass spectrometry and validation using surface plasmon resonance and isothermal titration calorimetry. J Mol Recognit 22:319–329

5. Daniel JRM, Friess SD, Rajagopalan S, Wendt S, Zenobi R (2002) Quantitative determination of noncovalent binding interactions using soft ionization mass spectrometry. Int J Mass Spectrom 216:1–27

6. Hossain BM, Simmons DA, Konermann L (2005) Do electrospray mass spectra reflect the ligand binding state of proteins in solution? Can J Chem 83:1953–1960

7. Ruotolo BT, Robinson CV (2006) Aspects of native proteins are retained in vacuum. Curr Opin Chem Biol 10:402–408

8. Van Duijn E (2010) Current limitations in native mass spectrometry based structural biology. J Am Soc Mass Spectrom 21:971–978

9. Mathur S, Badertscher M, Scott M, Zenobi R (2007) Critical evaluation of mass spectrometric measurement of dissociation constants: accuracy and cross-validation against surface plasmon resonance and circular dichroism for the calmodulin-melittin system. Phys Chem Chem Phys 9:6187–6198

10. Ashcroft AE (2005) Recent developments in electrospray ionisation mass spectrometry: noncovalently bound protein complexes. Nat Prod Rep 22:452–464

11. Freyer MW, Lewis EA (2008) Isothermal titration calorimetry: experimental design, data analysis, and probing macromolecule/ligand binding and kinetic interactions. In: Correia JJ, Detrich HW (eds) Methods in cell biology. Academic, San Diego, CA

12. Ghai R, Falconer RJ, Collins BM (2011) Applications of isothermal titration calorimetry in pure and applied research: survey of the literature from 2010. J Mol Recognit 25:32–52

13. Baranauskiene L, Petrikaite V, Matuliene J, Matulis D (2009) Titration calorimetry standards and the precision of isothermal titration calorimetry data. Int J Mol Sci 10:2752–2762

14. Duhr S, Braun D (2006) Why molecules move along a temperature gradient. Proc Natl Acad Sci U S A 103:19678–19682

15. Seidel SA, Dijkman PM, Lea WA, van den Bogaart G, Jerabek-Willemsen M, Lazic A, Joseph JS, Srinivasan P, Baaske P, Simeonov A, Katritch I, Melo FA, Ladbury JE, Schreiber G, Watts A, Braun D, Duhr S (2013) Microscale thermophoresis quantifies biomolecular interactions under previously challenging conditions. Methods 59:301–315

16. Cooper MA (2002) Optical biosensors in drug discovery. Nat Rev Drug Discov 1:515–528

17. Cunningham BT, Li P, Schulz S, Lin B, Baird C, Gerstenmaier J, Genick C, Wang F, Fine E, Laing L (2004) Label-free assays on the BIND system. J Biomol Screen 9:481–490

18. Cunningham BT (2009) Label-free optical biosensors: an introduction. In: Cooper MA (ed) Label-free biosensors techniques and applications. Cambridge University Press, Cambridge, UK

19. Nordin H, Jungnelius M, Karlsson R, Karlsson OP (2005) Kinetic studies of small molecule interactions with protein kinases using biosensor technology. Anal Biochem 340:359–368

20. Huber W, Perspicace S, Kohler J, Muller F, Schlatter D (2004) SPR-based interaction studies with small molecular weight ligands using hAGT fusion proteins. Anal Biochem 333:280–288

21. Fang Y, Ferrie AM, Fontaine NH, Yuen PK (2005) Characteristics of dynamic mass redistribution of epidermal growth factor receptor signaling in living cells measured with label-free optical biosensors. Anal Chem 77: 5720–5725

22. Halai R, Cooper MA (2012) Using label-free screening technology to improve efficiency in drug discovery. Expert Opin Drug Discov 7: 123–131

23. Karlsson R (2009) Experimental design. In: Cooper MA (ed) Label-free biosensors techniques and applications. Cambridge University Press, Cambridge, UK

24. Cooper MA (2009) Sensor surfaces and receptor deposition. In: Cooper MA (ed) Label-free biosensors techniques and applications. Cambridge University Press, Cambridge, UK

25. Rich RL, Myszka DG (2000) Advances in surface plasmon resonance biosensor analysis. Curr Opin Biotechnol 11:54–61

26. Malmqvist M (1999) BIACORE: an affinity biosensor system for characterization of biomolecular interactions. Biochem Soc Trans 27: 335–340

27. Myszka DG, Jonsen MD, Graves BJ (1998) Equilibrium analysis of high affinity interactions using BIACORE. Anal Biochem 265:326–330

28. Huber W (2009) Application of SPR technology to pharmaceutical relevant drug-receptor interactions. In: Cooper MA (ed) Label-free biosensors techniques and applications. Cambridge University Press, Cambridge, UK

29. Frostell-Karlsson A, Remaeus A, Roos H, Andersson K, Borg P, Hamalainen M, Karlsson R (2000) Biosensor analysis of the interaction between immobilized human serum albumin and drug compounds for prediction of human serum albumin binding levels. J Med Chem 43:1986–1992

Chapter 2

Label-Free Cell Phenotypic Profiling and Screening: Techniques, Experimental Design, and Data Assessment

Ye Fang

Abstract

Label-free biosensors enable novel cell phenotypic assays for drug discovery by providing a holistic view of drug action in native cells. The label-free cellular profiles of drug molecules permit the comprehension of their target(s), potency, efficacy, and safety. This chapter first discusses three essential components of label-free cell phenotypic assays, namely biosensors, cell phenotypes, and assays. Key considerations about experimental design, data quality assessment, and data analysis are then discussed.

Key words Assay robustness, Cell-based assay, Label-free biosensor, Mechanism of action, Phenotypic assay, Profiling, Screening

1 Introduction

The past decades have witnessed increasing number of label-free biosensors for both basic research and drug discovery. Many of these biosensors offer a single platform for both biochemical and cell-based assays. Early label-free biosensors, in particular surface plasmon resonance (SPR), were primarily used for biochemical assays [1, 2]. These assays are advantageous in that they not only detect different classes of compounds (e.g., orthosteric, allosteric, and bitopic binders) for a specific receptor, but also accurately determine binding kinetics and affinity. Equilibrium binding affinity was often used as an acceptable surrogate of the in vivo efficacy of drugs [3]; nonequilibrium mechanisms of action (MoA) are advantageous for developing efficacious drugs [4], and the drug residence time (the reciprocal of K_{off}) is a critical indicator for clinical features of drugs [5]. Therefore, it is not surprising to see the increasing adoption of label-free biosensors for in vitro affinity profiling and screening over the past decade.

However, it is the functional consequences of drug binding, rather than binding affinity and kinetics per se, that are directly related to in vivo effects. Owing to advances in cell engineering

Ye Fang (ed.), *Label-Free Biosensor Methods in Drug Discovery*, Methods in Pharmacology and Toxicology, DOI 10.1007/978-1-4939-2617-6_2, © Springer Science+Business Media New York 2015

17

and detection technologies, there has been a steady increase in cell-based assays for early drug discovery over the past decades. In recent years, several label-free biosensors have been becoming the basis of new-generation cell phenotypic assays for drug discovery [6–8]. The biosensor output signals of cells upon stimulation are integrative in nature, permitting label-free cell phenotypic assays to mirror the innate complexity of drug pharmacology, a significant advantage over traditional molecular assays which measure one specific molecule at a time [9, 10]. However, this also introduces obvious challenges to determine target engagement and MoA of drugs, thus slowing down the adoption of label-free assays in early drug discovery process. In this chapter common label-free techniques for cell phenotypic assays are first reviewed, and detailed guidance is provided about how to design experiments, assess data quality, and perform data analysis for drug profiling and screening.

2   Biosensors for Cell-Based Assays

Biosensor systems for cell phenotypic assays that are commercially available include electrical biosensor, resonant waveguide grating (RWG), quartz crystal microbalance with dissipation (QCM-D), surface acoustic wave (SAW), and SPR (Fig. 1).

2.1 Electric Biosensors

Electric biosensor employs the impedance of a cell-electrode system as the transduction mechanism for whole-cell sensing. Cells are brought to contact with a microelectrode array and exposed to sinusoidal voltages that are swept through a range of frequencies in a continuous wave mode. The changes in cellular impedance arising from the ionic redistribution surrounding the cells upon stimulation are monitored in real time and are calculated to obtain a dynamic cell index signal [11]. The impedance is a measure of changes in the electrical conductivity or permeability of the cell layer.

2.2 RWG

RWG uses its characteristic surface-bound electromagnetic wave, also known as evanescent wave, under resonance condition as the transduction mechanism for cell phenotypic assays. Cells are brought to contact with or in close proximity to a nano-grating waveguide structure, and exposed to a broadband light source. The changes in resonant wavelength arising from the dynamic mass redistribution (DMR) of cells upon stimulation are monitored in real time [12]. Grating coupler, photonic crystal biosensor, and optical waveguide lightmode spectroscopy (OWLS) all use similar 1D or 2D waveguide grating structure for biosensing [13, 14]. Spatially resolved RWG imagers enable single-cell analysis [15, 16], while high-frequency RWG allows for assessing compound-induced cardiotoxicity [17].

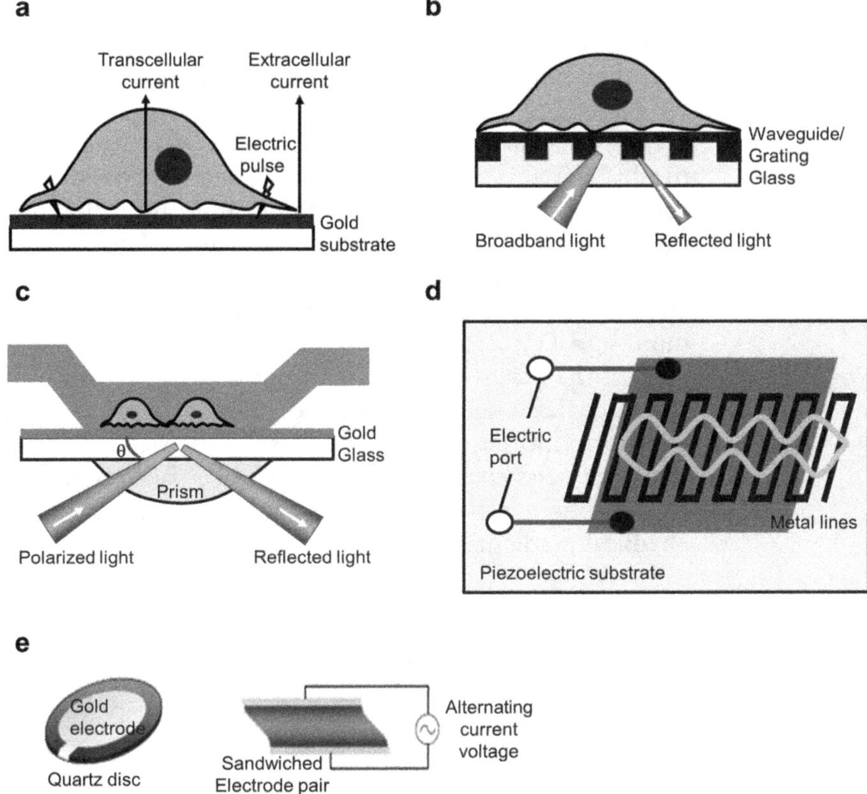

Fig. 1 Schematic drawing showing the principle of five different biosensors that are commonly used for label-free cell phenotypic profiling and screening. (**a**) Electric biosensor, (**b**) resonant waveguide grating biosensor, (**c**) surface plasmon resonance, (**d**) surface acoustic wave biosensor, (**e**) quartz crystal microbalance with dissipation

2.3 SPR

SPR employs light-excited surface plasmon polaritons as the transduction mechanism for whole-cell sensing. Cells are brought to attach onto the gold surface and exposed to a light source with varied angles. The changes in resonant angle are monitored in real time. Similar to RWG, SPR also detects changes in local refractive index, a function of local mass density, at the sensor surface [18, 19]. SPR mostly operates under microfluidics and in visible wavelength range. Extension of SPR to near- and mid-infrared wavelength range enables cell-based assays with long sensing depth [20].

2.4 QCM-D

QCM-D biosensor uses the excited frequency and energy dissipation of a quartz disc as the transduction mechanism for whole-cell sensing. Cells are brought to attach on the gold electrode, and exposed to an alternating current voltage across its paired electrodes, so a thin quartz disc sandwiched between the electrodes is excited to freely oscillate. The changes in resonant frequency and energy dissipation of cells upon stimulation are monitored in real time [21].

The energy dissipation signal is the change in the sum of all energy losses in the system per an oscillation cycle primarily arising from the alteration in the viscoelasticity of adherent cells.

2.5 SAW

SAW uses a surface mechanical acoustic wave as the transduction mechanism for whole-cell sensing and manipulation. Cells are brought to attach to a piezoelectric substrate which has an input interdigitated transducer on one side and a second, output interdigitated transducer on the other side, and exposed to a sinusoidal electrical input signal [22]. The transducer converts the electric input signal into a mechanical acoustic wave. The changes in amplitude of the acoustic wave are monitored in real time to determine the viscoelastic and conformational characteristics of cells upon stimulation, while the shifts in phase of the wave are used to determine the mass changes. SAW can also be used to manipulate cells and compounds, so assays can be performed under controlled chemical gradients [23, 24].

3 Cells and Cell Phenotypes

Label-free assays generally have high sensitivity to screen drugs using physiologically and/or clinically relevant cells including immortalized, primary, and stem cells [25–28]. This is unlike conventional target-based approaches that often use recombinant cell lines expressing a specific target to improve assay sensitivity. Furthermore, label-free imaging techniques such as SPR and RWG imagers permit assaying heterogeneous samples including tissue cells, differentiated stem cell products, or mixed populations of cells. In addition, a panel of cell lines can also be used for compound profiling and screening with a potential to determine target engagement of active compounds [29–31]. Large panels of disease-relevant cell lines annotated with both genetic and pharmacological data, as exemplified by NCI60 which consists of 60 (now 59) human cancer cell lines from nine different tissues [32], are powerful tools for drug discovery [33, 34]. Given that each cell line has unique expression pattern of functional receptors and signaling circuitry, the use of cell panels not only expands the number of addressable targets/pathways, but also offers confirmative information regarding to the potential MoA of active compounds identified in label-free screens [29, 30].

Label-free biosensors are generally sensitive to cell numbers, signaling, and morphological changes. This comes with advantages and disadvantages. On the one hand, these biosensors allow for drug profiling in the context of a great number of cellular phenotypes such as cell adhesion, cell-to-cell communication, death, infection, invasion, migration, proliferation, reprogramming, and receptor signaling [31, 35, 36]. The wide coverage in cellular process enables label-free assays to be an unprecedented means to match the diverse range of disease-relevant cellular phenotypes that may be associated with structural, morphological, or physiological abnormalities involving cells or cell components [37]. On the other hand, it is important to separate the background signals of different cell phenotypes from the net effects of drugs in specific label-free assays, given that cells at different phenotypes or states have different background signals [9].

4 Assay Design

Label-free offers great flexibility in assay formats due to its noninvasiveness in measurement, allowing for studying the acute and chronic effects of drugs on cells. However, the choice of assay formats is dependent on the purpose of drug profiling and screening. Besides cells and phenotypes studied, other common factors that should be considered for assay design include the choice of techniques, appropriate negative and positive controls, real-time kinetic profiling, and endpoint/multi-point screening.

4.1 Choice of Techniques

Label-free biosensors differ greatly in invasiveness, throughput, origin of biosensor output signals, and operational easiness. First, both SPR and RWG with or without gentle microfluidics are noninvasive, while electric biosensor, SAW, and QCM-D all use an electric input signal and thus are minimally invasive. Noninvasiveness is an important factor to be considered for studying targets, such as ion channels and electrogenic transporters, that are sensitive to the membrane potential [30, 38].

Second, SPR, QCM-D, and SAW all have low throughput, while electric biosensor enables assays up to 384-well microplates, and RWG permits assays up to 1,536-well microplates. High throughput is a critical factor for screening.

Third, all biosensors are mostly sensitive to cell-substratum interactions; in particular, SPR, RWG, SAW, and QCM-D all generally have short sensing depth (~100–200 nm), while infrared SPR and electric biosensors have long sensing depth. Although short sensing depth is sufficient for most cell-based assays, long sensing depth is critical to study certain cellular processes such as cell barrier functions and cell–cell communication [20, 35].

Fourth, the output signal is sensor dependent, although as common to all biosensors they measure an integrated cellular response. Both RWG and SPR measure the DMR arising from receptor signaling, which is often associated with protein trafficking, and remodeling of adhesion complexes, cytoskeletal structure, and morphology [12]. QCM-D measures energy dissipation which is mostly sensitive to remodeling of cell adhesion complexes [21]. Understanding of the origin of biosensor signals is essential to perform structure–activity analysis and elucidate the MoA of drugs.

Fifth, RWG, SAW, and electric biosensors all are made readily in microplate, so compound addition can be performed using automated liquid-handling devices. The ability to integrate with automation is essential to high-throughput screening (HTS). However, QCM-D requires sandwiching cells between two electrodes, and SPR generally operates with microfluidics, both of which require special care of sample addition. Of note, microfluidics may offer extra advantages, when spatial and temporal controls of chemicals exposed to cells are critical [39–43].

4.2 Negative and Positive Controls

Common to all cell-based assays, but more critical to label-free assays, is the inclusion of appropriate negative and positive controls. For most assays, negative controls are often the assay buffer. However, appropriate positive controls are dependent on the cell phenotype examined. For cell adhesion and proliferation, positive controls are cells at fixed or varied densities. For cell death, positive controls are known toxic compounds that cause cell apoptosis. For receptor signaling, positive controls are the agonists that are known to activate an endogenous and/or overexpressed receptor of interest. The agonists used as positive controls are often referred to probe molecules. Given the label-free nature of biosensor assays, the use of appropriate probe(s) is the most important factor determining the success of screens. In general, the probe molecule(s) should specifically activate the receptor of interest in the cell line examined.

Label-free is generally sensitive to three main environmental/operational factors, that is, temperature, solution composition, and assay parameters, all of which suggest the importance of positive and negative controls for ensuring assay quality. Temperature has dual effects on assay results. First, cell signaling and processes are known to be sensitive to assay temperature [15] (Fig. 2). The closer to physiological conditions the better. However, screening under physiological conditions may compromise throughput. Second, temperature mismatch between cell and compound solutions may introduce artifacts, which can be minimized by a pre-equilibrium step (usually about 1 h).

Solution composition also has dual effects on assay results. First, assay buffer can directly influence cell adhesion and signaling, which, in turn, could have an impact on cellular responses. Second, composition mismatch between cell and compound solutions may cause artifacts. This is particularly true when solvents such as dimethyl sulfoxide (DMSO) are used to prepare small-molecule compound solutions. DMSO is a high index of refraction solvent, is often considered a cytotoxic agent, and has complicated effects on cells. The common approach used to minimize the buffer effect is to perform assays using DMSO matching; that is, cell and compound solutions are made using the same buffer containing equal amount of DMSO. Alternatively, the background correction approach described below (*see* Section 6.1) can be used.

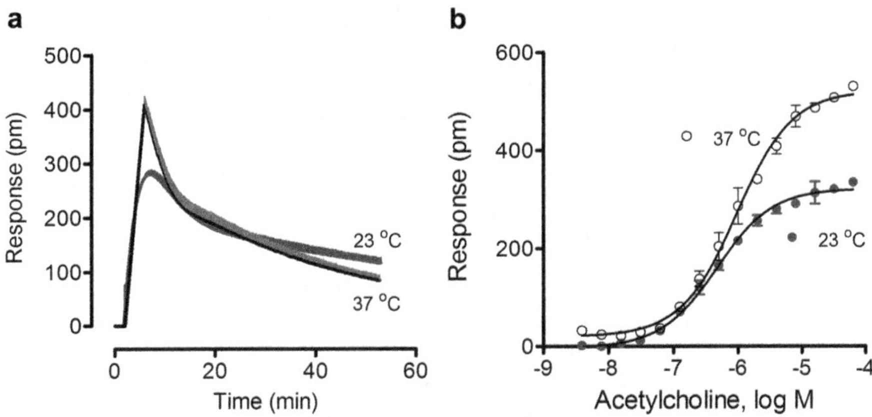

Fig. 2 Temperature dependency of the dynamic mass redistribution signal of acetylcholine in HEK293 cells. (**a**) The maximal DMR of 4 μM acetylcholine at room temperature versus 37 °C. (**b**) The dose–response curves of acetylcholine at room temperature versus 37 °C. Its DMR at 37 °C is faster with greater amplitude than that at room temperature. However, the potency is almost identical. Data represents mean ± s.d. ($n = 4$). Reprinted with permission from ref. [15], Copyright 2012, AIP Publishing LLC

Assay parameters may also influence biosensor output signals. First, fluidic movements or turbulence can generate undesired responses, given that many, if not all, cells are capable of mediating mechanical signal transduction [44]. There are several steps during label-free assays that fluidic movements could perturb results. For cell preparation, it is important to minimize solution turbulence using gentle wash and subsequent equilibrium step (usually 1 h). For compound addition, it is necessary to not only optimize liquid-handling parameters including dispensing height and speed, but also minimize the time gap between compound addition and data recording. For cell assays under microfluidics, it is important to use fluidic parameters below the threshold that could trigger mechanical responses of cells [39, 40]. Furthermore, optimal time resolutions also need to be predetermined.

4.3 Kinetic Profiling	Label-free kinetic measurements can provide rich textures for elucidating the MoA of drugs [45]. This is because biosensors often have wide coverage in targets and pathways ranging from G protein-coupled receptors to receptor tyrosine kinases, transporters, Toll-like receptors, immune receptors, enzymes, cell structural proteins, ion channels, and kinases [10, 31, 36]. The activation of different targets may trigger distinct kinetic profiles, leading to a unique fingerprint for each receptor.

The kinetic profiling of compounds is often performed in the context of a specific cellular process such as cell adhesion, death, growth, or signaling. The assay window and duration are dependent on the cell phenotype examined. For screening drugs that interfere with cell adhesion, compounds are preferably pre-incubated with cells and the assay duration is about 1–4 h [46]. For screening drugs that influence cell proliferation, compounds are often introduced after cell adhesion and the assay duration is at least 1–2 cell doubling time [47, 48]. For receptor signaling, compounds are often introduced after cells reach high confluency and the assay duration can be short (~30 min) or long (~days) [9, 10]. For other long-term effects such as cell death and infection, compounds or pathogens are introduced after cells reach high confluency and the assay duration is approximate to the length of the cellular process itself [49].

Interestingly, multiple combinations of compounds and probe molecules can be used to determine different biological effects (e.g., long- and short-acting antagonism, agonism, allosteric modulation, pathway modulation) of compounds [42]. For instance, for one-step agonism assay the cells are directly stimulated with a ligand. For one-step competitive antagonism assay the cells are stimulated with an agonist together with a known antagonist for the same receptor. For two-step antagonism/desensitization assay a ligand is introduced before stimulation with an agonist, so an agonist ligand for the same receptor desensitizes the cells responding to the subsequent agonist stimulation, but an antagonist ligand blocks the agonist response. For two-step pathway deconvolution assay the cells are first treated with a pathway modulator, followed by the stimulation with an agonist. For three-step ligand washout assay the cells are first treated with a ligand, followed by the removal of the ligand through washing or perfusion with a microfluidic device, and finally the stimulation with an agonist. For two-step antagonist reverse assay the cells are first stimulated with an agonist for a receptor, followed by the treatment with an antagonist for the same receptor. A washout or perfusion step can also be applied between the two treatments.

4.4 Endpoint/Multipoint Screening

Endpoint or multipoint measurements are commonly used to screen drugs with high throughput for a specific target [50]. The assay for the receptor of interest is first optimized using a probe molecule (often a cognate agonist), or a small set of ligands including agonists and antagonists. The biosensor signal of the probe is then used as the reference to select specific time point(s) for compound screening [50–52]. Screening distinct classes of ligands for the same receptor can be performed using different assay formats. One-step assay is useful for discovering agonists, wherein the cells are stimulated individually with different compounds. Given the wide pathway coverage of biosensors as well as the presence of compensatory signaling pathways, the one-step agonist screen may result in relatively high false positives for the receptor of interest. Such false positives can be minimized using two-step endpoint screens, wherein the cells are stimulated with compounds first, followed by stimulation with a cognate agonist specific to the receptor. This two-step assay allows for separation of agonists from antagonists and pathway modulators [51]. In addition, a three-step assay can also be performed to identify specific types of ligands.

For instance, a compound washout step that is introduced between compound and receptor cognate agonist stimulation steps can be used to identify long-acting antagonists or agonists [39–42]. Alternatively, a three-step assay that consists of compound and a cognate agonist at its EC_{20} and EC_{80}, respectively, would be useful to identify antagonists, allosteric modulators, and agonists for the same receptor within a single screen [53].

Multi-point assays can be used for high-throughput/content screening. Receptor signaling is encoded by the coupling of temporal dynamics with spatial gradients of signaling activities, and may come in multiple pathways and waves [42, 54, 55]. Given that label-free biosensors can noninvasively track the dynamics and multiple waves/phases of receptor signaling, multi-point profiling and screening may offer additional information regarding the specificity and MoAs of hits for the receptor of interest.

5 Data Quality Assessment

Critical to all cell-based assays is to ensure high quality of data acquired. Given that most data are generated from target-based profiling and screening, this section is primarily focused on how to assess data quality for these data.

First, negative controls (i.e., the assay buffer) should give rise to no or little signals, given that the baseline of confluent cells is typically steady. Positive controls (i.e., the cognate probe agonist) should give rise to expected signals with reproducible kinetic characteristics. For the maximal signal of positive controls the coefficient of variance (CV), defined as the ratio of the standard deviation to the mean, can be calculated for each plate or entire screen. The smaller the CV the better the assay quality is. Given that the signals of positive controls are usually large, the CV obtained is generally less than 10–15 %, below the acceptable value of less than or equal to 20 % [50, 51].

Second, the assay needs to be optimized and validated before actual screen. This is done through plate uniformity and replicate-experiment studies. Plate uniformity tests are typically performed over the course of several days to assess uniformity and separation of positive and negative signals. Replicate-experiment studies are performed to evaluate the within-run assay variability based on the minimum significant ratio (MSR), the smallest ratio between the potencies of two compounds that is statistically significant and should be less than 3.0. The minimum significant ratio is calculated as $MSR = 10^{2\sqrt{2}s}$, where s is an estimate of the standard deviation of a log potency for one compound [56].

Third, assay robustness, defined as a Z' factor (Z') [57], is the most commonly used parameter in HTS campaigns and is calculated based on the means and standard deviations of both positive

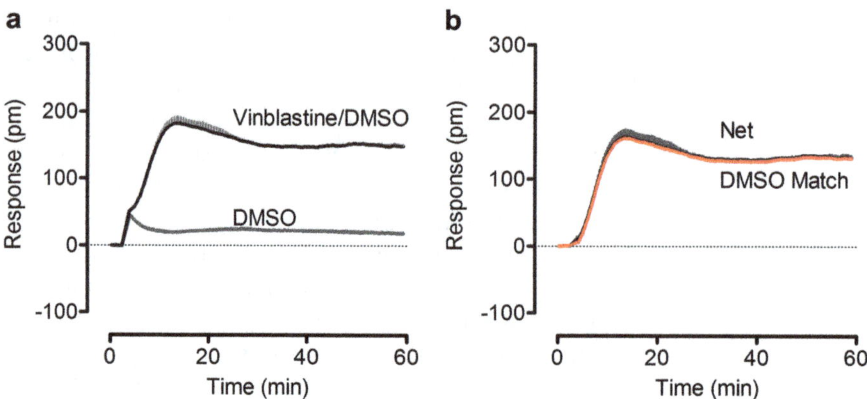

Fig. 3 Background correction of the label-free signals of vinblastine in HEK293 cells. (**a**) The DMR of 0.1 %
dimethyl sulfoxide (DMSO) and 10 μM vinblastine in the presence of 0.1 % DMSO. (**b**) The net DMR of vinblastine after background correction versus that obtained using DMSO matching condition. Both are identical. Data
represents mean ± s.d (*n* = 4)

and negative controls. For HTS, the Z′ value should be between
0.4 and 1.0, and can be calculated for each plate or entire screen.
This is to ensure that the probe potency and hit selection are consistent throughout the campaign.

Fourth, once hits are selected based on the response threshold
predefined, hits need to be confirmed. Secondary screens using the
same engineered cell line and/or its parental native line can be
used to determine the specificity of hits to the receptor of interest
[58, 59]. Dose responses can further be used to determine the
potency and efficacy of the confirmed hits.

6   Data Analysis

6.1   Background Correction

The biosensor signal of a compound may contain nonspecific signal
due to the environmental/operational factors (*see* Section 4.2).
These nonspecific signals, including the one induced by DMSO mismatch, can be background corrected. Subtracting the signal of the
negative control from that of a compound generally leads to the net
response of the compound, given that the negative control and the
compound solution contain equal amount of DMSO (Fig. 3). Due
to the presence of certain variability multiple negative controls
are included in the same plate, and their averaged response is used
for background correction. However, for certain cell lines that are
highly sensitive to DMSO, it is recommended to use the DMSO
match approach to minimize nonspecific responses.

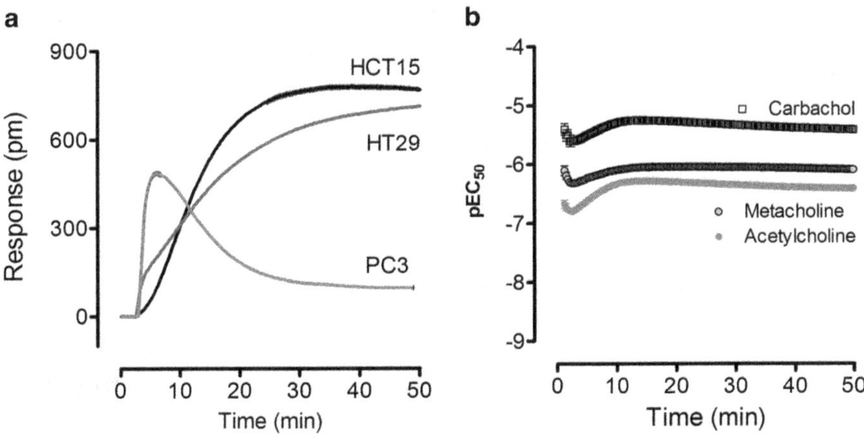

Fig. 4 Cell background and stimulation duration-dependent potency and efficacy of endogenous muscarinic M_3 receptor. (**a**) The maximal DMR of acetylcholine in three distinct cell lines, HT29, HCT15, and PC3, all endogenously expressing M_3 receptor. (**b**) The stimulation duration-dependent logEC$_{50}$ of three M_3 receptor agonists as a function of time in HT29 cells. Data represents mean ± s.d ($n=4$). Reprinted with permission from ref. [60], Copyright 2013, Elsevier Limited

6.2 Potency and Efficacy Analysis

Potency is a measure of drug activity expressed in terms of the amount required to produce an effect of given intensity. Potency depends on both affinity and efficacy. Affinity is the ability of the drug to bind to a receptor, while efficacy refers to the maximum response (E_{max}) achievable from a drug. The efficacy is the relationship between receptor occupancy and the ability to initiate a response. Historically, efficacy and affinity were considered to be totally independent properties of drugs [61]. Advances in pharmacological assays in the past decades have led to the comprehension that efficacy is vectorial (positive and negative cell activation) and pluridimensional (assay readout dependent), instead of being linear in controlling different receptor behaviors [62].

Label-free potency and efficacy of drugs are often dependent on cell background. The cell background dependency is due to the fact that different cell lines have distinct cell signaling circuitries; a receptor can activate multiple pathways; label-free has wide pathway coverage, enabling a holistic representation of receptor signaling [60].

Label-free potency and efficacy of drugs may also depend on stimulation duration (Fig. 4). This is originated from the fact that many active compounds are capable of triggering rapid-onset biosensor responses, suggesting that receptor signaling proceeds right after agonist binding but long before reaching equilibrium binding [60]. Under such a nonequilibrium condition ligand potency is expected to depend on stimulation duration. Common to all cell-based assays for determining the potency of a drug is to calculate its EC_{50} value from its dose response based on specific time point post-stimulation. For label-free profiling, the time to reach its maxima is often used to determine the potency and efficacy of drugs. Furthermore, analysis of the time-dependent potency may also offer extra information such as biased agonism [60]. This is in part due to the fact that receptor signaling is known to consist of a series of spatial and temporal events and pathways, each with its own characteristics such as kinetics, dynamics, amplitude, and location. Many of these events and pathways not only can contribute to the DMR arising from the receptor activation, but also can be encoded in different time domains of the DMR [9]. Of note, the time-dependent potency may also be due to distinct binding kinetics, in particular on-rates.

6.3 Kinetics Parameter Analysis

The ability of label-free to measure the cellular responses in real time enables the extraction of multiple kinetic parameters for analyzing drug pharmacology. For a panel of agonists for the same receptor, multiparameter analysis is useful to examine biased agonism [63]. Here, the real-time biosensor signals of a panel of agonists are recorded using the one-step agonist assay. Multiple kinetics parameters are extracted. These parameters include the transition time from one to another biosensor event, and the amplitudes, duration, and kinetics of each event. Of note, given that the binding kinetics of ligands may influence the functional responses of cells [60, 64] and at least the early biosensor response is obtained under nonequilibrium condition [60], the biosensor kinetic parameters may not directly correlate with ligand bias. However, the use of multiple parameters and similarity analysis can be used to relate a kinetic parameter to a specific signaling event [63], and manifest divergent pharmacology and MoAs of a panel of structurally similar ligands at the receptor [65].

6.4 Kinetics Similarity Analysis

Label-free kinetic responses of cells upon drug stimulation contain target- and pathway-specific information [9, 10]. Target engagement determination is vital to guide lead optimization and to understand potential toxicity. For target-based screen, target hypothesis is predefined by the reference agonist cognate to the receptor of interest, so target engagement can be confirmed using direct binding assays or counter profiling using another cell line that does not express the target receptor. For phenotypic screens, clustering of phenotypes, or label-free kinetic profiles, is generally the first step in understanding how a class of compounds behaves similarly to reference molecules with known MoAs in a biological system, the similarity of which can be used to generate target hypotheses [47, 48, 66, 67]. Traditional approaches including proteomics-, genetics-, and bioinformatics-based approaches can then be used

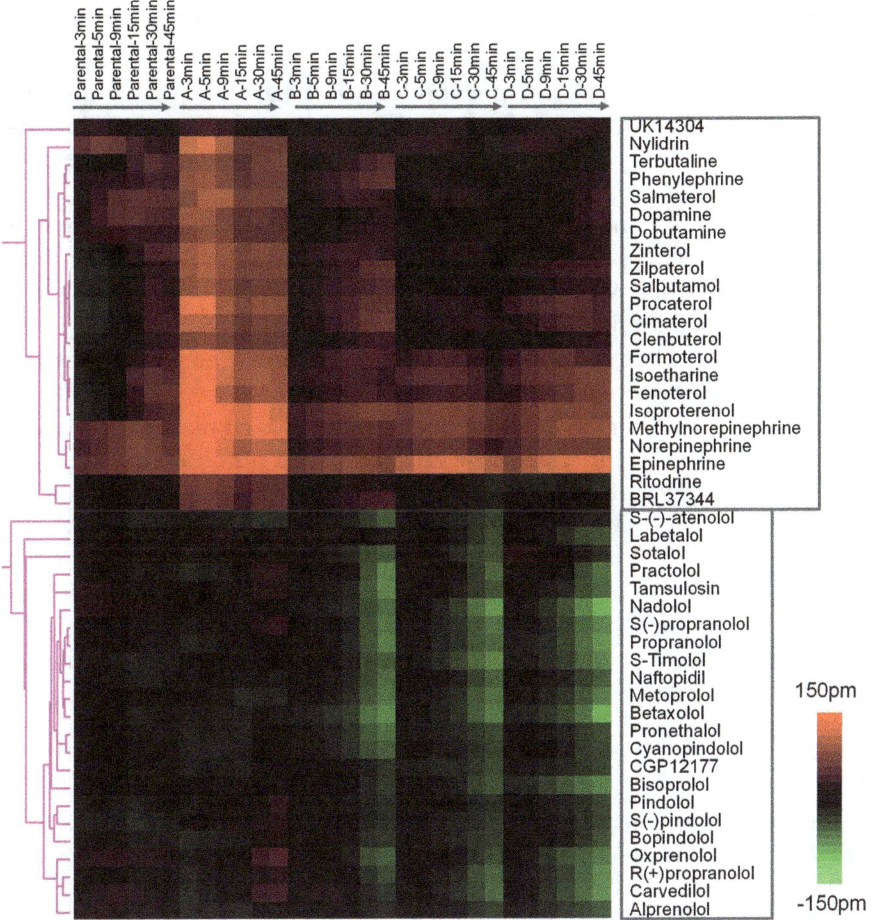

Fig. 5 DMR agonist heat map of adrenergic receptor ligands in HEK293 and four subclones, all expressing β₂-adrenergic receptors. The heat map obtained using DMR agonist profiling of the ligands in the five cell lines, followed by similarity analysis using the Ward hierarchical clustering algorithm and Euclidean distance metrics. The cell lines from left to right were the parental HEK293 (parental), and the four stable subclones (A, B, C, D). For each ligand in a cell line, its real DMR responses at six time points (3, 5, 9, 15, 30, and 45 min post-stimulation) were grouped together in a time series from left to right, so its kinetic signature can be directly visualized. False-colored scale bar is included to assist the data visualization. This figure is adapted from ref. [70] through the Creative Commons Attribution License

for determining target engagement [68]. For instance, similarity analysis of cellular impedance signals has led to identification of novel molecules that influence cell proliferation [47, 48], while analysis of DMR signals in different cellular backgrounds has revealed target selectivity and biased agonism of ligands for the same receptor [69, 70] (Fig. 5).

7   Future Perspectives

Label-free cell phenotypic assays have been adopting in early drug discovery in the past decade. As a kinetic profiling tool SPR is now integrated part of lead optimization. As an HTS tool RWG in microplate has been gaining attraction for primary and secondary screening. The increasing number of label-free techniques has opened new possibilities to investigate cell biology and drug pharmacology that were considered to be impossible in the past. However, the adoption rate of these assays remains to be slow, mostly due to relatively high cost and lacking comprehension about the origin of biosensor signatures.

Label-fee cell phenotypic assays emulate the innate complexity of the interaction with targets and functions of drugs. Combining label-free with chemical biology, molecular genetics and chemoinformatics is a rational strategy to determine the MoAs of active compounds. The potential of label-free in drug discovery is far from full realization. Advances in label-free methodologies including biosensor techniques, assay design, and data analysis would be essential to drive the wide adoption of these techniques in drug discovery.

References

1. Cooper MA (2002) Optical biosensors in drug discovery. Nat Rev Drug Discov 1:515–528. doi:10.1038/nrd838

2. Fang Y (2013) Ligand-receptor interaction platforms and their applications for drug discovery. Exp Rev Drug Discov 7:969–988. doi:10.1517/17460441.2012.715631

3. Nunez S, Venhorst J, Kruse CG (2012) Target-drug interactions: first principles and their application to drug discovery. Drug Discov Today 17:10–22. doi:10.1016/j.drudis.2011.06.013

4. Swinney DC (2004) Biochemical mechanisms of drug action: what does it take for success? Nat Rev Drug Discov 3:801–808. doi:10.1038/nrd1500

5. Copeland RA, Pompliano DL, Meek TD (2006) Drug-target residence time and its implications for lead optimization. Nat Rev Drug Discov 5:730–739. doi:10.1038/nrd2082

6. Fang Y (2006) Label-free cell-based assays with optical biosensors in drug discovery. Assay Drug Dev Technol 4:583–595. doi:10.1089/adt.2006.4.583

7. Rocheville M, Jerman JC (2009) 7TM pharmacology measured by label-free: a holistic approach to cell signalling. Curr Opin Pharmacol 9:643–649. doi:10.1016/j.coph.2009.06.015

8. Rocheville M, Martin J, Jerman J, Kostenis E (2013) Mining the potential of label-free biosensors for seven-transmembrane receptor drug discovery. Prog Mol Biol Transl Sci 115:123–42. doi:10.1016/B978-0-12-394587-7.00003-8

9. Fang Y (2011) The development of label-free cellular assays for drug discovery. Exp Opin Drug Discov 6:1285–1298. doi:10.1517/17460441.2012.715631

10. Fang Y (2013) Troubleshooting and deconvoluting label-free cell phenotypic assays in drug discovery. J Pharmacol Tox Methods 67:69–81. doi:10.1016/j.vascn.2013.01.004

11. McGuinness R (2007) Impedance-based cellular assay technologies: recent advances, future promise. Curr Opin Pharmacol 7:535–540. doi:10.1016/j.coph.2007.08.004

12. Fang Y, Ferrie AM, Fontaine NH, Mauro J, Balakrishnan J (2006) Resonant waveguide grating biosensor for living cell sensing. Biophys J 91:1925–1940. doi:10.1529/biophysj.105.077818

13. Shamah SM, Cunningham BT (2011) Label-free cell-based assays using photonic crystal optical biosensors. Analyst 136(6):1090–1102. doi:10.1039/c0an00899k

14. Aref A, Horvath R, McColl J, Ramsden JJ (2009) Optical monitoring of stem cell-substratum interactions. J Biomed Opt 14:010501. doi:10.1117/1.3065541

15. Ferrie AM, Deichmann OD, Wu Q, Fang Y (2012) High resolution resonant waveguide grating imager for cell cluster analysis under physiological condition. Appl Phys Lett 100:223701. doi:10.1063/1.4723691

16. Febles NK, Ferrie AM, Fang Y (2014) Label-free single cell quantification of the invasion of spheroidal colon cancer cells through 3D Matrigel. Anal Chem 86:8842–8849. doi:10.1021/ac502269v

17. Ferrie AM, Wu Q, Deichmann O, Fang Y (2014) High frequency resonant waveguide grating imager for assessing drug-induced cardiotoxicity. Appl Phys Lett 104:183702. doi:10.1063/1.4876095

18. Hide M, Tsutsui T, Sato H, Nishimura T, Morimoto K, Yamamoto S, Yoshizato K (2002) Real-time analysis of ligand-induced cell surface and intracellular reactions of living mast cells using a surface plasmon resonance-based biosensor. Anal Biochem 302:28–37. doi:10.1006/abio.2001.5535

19. Bourassa P, Tudashki HB, Pineyro G, Grandbois M, Gendron L (2014) Label-free monitoring of μ-opioid receptor-mediated signaling. Mol Pharmacol 86:138–149. doi:10.1124/mol.114.093450

20. Yashunsky V, Lirtsman V, Golosovsky M, Davidov D, Aroeti B (2010) Real-time monitoring of epithelial cell-cell and cell-substrate interactions by infrared surface plasmon spectroscopy. Biophys J 99:4028–4036. doi:10.1016/j.bpj.2010.10.017

21. Chen JY, Shahid A, Garcia MP, Penn LS, Xi J (2012) Dissipation monitoring for assessing EGF-induced changes of cell adhesion. Biosens Bioelectron 38:375–381. doi:10.1016/j.bios.2012.06.018

22. Saitakis M, Gizeli E (2012) Acoustic sensors as a biophysical tool for probing cell attachment and cell/surface interactions. Cell Mol Life Sci 69(3):357–371. doi:10.1007/s00018-011-0854-8

23. Ding X, Lin S-C, Lapsley M, Li S, Guo X, Chan CYK, Chiang I-K, Wang L, McCoy JP, Huang TJ (2012) Standing surface acoustic wave (SSAW) based multichannel cell sorting. Lab Chip 12:4228–4231. doi:10.1039/c2lc40751e

24. Ahmed D, Muddana H, Lu M, French J, Ozcelik A, Fang Y, Butler P, Benkovic S, Manz A, Huang TJ (2014) Acoustofluidic chemical waveform generator and switch. Anal Chem 86(23):11803–11810. doi:10.1021/ac5033676

25. Hennen S, Wang H, Peters L, Merten N, Simon K, Spinrath A, Blättermann S, Akkari R, Schrage R, Schröder R, Schulz D, Vermeiren C, Zimmermann K, Kehraus S, Drewke C, Pfeifer A, König GM, Mohr K, Gillard M, Müller CE, Lu QR, Gomeza J, Kostenis E (2013) Decoding signaling and function of the orphan G protein-coupled receptor GPR17 with a small-molecule agonist. Sci Signal 6:ra93. doi:10.1126/scisignal.2004350

26. Bagnaninchi PO, Drummond N (2011) Real-time label-free monitoring of adipose-derived stem cell differentiation with electric cell-substrate impedance sensing. Proc Natl Acad Sci U S A 108:6462–6467. doi:10.1073/pnas.1018260108

27. Pai S, Verrier F, Sun H, Hu H, Ferrie AM, Eshraghi A, Fang Y (2012) Dynamic mass redistribution assay decodes differentiation of a neural progenitor stem cell. J Biomol Screen 17:1180–1191. doi:10.1177/1087057112455059

28. Carter RL, Grisanti LA, Yu JE, Repas AA, Woodall M, Ibetti J, Koch WJ, Jacobson MA, Tilley DG (2014) Dynamic mass redistribution analysis of endogenous β-adrenergic receptor signaling in neonatal rat cardiac fibroblasts. Pharmacol Res Perspect 2:24. doi:10.1002/prp2.24

29. Zhang X, Deng H, Xiao Y, Xue X, Ferrie AM, Tran E, Liang X, Fang Y (2014) Label-free cell phenotypic profiling identifies pharmacologically active compounds in two traditional Chinese medicinal plants. RSC Advances 4:26368–26377. doi:10.1039/C4RA03609C

30. Sun H, Wei Y, Xiong Q, Li M, Lahiri J, Fang Y (2014) Label-free cell phenotypic profiling decodes the composition and signaling of an endogenous ATP-sensitive potassium channel. Sci Rep 4:4934. doi:10.1038/srep04934

31. Fang Y (2014) Label-free drug discovery. Front Pharmacol 5:52. doi:10.3389/fphar.2014.00052

32. Shoemaker RH (2006) The NCI60 human tumour cell line anticancer drug screen. Nat Rev Cancer 6:813–823. doi:10.1038/nrc1951

33. Garnett MJ, Edelman EJ, Heidorn SJ, Greenman CD, Dastur A, Lau KW (2012) Systematic identification of genomic markers of drug sensitivity in cancer cells. Nature 483:570–575. doi:10.1038/nature11005

34. Barretina J, Caponigro G, Stransky N, Venkatesan K, Margolin AA, Kim S et al (2012) The cancer cell line Encyclopedia enables predictive modelling of anticancer drug sensitivity. Nature 483:603–607. doi:10.1038/nature11003

35. Fang Y (2011) Label-free biosensors for cell biology. Intl J Electrochem 2011:e460850. doi:10.4061/2011/460850

36. Fang Y (2014) Label-free cell phenotypic drug discovery. Comb Chem High Throughput Screen 17:566–578. doi:10.2174/138620731 7666140211100000

37. Hoehndorf R, Harris MA, Herre H, Rustici G, Gkoutos GV (2012) Semantic integration of physiology phenotypes with an application to the cellular phenotype ontology. Bioinformatics 28:1783–1789. doi:10.1093/bioinformatics/bts250

38. Wong S-H, Gao A, Ward S, Henley C, Lee PH (2012) Development of a label-free assay for sodium-dependent phosphate transporter NaPi-IIb. J Biomol Screen 17:829–834. doi:10.1177/1087057112442961

39. Goral V, Wu Q, Sun H, Fang Y (2011) Label-free optical biosensor with microfluidics for sensing ligand-directed functional selectivity on trafficking of thrombin receptor. FEBS Lett 585:1054–1060. doi:10.1016/j.febslet.2011.03.003

40. Goral V, Jin Y, Sun H, Ferrie AM, Wu Q, Fang Y (2011) Agonist-directed desensitization of the β_2-adrenergic receptor. PLoS One 6:e19282. doi:10.1371/journal.pone.0019282

41. Deng H, Wang C, Su M, Fang Y (2012) Probing biochemical mechanisms of action of muscarinic M_3 receptor antagonists with label-free whole-cell assays. Anal Chem 84:8232–8239. doi:10.1021/ac301495n

42. Ferrie AM, Wang C, Deng H, Fang Y (2013) Label-free optical biosensor with microfluidics identifies an intracellular signalling wave mediated through the β_2-adrenergic receptor. Integr Biol 5:1253–1261. doi:10.1039/c3ib40112j

43. Deng H, Wang C, Fang Y (2013) Label-free cell phenotypic assessment of the molecular mechanism of action of epidermal growth factor receptor inhibitors. RSC Advances 3:10370–10378. doi:10.1039/C3RA40426A

44. Sen S, Kumar S (2010) Combining mechanical and optical approaches to dissect cellular mechanobiology. J Biomechanics 43:45–54. doi:10.1016/j.jbiomech.2009.09.008

45. Kenakin T (2009) Cellular assays as portals to seven-transmembrane receptor-based drug discovery. Nat Rev Drug Discov 8:617–626. doi:10.1038/nrd2838

46. Orgovan N, Peter B, Bősze S, Ramsden JJ, Szabó B, Horvath R (2014) Dependence of cancer cell adhesion kinetics on integrin ligand surface density measured by a high-throughput label-free resonant waveguide grating biosensor. Sci Rep 4:4034. doi:10.1038/srep04034

47. Abassi YA, Xi B, Zhang W, Ye P, Kirstein SL, Gaylord MR, Feinstein SC, Wang X, Xu X (2009) Kinetic cell-based morphological screening: prediction of mechanism of compound action and off-target effects. Chem Biol 16:712–723. doi:10.1016/j.chembiol.2009.05.011

48. Fu H, Fu W, Sun M, Shou Q, Zhai Y, Cheng H, Teng L, Mou X, Li Y, Wan S, Zhang S, Xu Q, Zhang X, Wang J, Zhu J, Wang X, Xu X, Lv G, Jin L, Guo W, Ke Y (2011) Kinetic cellular phenotypic profiling: prediction, identification, and analysis of bioactive natural products. Anal Chem 83:6518–6526. doi:10.1021/ac201670e

49. Owens RM, Wang C, You JA, Jiambutr J, Xu AS, Marala RB, Jin MM (2009) Real-time quantitation of viral replication and inhibitor potency using a label-free optical biosensor. J Recept Signal Transduct Res 29:195–201. doi:10.1080/10799890903079919

50. Dodgson K, Gedge L, Murray DC, Coldwell M (2009) A 100K well screen for a muscarinic receptor using the Epic label-free system: a reflection on the benefits of the label-free approach to screening seven-transmembrane receptors. J Recept Signal Transduct Res 29:163–172. doi:10.1080/10799890903079844

51. Tran E, Fang Y (2008) Duplexed label-free G protein-coupled receptor assays for high throughput screening. J Biomol Screen 13:975–985. doi:10.1177/1087057108326141

52. Verrier F, An S, Ferrie AM, Sun H, Kyoung M, Deng H, Fang Y, Benkovic S (2011) GPCRs regulate the assembly of a multienzyme complex for purine biosynthesis. Nat Chem Biol 7:909–915. doi:10.1038/nchembio.690

53. Gitschier HJ, Bergeron AB, Randle, DH, Bacon CE, Baez M, Yang P, Broad LM, Goldsmith PJ, Felder CC, Schober DA (2015) Triple-addition label-free assays for high throughput screening of agonists, antagonists and allosteric modulators of muscarinic m1 receptor. Methods Pharmacol Tox (Chapter 11). doi: 10.1007/978-1-4939-2617-6_11

54. Kholodenko BN (2006) Cell signaling dynamics in time and space. Nat Rev Mol Cell Biol 7:165–176. doi:10.1038/nrm1838

55. Lohse MJ, Calebiro D (2013) Cell biology: receptor signals come in waves. Nature 495:457–458. doi:10.1038/nature12086

56. Eastwood BJ, Farmen MW, Iversen PW, Craft TJ, Smallwood JK, Garbison KE, Delapp N, Smith GF (2006) The minimum significant ratio: a statistical parameter to characterize the reproducibility of potency estimates from concentration-response assays and estimation by replicate-experiment studies. J Biomol Screen 11:253–261.doi:10.1177/1087057105285611

57. Zhang J, Chung TDY, Oldenburg KR (1999) A simple statistical parameter for use in

evaluation and validation of high throughput screening assays. J Biomol Screen 4:67–73. doi:10.1177/108705719900400206

58. Morse M, Tran E, Levension RL, Fang Y (2011) Ligand-directed functional selectivity at the mu opioid receptor revealed by label-free on-target pharmacology. PLoS One 6:e25643. doi:10.1371/journal.pone.0025643

59. Morse M, Sun H, Tran E, Levenson R, Fang Y (2013) Label-free integrative pharmacology on-target of opioid ligands at the opioid receptor family. BMC Pharmacol Tox 14:17. doi:10.1186/2050-6511-14-17

60. Deng H, Sun H, Fang Y (2013) Label-free cell phenotypic assessment of the biased agonism and efficacy of agonists at the endogenous muscarinic M_3 receptors. J Pharmacol Tox Methods 68:323–333. doi:10.1016/j.vascn.2013.07.005

61. Onaran HO, Costa T (2012) Where have all the active receptor states gone? Nature Chem Biol 8:674–677. doi:10.1038/nchembio.1024

62. Kenakin T (2013) New concepts in pharmacological efficacy at 7TM receptors: IUPHAR review 2. Br J Pharmacol 168:554–575. doi:10.1111/j.1476-5381.2012.02223.x

63. Fang Y, Ferrie AM (2008) Label-free optical biosensor for ligand-directed functional selectivity acting on β_2-adrenoceptor in living cells. FEBS Lett 582:558–564. doi:10.1016/j.febslet.2008.01.021

64. Guo D, Mulder-Krieger T, Ijzerman AP, Heitman LH (2012) Functional efficacy of adenosine A_{2A} receptor agonists is positively correlated to their receptor residence time. Br J Pharmacol 166:1846–1959. doi:10.1111/j.1476-5381.2012.01897.x

65. Fang Y (2010) Label-free receptor assays. Drug Discov Today Technol 7:e5–e11. doi:10.1016/j.ddtec.2010.05.001

66. Young DW, Bender A, Hoyt J, McWhinnie E, Chirn GW, Tao CY, Tallarico JA, Labow M, Jenkins JL, Mitchison TJ, Feng Y (2008) Integrating high-content screening and ligand-target prediction to identify mechanism of action. Nat Chem Biol 4:59–68. doi:10.1038/nchembio.2007.53

67. Schenone M, Dančík V, Wagner BK, Clemons PA (2013) Target identification and mechanism of action in chemical biology and drug discovery. Nat Chem Biol 9:232–240. doi:10.1038/nchembio.1199

68. Ziegler S, Pries V, Hedberg C, Waldmann H (2013) Target identification for small bioactive molecules: finding the needle in the haystack. Angew Chem Int Ed Engl 52:2744–2792. doi:10.1002/anie.201208749

69. Ferrie AM, Sun H, Fang Y (2011) Label-free integrative pharmacology on-target of drugs at the β_2-adrenergic receptor. Sci Rep 1:33. doi:10.1038/srep00033

70. Ferrie AM, Sun H, Zaytseva N, Fang Y (2014) Divergent label-free cell phenotypic pharmacology of ligands at the overexpressed β_2-adrenergic receptors. Sci Rep 4:3828. doi:10.1038/srep03828

Chapter 3

Surface Plasmon Resonance for Therapeutic Antibody Characterization

S. Nicole Davidoff, Noah T. Ditto, Amanda E. Brooks, Josh Eckman, and Benjamin D. Brooks

Abstract

The use of Surface Plasmon Resonance (SPR)-based optical biosensors contributes extensively to discovery and development of therapeutic monoclonal antibodies, owing to its ability to real-time analyze interactions of an antigen with an antibody without intrinsic or extrinsic labels. SPR has been a mainstay in pharmaceutical companies for almost two decades, and its role in drug discovery has experienced significant growth with the expanded number of therapeutic antibodies. Additionally, the burgeoning field of biosimilars depends on SPR to ascertain comparability to innovator mAbs. While the promise of the technology is exciting, the full role of SPR has yet to be realized. SPR has historically been hampered by limited throughput; however, new instruments and methods have emerged that allow for the analysis of up to thousands of biomolecular interactions per day. Here, we detail the use of traditional and emerging SPR techniques for characterizing monoclonal antibodies such as antigen/antibody kinetics, epitope profiling, and immunogenicity screening. In conjunction with efforts to improve throughput and sensitivity, SPR is expected to continue in its growth as a central technique in pharmaceutical discovery and development.

Key words Affinity, Antibodies, Binding, Biologics, Biosensor, Detection, Diagnostics, Drug discovery, Epitope binning, Fc-gamma receptor, High throughput, Immobilization, Kinetics, Label-free binding, Ligand, Off-rate, Protein, Protein profiling, Regeneration, Screening

1 Introduction

The pharmaceutical industry is in the midst of a "biologics boom" with antibodies leading the charge (*1x*). While monoclonal antibodies (mAb) are commonly used in life science research, their use has exploded as therapeutics for treatment of leukemia, cancer, asthma, psoriasis, Crohn's disease, arthritis, and transplant rejection [1]. Technological advances have dramatically improved the engineering, expression, and purification tool sets available for the production of therapeutic antibodies with better safety and efficacy. These advances have allowed the pharmaceutical industry to release new and improved antibody-based drugs for the treatment of

Ye Fang (ed.), *Label-Free Biosensor Methods in Drug Discovery*, Methods in Pharmacology and Toxicology, DOI 10.1007/978-1-4939-2617-6_3, © Springer Science+Business Media New York 2015

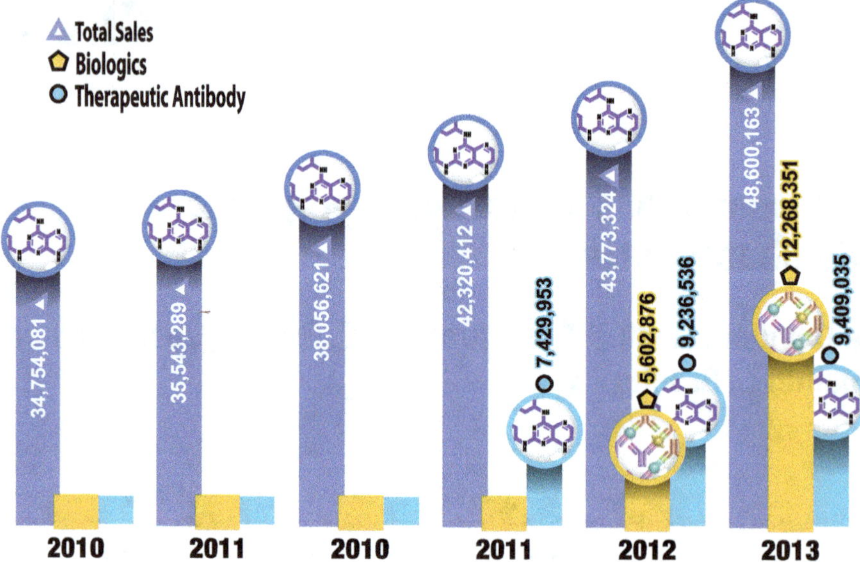

Fig. 1 Drug revenues by year. Chart detailing the annual drug revenues from biologics and small molecules

disease [2]. Subsequent to the expansion of therapeutic mAbs is the growing effort to generate biosimilars by the time an innovator mAb's patents expire [3]. Biosimilar studies require multiple physiochemical and functional assays to ascertain comparability to the innovator mAb, due in large part to the complications of manufacturing requirements in living cells. In contrast, production of small molecule generics is a much less analytically intensive process due to highly streamlined manufacturing with a much lower cost of goods [4].

Small molecules still account for the majority of pharmaceutical revenues; however projected revenue from biologics, in particular antibodies, will in a few years outpace projected small molecule revenues (Fig. 1) [5]. The surge in revenue from biologics is attributed to increased prescription use of existing biologics and the large number of new biologic drugs approved for use (Fig. 2). By 2016, biologics are projected to capture ~17 % of total global spending of pharmaceutics with an overall market value reaching to $210 billion [6]. Even more telling is the projection that seven of the top ten drugs will be biologics within 5 years [6].

Biosensors, and in particular Surface Plasmon Resonance (SPR), are an important tool in biologic drug discovery. Historically, biosensor technology has been used for the characterization of the kinetics of macromolecular interactions; however, the application of biosensors has been expanded to support drug screening, early absorption, distribution, metabolism, and excretion (ADME), target characterization, lead optimization, compound screening, clinical trials, and biopharmaceutical production (Table 1) [7–9].

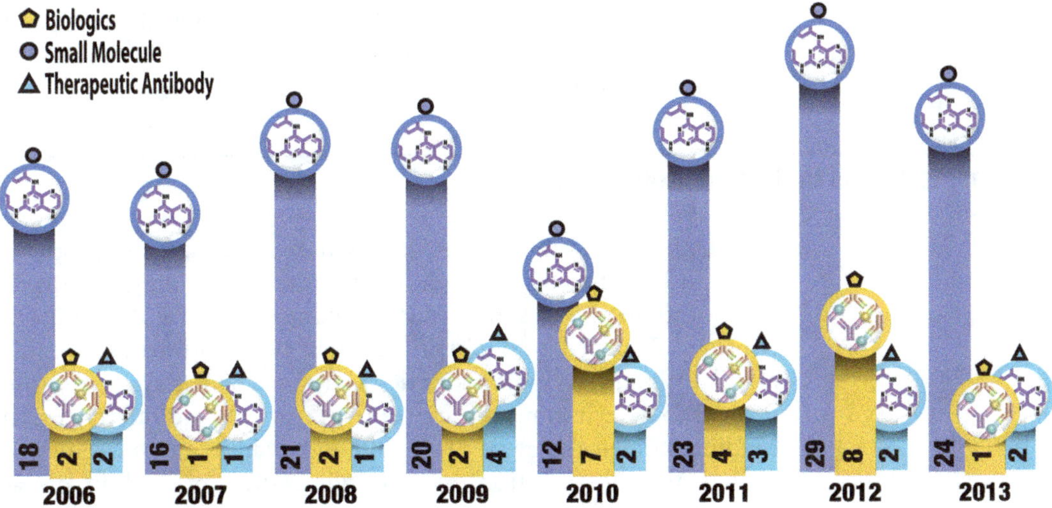

Fig. 2 FDA drug approvals by year. Chart detailing the yearly drug approvals broken down into biologics and small molecules

Table 1
SPR biosensor applications

Qualitative	Quantitative
Follow purification	Active concentration
Specificity	Kinetics (k_a, k_d)
Epitope mapping	Equilibrium constants (K_D)
Molecular assembly	Thermodynamics (ΔH *van't Hoff*)
Small molecule screening	Mechanism

Biosensor technologies are starting to compete with existing drug discovery technologies on the grounds of "low cost, ease of use, robustness, sensitivity, and stability" [9, 10]. In addition, SPR presents an attractive alternative to traditional label-based techniques such as ELISA, since labels may compromise protein function [11] and SPR also enables the determination of association and dissociation rates of interacting molecules [12]. SPR biosensors have the capacity to provide label-free information across a wide range of applications.

This chapter reviews both existing and developing SPR techniques for characterizing mAbs, including antigen/antibody kinetics, epitope profiling, Fc receptor binding, formulation and stability, condition scouting, immunogenicity screening, and SPR in whole cells. Additional attention will be given to current commercially available SPR platforms as well as other platforms for label-free detection. These techniques and platforms represent indispensable means for determining protein/protein and protein/ligand binding in order to achieve regulatory approval of a therapeutic mAb.

2   Considerations in SPR Method Design

Although SPR overall is a relatively user-friendly technology and data can be acquired with a limited degree of training, numerous key points in the design of SPR experiments exist that must be considered in order to obtain accurate data and avoid common pitfalls. When developing kinetics assays, particular attention must be paid to determining the appropriate controls and references, the binding stoichiometry of the ligand and analyte, the movement of analyte in bulk solution, the coupling strategy, and in certain instances, the approach to overcoming regeneration challenges. This section highlights these issues and offers a number of approaches to maximize the data quality and overall success of SPR studies.

2.1 Coupling of Ligand to the Chip Surface

Ligand coupling is one of the more challenging aspects of an SPR experiment. Ligand coupling can be direct by covalently immobilizing the ligand to the surface or indirect by capturing the ligand through another covalently coupled molecule (Fig. 3). Most proteins can be directly covalently attached through one of four major chemistries, amine, thiol, maleimide, or aldehyde. One of the most commonly used chip surfaces has a hydrophilic dextran surface

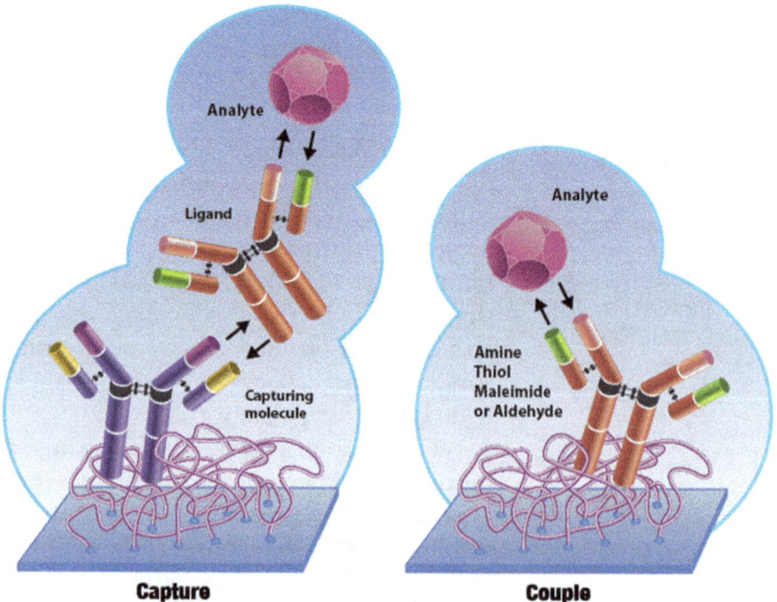

Fig. 3 Immobilization schemes for SPR analysis

with exposed carboxylic end groups that are activated as *N*-hydroxy succinimide esters, thereby immobilizing the ligand by an amide bond [13–15]. Direct immobilization does require the protein to be relatively pure (>50 %) and have a pI greater than 3.5. Coupling in this fashion is sometimes ineffective because the chemistries are not discriminative of its location on the protein; in other words, the chemistries can bind at multiple sites on a protein leaving the orientation and the densities of the protein on the surface random [16, 17]. In worst-case scenarios, the protein can have the binding site completely obscured due to orientation of the protein on the surface either by the surface or a neighboring protein [18, 19], or be denatured entirely [20].

Indirect immobilization overcomes many limitations of direct immobilization. Capture approaches often are used to take advantage of affinity purification tags, or in the case of antibodies, the capture molecule is another antibody which bind the Fc region of the antibody of interest. Ligand capture is commonly accomplished using a nickel-NTA surface to capture His-tagged proteins, a streptavidin or neutravidin surface to capture biotinylated molecules, a hydrophobic surface to capture lipids, anti-Fc antibody or protein A to capture IgG antibodies. The protein sample does not have to be purified. Using this approach, the antibody is often presented on the surface in a consistent and presentable orientation that is readily available for binding. As a result, antibodies can be captured from crude samples [21, 22]. Capture of the ligand also allows for regeneration of the SPR surface because the bonds created by capture are not as strong as the covalent bonds utilized in direct immobilization. However, these weaker bonds can create an unstable surface allowing ligands to dissociate from the surface. The one exception to this is the streptavidin–biotin capture whose bonds are stable and almost as strong as covalent bonds [23]. Lastly, capture methods are conducive to regeneration, except for the streptavidin–biotin bond as it is almost impossible to remove the biotinylated ligand from streptavidin under standard conditions [24].

2.2 Mass Transport Limitation

In kinetic experiments conducted on biosensors, minimizing the limitations of mass transport is critical for accurate data acquisition. The problem arises when the concentration of the analyte is different between the bulk solution and the area near surface, resulting in the analyte concentration exhibiting either a localized retention area or depletion area in the unstirred layer on the biosensor chip surface (Fig. 4) [25]. These mass transport limitations are more likely to occur when an antibody has a high k_a (>10^6–10^7 M^{-1} s^{-1}) and suffers from rebinding effects [26]. The result arising from mass transport issues manifests as linear regions in the association component of the sensorgram. SPR is susceptible to this effect when the flow rates of the flow cell are slow (<30 μL/min) or the

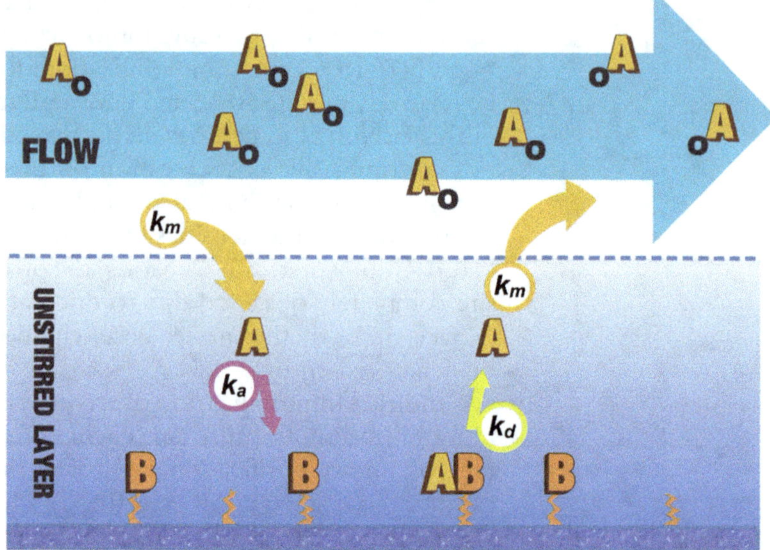

Fig. 4 Mass transport. Schematic shows the interactions at the biosensor surface. The surface-attached antibody (B) or ligand interacts with the target antigen (A) or analyte during the association phase (*ka*). The mass transport coefficient (*km*) describes the diffusion of the analyte through the unstirred layer. The dissociation (*kd*) phase describes when the flow does not contain the analyte

surface capacity of the ligand is high (>100 RU) [27]. To overcome the problems of mass transport, the following guidelines are suggested: (1) use high flow rates, around 100 µL/min; (2) immobilize small amounts of antibody on the surface such that the antigen binding will be limited to around 50 RU; (3) fit the data with a standard 1:1 interaction model; and (4) inject a wide range of antigen concentrations ranging from 10- to 100-fold above and below the K_D. Detailed treatment of more challenging mass transport problems on the biosensor is available [26–30].

2.3 Replicate Controls

One component of effectively validating an experiment is to demonstrate reproducibility. As most SPR instruments are automated, replicates should be a standard practice; however, this is still commonly not performed [51]. Replicates give information on experimental noise, antibody/antigen activity across the experiment, and regeneration efficiency. Ideally the location of replicates should also be randomized on the biosensor chip to remove locational and timing bias. To further validate the experiment, injecting the analyte with a small number of concentrations covering a wide range, with replicates of each concentration (>100 fold concentration range with at least three replicates at each concentration), is more beneficial than single injections of more concentrations.

2.4 Referencing

SPR experiments use referencing to correct for system artifacts such as instrument noise, baseline drift, and bulk refractive index changes [31]. Myszka et al. proposed a double referencing control, which is widely accepted as one mark of high-quality SPR data. The first reference should be a surface exposed to the same analyte conditions as the experimental flow cell or sample spot. Ideally this reference surface should contain a reference ligand that does not bind the analyte. The second reference is a "blank" injection of buffer across the reaction surface. The signal from both the reference surface and "blank" injection are subtracted from the reaction surface analyte binding traces [27, 32, 33]. In traditional SPR instruments with sequential flow cells, the reference surface is often selected as the first in the flow path, whereas with SPR array-type platforms reference surfaces (termed interspots) are commonly placed in close proximity to each ligand spot. Low surface capacities with double referencing can salvage an experiment that has poor signal to noise.

2.5 Avidity

Avoiding avidity effects is an important factor in experimental design. Antibodies, due to their bivalency, should be immobilized on the surface in order to reduce the effects of avidity in kinetics studies [32]. Binding the bivalent molecule on the surface better ensures a simple 1:1 kinetic binding model where the association and dissociation can be reliably calculated. If a monovalent ligand has a bivalent analyte flowed across it, each binding site on the analyte can interact independently with the ligand surface and dissociation rates can be artificially slow resulting in erroneous values reported for both k_d and K_D. Kinetic fitting then becomes more challenging because the data modeling is likely to be ambiguous [53]. Ideally, in this instance the experiment should be designed with low ligand density to minimize analyte binding sites from engaging multiple ligands simultaneously [32]. Equilibrium-based measurements are advised for situations where accurate numbers are necessary [26].

2.6 Surface Selection

Choosing the appropriate chip surface is critical for a well-designed and controlled experiment. Early SPR surfaces employed two-dimensional (2D) chemistry coatings for biomolecule attachment. These planar coatings were applied on top of the thin (50 nm) gold transducer layer. Planar coatings offer multiple surface chemistries for coupling and can provide a good option for immobilization when ligand surface density needs to be controlled to a low level [34]. As surface chemistry technologies matured, researchers experimented with thin hydrogels, commonly referred to as three-dimensional (3D), to decrease non-specific binding, and to provide molecular flexibility, high binding capacity, and custom coupling chemistries [35]. Over time, Biacore's CM5 carboxy-methyl dextran hydrogel surface has

Table 2
Surfaces for antibody studies using SPR

Surface	Application	Example
Gold	User customizable	AU[a]
Low-capacity hydrogel		
Normal matrix (100 nm)	Cell extracts, serums, membranes	CM4[a], HCLx[b]
Normal-capacity hydrogel		
Short matrix (30 nm)	Cell extracts, serums, membranes	CM3[a], GLC[c], CMD50[b],HC30[b]
Normal matrix (100 nm)	High immobilization of ligand	CM5[a], GLM[c], CMD200[b], CMD500[b], HC200[b]
High-capacity hydrogel		
Normal matrix	High immobilization of ligand	CM7[a], CMD5000D[b], HC1500M[b]
Streptavidin	Biotinylated protein, homogenous surface applications	SA[a], NLC[c], SADxx[b], SAHCx[b], BDx[c]
NTA	HIS tagged capture	NTA[a], HTG/HTE[c], NiHC1000M[b]
Hydrophobic	Membrane biochemistry and membrane-bound receptors	HPA[a], HPP[b]

[a]Biacore
[b]Xantec
[c]Bio-Rad

emerged as one of the most commonly used surfaces for SPR. More recently, chip surfaces are available from a number of different vendors. Table 2 highlights select surface chemistries available and provides general guidelines for surface selection.

2.7 Regeneration Techniques

Surface regeneration is the process of removing the bound analyte from the immobilized ligand, allowing it to rebind new analyte on a subsequent injection. Regenerating the ligand for sequential analyte binding is crucial for assay development [32, 33] and may depend in part on the stability of binding between the ligand and the surface. There are four general categories of regeneration solutions: chelators, high/low pH, high ionic strength, and detergents. For additional detail, van der Merwe has developed a thorough list of regeneration solutions under these groupings [36]. Notably there are no good quality control systems for surface regeneration.

Regeneration between antigen injection cycles is necessary because it is normally impractical to wait for the dissociation phase of a kinetic sensorgram to decay back down to the baseline, especially when studying highly stable antigen–antibody complexes with antibody covalently coupled to the biosensor surface. Randomly injecting antigen concentrations in duplicate or triplicate provides assurance that a sensorgram generated early in the experiment is reproduced several cycles later with the identical antigen concentration. This is only possible when the optimal surface regeneration conditions have been determined and the surface is stable for the duration of a full kinetic experiment.

For capture experiments where antigen is injected over antibody captured to a high-density covalently immobilized antispecies polyclonal antibody surface, one to two short 15 s pulses of ~146 mM phosphoric acid or glycine-HCl, pH 1.7 usually works well to remove all captured antibody while maintaining a reproducible capture surface. Certainly no "magic" regeneration formula exists that can be applied to all covalently immobilized antibody surfaces; however, to scout regeneration conditions, reagents of either low pH (i.e., phosphoric acid, glycine-HCl) or high pH (i.e., NaOH) should be injected at relatively short pulses of ~10–30 s each. Often multiple pulses of a regeneration reagent may be needed. Researchers often make the mistake of attempting to match the baseline before an antigen injection cycle with the post-regeneration baseline to assess regeneration success [36–38]. However, the fluid-like dextran matrix on the biosensor surface can swell as a result of certain regeneration solutions, causing discrepancies in the post-injection baseline signal, and necessitating a stabilizing period after regeneration in order to allow the signal to return to baseline. A successful regeneration scheme is achieved when multiple, properly referenced sensorgrams of identical antigen concentrations are reproducible. Drake and Klakamp (2011) recently detailed the Drake–Klakamp Method as a systematic, seven step experimental approach to more efficiently determine the optimal regeneration conditions for Biacore surfaces with covalently coupled proteins [39]. Finally, an injection of sample buffer should always be flowed over the flow cells at the start of an antigen injection cycle and immediately after the regeneration injections to wash out the microfluidic system.

2.8 General SPR System Maintenance

High-quality data requires that the SPR instrument is kept in good working condition, which includes instrument cleaning. It has been recommended that SPR instruments be cleaned with each of the following solutions, in order: (1) 0.5 % SDS, (2) 6 M urea, (3) 1 % acetic acid, and (4) 0.2 M $NaHCO_3$ [32]. Additional water rinsing is important to reduce the salt build-up in the flow system. To ensure the proper functionality of the instrument, a baseline must also be conducted as a quality control check. Generally, this is done by injecting the same running buffer as will be used for the experiment in order to initialize the system. Ideally there would be a stable baseline near 0 RU; however, it is more common that a low bulk refractive index change is observed that can then be subtracted from the experimental data with proper referencing [32].

3   Applications of SPR in Therapeutic mAb Development

3.1   Antigen-mAb Kinetics and Affinity

As SPR sensors can measure complex formation or dissociation, one of the primary uses of the instrument is for kinetic measurements [40]. Kinetic analysis of antibody interactions determines association and dissociation rate constants for interactions in real time. Most commercial SPR instruments have the ability to perform kinetic measurements "out of the box."

Biacore Inc. (now GE Healthcare) pioneered the use of SPR for kinetic analysis and to this day remains the market leader in this area [33, 41]. Several research papers provide a detailed description of performing kinetic analysis [21, 42–44] or a high level review of the topic [45]. In traditional kinetics experiments, a "ligand" (commonly the antibody) is attached to a biosensor chip surface followed by microfluidic injection of an "analyte" (commonly the antigen or target) over the surface [41]. In an experiment, the analyte associates and dissociates from the ligand over time, which generates an optical signal recorded in arbitrary resonance units (RUs). The accumulated signal trace as a function of time, or sensorgram, is in direct proportion to the amount of bound protein [21, 41–44]. Kinetics experiments commonly have four phases: (1) buffer injection phase where buffer is injected across the chip to prepare the surface and provide a baseline; (2) association phase where antigen is flowed over the surface; (3) dissociation phase where buffer alone is flowed across the surface to determine the dissociation of the antigen/antibody complex; and (4) regeneration where a regeneration buffer strips off the antigen to return to signal baseline. At this point, another experiment is conducted beginning at the buffer injection phase. Figure 5 shows an idealized sensorgram in which an antigen is injected over an immobilized antibody [33]. Typical experiments are represented by the following two state conformational change equation:

$$A + B \rightleftharpoons AB \rightleftharpoons (AB)^{*} \tag{1}$$

where A commonly represents the antigen (analyte), B represents the antibody (ligand), and AB represents the antigen/antibody complex [46].

In a well-designed affinity experiment, at least five analyte concentrations should be used that are below and above the K_D by at least tenfold if possible. In SPR experiments, $[AB]$ and $[B]$ are not approached as concentrations in solution, but as amounts at the surface expressed as an SPR signal [47].

As SPR data are recorded in real time, the kinetics constants for the binding interactions between the antigen and antibody can be derived. The kinetics modeling of the real-time sensor data represents the primary advantage of the biosensor. Three methods are

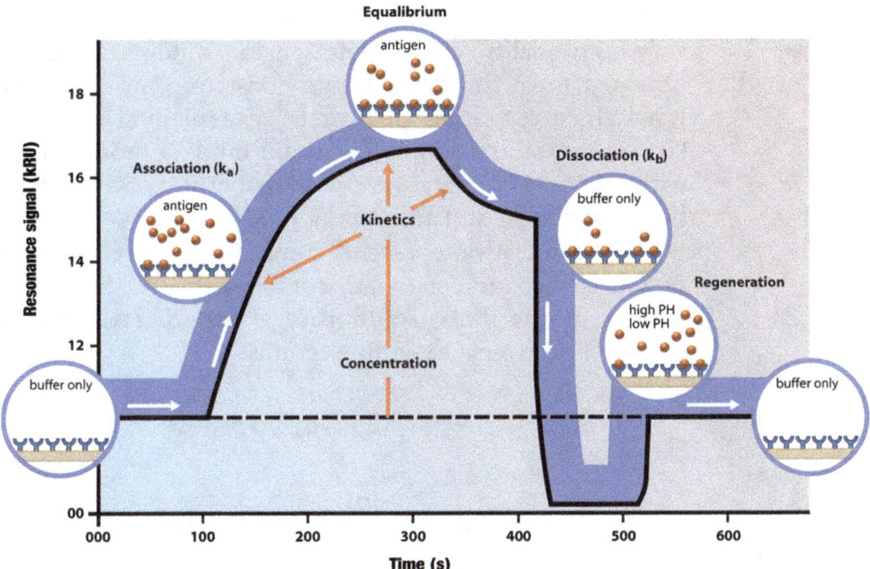

Fig. 5 Real-time binding with SPR enables measurement of concentration, affinity, and kinetics

currently used for calculating kinetic rate constants: (1) linearization, (2) curve fitting with analytical integration, and (3) curve fitting with numerical integration [46]. Linearization and curve fitting with analytical integration historically were popular providing a "reasonable estimate" for simple systems [46]. Initially, kinetic information was extracted from SPR biosensor data by fitting straight lines to portions of the transformed binding responses [28]. This method is extremely subjective when transformed data are inherently nonlinear [48] and can only be used to interpret a simple one-to-one interaction. The next approach developed was to directly fit response data using nonlinear least squares analysis by fitting an integrated rate equation for a simple one-to-one interaction model (Eq. 1) [48]. Unfortunately, most researchers found their experimental data were not described by a single integrated rate equation. Invariably, they discovered their data were described very well by fitting it to the sum of two integrated rate equations [48–57]; however, it has been demonstrated that this method of analysis can lead to misinterpretations of the true binding mechanism [46]. Multiple rate equations model only independent binding sites on the sensor surface. However, almost any response curve can be described by the sum of two or more of these equations, regardless of the underlying binding mechanism. The problem lies in the fact that there is not enough information in a single sensorgram to discriminate between different mechanisms. It has been shown that fitting association and dissociation phase data for a series of concentrations simultaneously (referred to as global analysis) can be used to discriminate between different reaction mechanisms [46]. In practice, however, global analysis requires very-high-quality experimental data. Binding affinities can be obtained from the ratio of rate constants, yielding a straightforward characterization of protein–protein interaction. To obtain kinetic constants a simple Langmuir binding model can be applied with numerical integration and global fitting of the data, providing the most robust and accurate fit [33, 46, 47].

The association constant, commonly referred to as on rate, k_a or k_{on}, is the number of AB complexes formed per second/unit volume in one molar solution of A and B. The units of this are (M^{-1} s^{-1}) or inverse molarity-seconds.

$$A + B \xrightarrow{k_{on}} AB \tag{2}$$

$$K_A = \frac{[AB]}{[A][B]}, \text{ with } K_A \text{ in } 1\,\text{mol}^{-1} \tag{3}$$

This value is determined during the association phase of the experiment. The k_{on} can be determined using the below equation:

$$R = \frac{[A]k_{on}R_{max}\left[1 - e^{-}\right]}{\left([A]k_{on} + k_{off}\right)} \tag{4}$$

The dissociation constant, commonly referred to as off rate, $k_{d,}$ or k_{off}, measures the inertness of AB complex and represents the fraction of complexes that decay per second. The units of the dissociation constant are inverse seconds or s^{-1}. The rate of the dissociation is described by the differential rate law or a simple exponential decay equation:

$$AB \xrightarrow{k_{off}} A + B \tag{5}$$

The equilibrium dissociation constant, referred to as affinity or K_D, has units of molarity. The equilibrium dissociation constant can be described in the following equation:

$$\frac{[A][B]}{[AB]} = \frac{k_{off}}{k_{on}} = K_D \tag{6}$$

$$K_D = \frac{[A][B]}{[AB]}, \text{ with } K_D = \frac{1}{K_A} \text{ in mol}\,1^{-1} \tag{7}$$

Beyond the modeling of the data, several factors remain challenging when measuring kinetic constants for mAbs: (1) long equilibrium times (days to reach), (2) fast association rates (ka >10^7 M^{-1} s^{-1}),

(3) slow dissociation times ($k_a < 1\mathrm{e}^{-5}$), and (4) very rapid dissociation time ($> 1\mathrm{e}^{-2}$). In these situations, utility of SPR instruments becomes somewhat limited, and other techniques such as the KinExA and fluorescence polarization anisotropy may be more appropriate. Affinities ranging from 1 nM to less than 10 pM should be readily measurable using most SPR units when utilizing kinetics constants.

3.2 Equilibrium Binding Analysis

As indicated above, for instances where association and dissociation rates become very rapid, data collection rates on most SPR instruments are insufficient to capture enough data points for accurate fitting. Potentially further complicating affinity determination using kinetics rates are mass transport limitations, multivalency of the proteins in question, and issues with analyte re-binding to the sensor surface. In these situations, although rates cannot be accurately measured, opportunities still exist to quantitate affinity by fitting the SPR responses to steady-state equations using equilibrium binding analysis.

Binding responses corresponding to formation of AB complex at equilibrium, previously described in Eq. (2), are correlated with injected analyte concentrations. In practice this can be modeled as follows, where R_{eq} is the analyte response at equilibrium:

$$R_{\mathrm{eq}} = \frac{C^A * \mathrm{Max}}{C^A + K_D} \tag{8}$$

Max is a variable denoting the maximum analyte binding capacity of the surface, with C_A as the concentration of injected analyte.

Fitting of the data using a nonlinear curve equation yields Max and K_D. Models should reflect 1:1 Langmuir binding. Ideally the plotted responses span a range at least two to three orders of magnitude above and below the estimated K_D with the higher responses beginning to approach saturating levels on the surface to ensure sufficient curvature for fitting. Equilibrium binding analysis is largely unaffected by high levels of ligand, in contrast to binding kinetics. Experimental conditions having the highest impact on accuracy of calculated K_D values for equilibrium binding analysis are fractional activity of analyte and surface coupled ligand, the latter of which must remain consistent during the course of the analyte injections.

3.3 Low-Resolution Screening

Traditionally, low-resolution screening on an SPR sensor has involved coupling the target antigen on the surface followed by flowing antibodies over the antigen, with an emphasis on increasing sample throughput, while minimizing time and reagent resources. Relative ranking of off-rates is often sufficient for assessing candidate mAbs and does not require accurate knowledge regarding the active concentration of mAb. This is particularly useful if the samples are crude hybridoma supernatants. Less common, but still an option is injection of a mAb concentration series, in order to obtain a series of sensorgrams for kinetics fitting, albeit with diminished throughput. However, as discussed in the Considerations section of this chapter, immobilizing antigen and then injecting the antibody as an analyte is not ideal due to avidity effects and poorly determined affinity.

Avoiding these avidity issues, Canziani et al. screened 24 antibodies from crude supernatant against their antigen with an Fc-specific capture surface using Biacore 2000 and 3000 optical biosensors [12]. Additionally, screening from crude mixtures against captured mouse anti-lysozyme monoclonal antibodies was performed using a continuous flow microspotter (CFM) to create a 4×12 array of 48 samples that were then analyzed in real-time for binding kinetics using a Biacore Flexchip instrument [22]. To facilitate the visualization of large amounts of kinetic data, it is convenient to plot the association and dissociation rates against one another. This analysis currently can be performed using the Ibis MX96 instrument and CFM with 96 mAbs. This type of presentation provides what is termed a kinetic distribution plot and quickly allows the identification of the antibodies with the desired affinity and kinetic characteristics.

3.4 High-Resolution Kinetics

SPR is widely regarded as the gold standard for antibody characterization because of the high-quality kinetic and affinity data that can be generated [58]. High-resolution SPR experiments require thoroughly addressing all of the issues discussed in the Considerations section of this chapter [59]. High-quality reagents (and hopefully well characterized reagents) are diluted across a range ideally spanning at least tenfold above and below the estimated K_D, resulting in seven to eight injections with three technical replicates [39]. Assuming the data generated are of sufficient quality, including little to no nonspecific binding to reference surfaces and curvature in sensorgram association profiles indicative of approaching surface saturation, the sensorgram curves should be globally fit. Data should be treated with caution, particularly if dissociation rates approach $1E^{-5}$ per second or slower, which is the limit of measure for most SPR sensors in typical experimental timeframes.

Generally speaking, high-quality kinetics is reproducible across multiple platforms by multiple users. As an example, a study was conducted involving 22 users, all measuring the binding of prostate-specific antigen (PSA) to a monoclonal antibody [42]. Kinetic characterization was performed by immobilizing the monoclonal antibody on the sensor chip surface at three different densities and then flowing the PSA over the surface at different concentrations to determine association and dissociation rate constants. Overall, the experimental standard error across all 22 studies for the values of the rate constants was only ~14 % [42], indicating a high reproducibility of kinetics data.

Although the above study nicely demonstrates a reproducible measure and speaks to the quality of data achievable when kinetics experiments are well thought out, it is low throughput in nature due to the limited sensor surfaces available on the instruments used. The next challenge for SPR kinetics is the development of new technologies that deliver the kinetics quality of current SPR systems in a robust, high-throughput manner. While throughput over the years has increased, an order of magnitude increase in throughput remains the elusive dream of long time SPR users [60].

4 Epitope Profiling

4.1 Epitope Binning

In addition to kinetics, another highly utilized application of SPR for antibody characterization is epitope binning [61]. Epitope binning is a pairwise competitive immunoassay that screens a library of antibodies to assess the ability of mAb pairs to block one another's binding to their antigen. Two antibodies that compete for the same or closely overlapping epitopes on the target antigen are said to "block" one another. Conversely, two antibodies that bind non-overlapping epitopes on the target antigen are said to "not compete with" or "not block" one another or "form a sandwich complex", because the two antibodies can bind the antigen at the same time. The blocking information from these experiments determines the family or "bin" into which the antibodies are placed. A blocking profile for each antibody relative to the others in the panel is calculated and antibodies with similar epitopes are binned together [62].

Recently, due to improvements in system throughput, the approach has been adapted to SPR and related biosensor technologies [63, 64]. Abdiche et al. outlined different assay formats in which an epitope binning assay can be performed using label-free biosensors (Fig. 6) [61, 65]. In the classical sandwich binning assay an immobilized antibody is used to capture the antigen followed by the addition of another antibody to test for binding to (or "sandwiching with") the preformed antibody/antigen complex. In the premix binning assay, immobilized antibody is tested for binding to a solution of the antigen that has been premixed with a saturating concentration of another antibody. In an in tandem assay, two antibodies are bound, one after another, to an immobilized antigen, to test whether the first antibody blocks binding of the second antibody. These binning assay formats complement one another as each has its unique applications and uses [61, 65]. Array-based SPR technology can be used to conduct epitope binning experiments with minimal sample amounts in either a classical sandwich assay or premix assay format, since both can be performed on an array of immobilized antibodies.

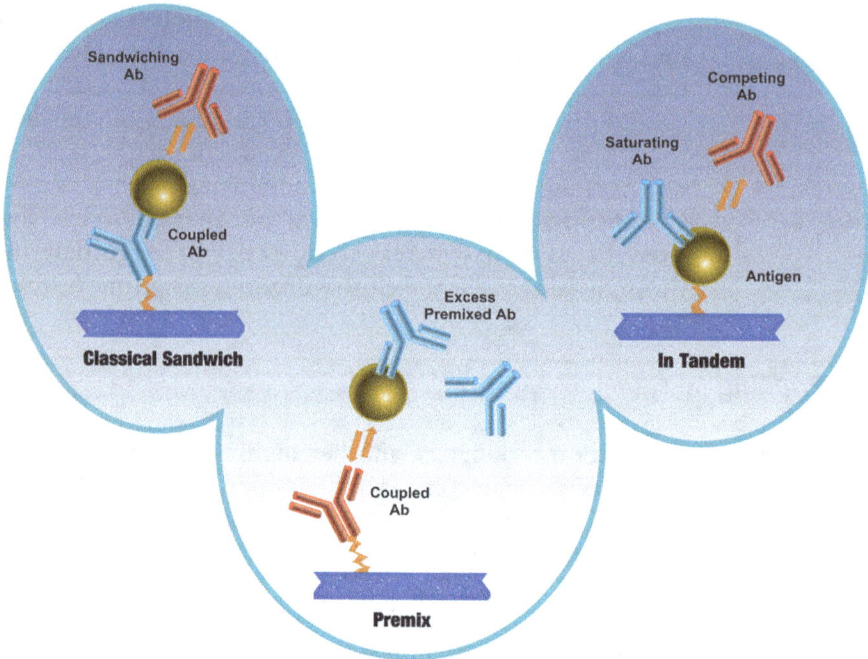

Fig. 6 Epitope binning. The three main assay formats in which an epitope binning assay can be performed using label-free biosensors

The limited throughput and high cost of performing epitope binning on SPR has resulted in the scientific community, using ELISA to conduct epitope binning assays. Traditionally, epitope binning methods have been performed using ELISA [44, 66] or Luminex [67] for higher throughput or Biacore or other SPR instruments for lower throughput [33]. Commonly, binning has been done later in the drug discovery process [61]. The Biacore 4000, ForteBio HTX, Ibis MX96, Sierra MASS-1, and Bio-Rad ProteOn XPR36 biosensor array systems each provide higher throughput with unique advantages [39]. Abdiche et al. detailed these advantages thoroughly [61, 62]. The importance of throughput cannot be understated for epitope binning [12, 13]. A comprehensive competitive pairwise epitope binning experiment of 96 antibodies would require up to 10,000 interactions, which is not easily accomplished with most commercial label-free biosensors in terms of time, cost, and sample requirement [4]. Also, software tools for the analysis of large epitope binning experiments are immature on most commercial platforms, with users routinely performing epitope binning analyses manually in external statistical software packages [68]. High-throughput epitope analysis tools are among the most critical to develop [68]. In this environment, epitope binning is emerging as an important new analytical tool.

Epitope binning reduces epitope bias and enables the maintenance of epitope diversity, which is highly desirable in the drug discovery process. The target antigen's epitopes may possess undesirable properties that current engineering practices cannot address; however, engineering an antibody's affinity is standard practice [69]. Thus, epitope selection may be of more importance in the early stages of discovery than affinity selection; moreover, performing epitope binning early in the process on large panels of antibodies to narrow it down to a few leads reduces the number of functionally inert clones or "dead-ends" that waste valuable time and resources [11]. Early epitope binning gives the researcher more biologically relevant candidates earlier and promising candidates are not missed that could be affinity-matured (Fig. 7) [61, 62, 66]. Epitope binning information can be merged with other data such as kinetic rate constants and activity in functional assays, allowing a more comprehensive view of a target antigen's epitope profile. Ultimately, epitope binning provides epitope diversity in a target and increases the number of promising candidates, thereby

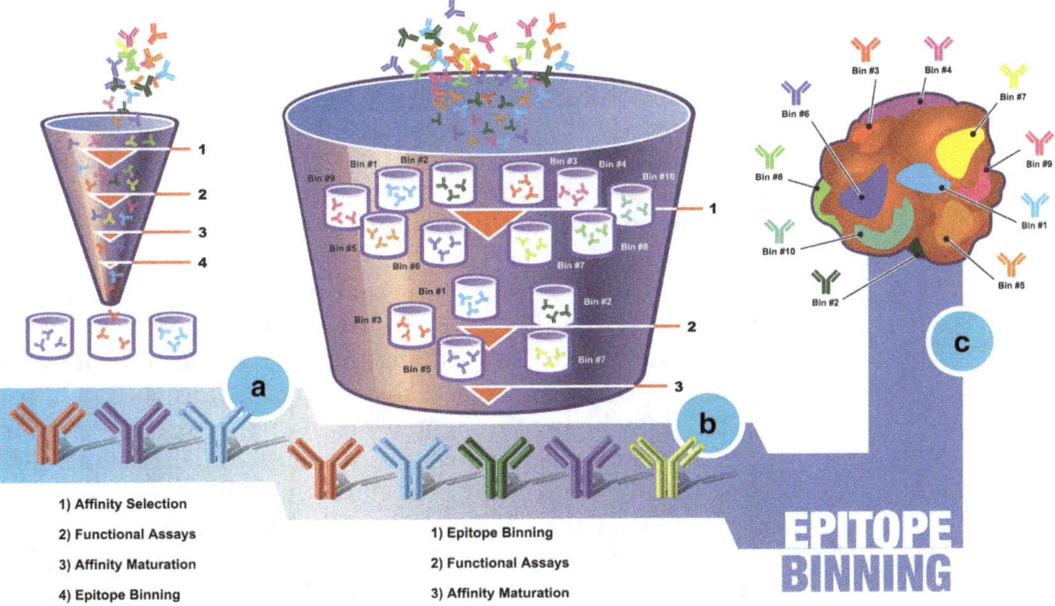

Fig. 7 Schematic illustrating the advantages of epitope binning early in the screening process. (**a**) Affinity-selection often leads to epitope bias as only a few of the high-affinity antibodies may bind functional epitopes. As a result, the probability that functional epitopes are represented in the selected panel is smaller as lower-affinity candidates are sometimes overlooked even though they possess the interaction with functional epitopes. (**b**) Epitope-based selection of the antibodies maintains epitopic diversity and increases the probability of finding therapeutically active antibody candidates. Once an antibody is identified with the desired functional activity it is likely to have "bin buddies" that exhibit a similar functional activity, thereby providing multiple leads to choose from. (**c**) Graphic illustrating where epitopes may fall on a 3D topology of an antigen surface; this graphic is meant only for illustration purposes, because binning does not identify or map the specific contact residues involved at the antigen/antibody binding interface

potentially reducing overall costs and increasing R&D productivity [11]. Beyond identifying different functional epitopes, binning also provides intellectual property value as well [62].

Epitope binning is also a relatively low cost assay that requires only the antigen and the antibodies, thus it is an ideal assay to begin the characterization of a large antibody panel [15]. Lastly, binning can help in characterizing antigens that possess antigen heterogeneity, which can be difficult to identify by other analytical methods [9]. Due to the benefits of real-time analysis and small sample consumption, high-throughput array-based SPR is poised to be a "game changer" for epitope binning. Further functional tests in combination with epitope binning data can provide more biologically and therapeutically relevant information earlier in the drug discovery process.

4.2 Epitope Mapping

Similar to epitope binning, but designed to more explicitly elucidate amino acid residues key to binding energetics, *epitope mapping* provides a much higher degree of resolution around the binding interfaces between antigens and monoclonal antibodies. Classic epitope mapping experiments involve the use of small peptide fragments and ELISAs [70, 71]. One of the more obvious challenges to the ELISA approach is the lack of real-time binding data, as an end-point-based measure is all the technique provides. For example, weaker epitopes may be missed if the binding signal, due to rapid dissociation, is below the limit of detection when the assay read-out is collected [62].

In the context of SPR, there are two potential assay formats for epitope mapping and both, in contrast to ELISA, enable real-time monitoring of both association and dissociation profiles. In the first format, antibodies are either immobilized or captured on the chip surface followed by probing the antibody ligands with overlapping peptide sequences of the antigen. In this approach, particularly in a higher-throughput array type format, an extensive number of antibodies on the surface could be interrogated against sequential injections of antigen peptides, providing high-resolution mapping for a large number of candidate antibodies.

In the alternate configuration, but still taking advantage of the power of an SPR array format, peptide libraries can be immobilized or captured on the chip surface followed by subsequent injections of antibody. Immobilization of the antigen peptides is less desirable due to the limited and varied reactive sites available as well as the potential for masking or otherwise compromising epitopes. Capture, via synthesis of a tag on the amine or carboxyl termini during peptide generation, is the preferred format to better ensure the most optimal presentation of the potential epitopes. Additionally a high affinity capture such as biotin-streptavidin would ensure a stable surface with no appreciable decay. Utilizing an SPR array approach, it is possible to screen high numbers of antibodies specific to different epitopes present on the antigen. With either of the aforementioned formats, one could envision the potential value in rapidly comparing epitope maps of in-house generated antibodies against competitor molecules to better ascertain freedom to operate in an intellectual property space.

A potential limitation of SPR epitope mapping is the under-representation of conformational epitopes [85]. Presence of a conformational epitope may however be inferred if epitope mapping experiments indicate no binding of a mAb to antigen peptides despite having demonstrated binding in other SPR formats with the intact antigen. If site-directed mutagenesis is performed and the antigen mutations are characterized, conformational epitopes can be characterized; however, under these circumstances additional inputs of expression and purification resources may make other techniques such as nuclear magnetic resonance (NMR) imaging more practical than SPR, albeit at a much reduced level of throughput, higher sample requirements, and the requirement of molecular weights less than 25 kDa [72]. Issues with sample requirements and molecular weight in NMR can be overcome using the more recently developed hydrogen-deuterium exchange mass spectrometry (HDX-MS), which monitors solvent accessible regions of a protein [73]. Similar to NMR, however, HDX-MS does not possess near the level of throughput achieved by SPR array epitope mapping, largely limiting the utility of HDX-MS in a screening setting.

4.3 Fc Receptor Binding

Although the antigen-binding (Fab) domain of a mAb garners significant attention from a drug discovery and development standpoint, the fragment crystallizable (Fc) region can potentially interact with receptor pathways independent of the Fab domain (Fig. 8). Specifically, the Fc-gamma receptors (Fc𝛾Rs) and neonatal receptor (FcRn) pathway are two avenues for modulating effector functions and circulation half-life, respectively.

In humans, there are four Fc𝛾Rs: Fc𝛾RIA, Fc𝛾RIIA, Fc𝛾RIIB, Fc𝛾RIIIA, and Fc𝛾IIIB. Figure 8 depicts the effector functions stimulated by Fc𝛾Rs binding to the various Ig isotypes. Excitatory receptors include Fc𝛾RI, Fc𝛾RIIA, and Fc𝛾RIIIB, of which Fc𝛾RIIIA is the most clinically relevant for induction of antibody dependent cellular cytotoxicity (ADCC) [74, 75]. The remaining receptors Fc𝛾RIIB and Fc𝛾RIIIB, are considered inhibitory based on their tendency to temper immune response [74, 75]. In addition to the specific immune functions that each of these receptors trigger, all induce phagocytosis. Also, it is worth pointing out the presence of multiple polymorphisms of Fc𝛾Rs in humans, which can significantly impact therapeutic responses [76]. Some of the more therapeutically relevant IgG-containing biologics have traditionally acted through Fc-mediated mechanisms to trigger anti-tumor responses [77]. More recently, oncology, immunology, and

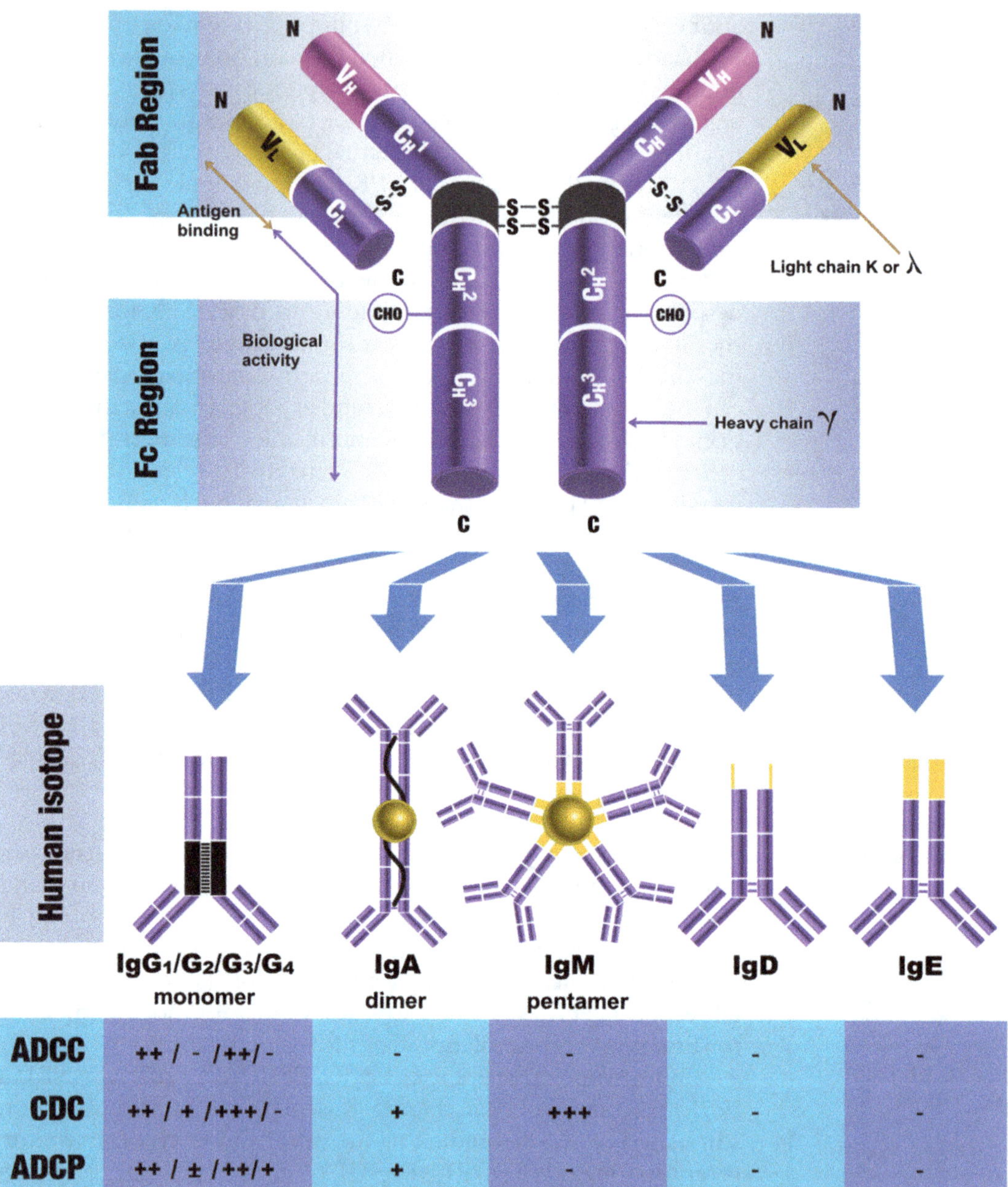

	IgG₁/G₂/G₃/G₄	IgA	IgM	IgD	IgE
ADCC	++ / - /++/ -	-	-	-	-
CDC	++ / + /+++/ -	+	+++	-	-
ADCP	++ / ± /++/ +	+	-	-	-

Fig. 8 Antibody structure based on isotype. Isotypes exhibit distinct structural and effector properties. Effector characteristics are critical when choosing the backbone for a therapeutic antibody

virology strategies have focused on enabling immune system recognition of disease where it otherwise would evade surveillance [78]. In both cases the selection and potential engineering of the IgG is critical towards optimizing the FcγR binding profile to achieve the most therapeutically beneficial response. To this end, modifications of the IgG Fc region can encompass both changes in primary sequence as well as altering the glycosylation profile [79, 80].

FcRn binding is also an important trait for mAbs as it is largely attributed to the long half-lives they enjoy in circulation [81]. FcRn binds to mAbs during endocytosis in the low pH (<6.0) endosomal compartment and recycles them to cell surface where they are released back into the more basic pH of the circulatory system. Efforts to design longer half-life mAbs with higher Fc-mediated affinity towards FcRn have met with limited success due to the requirement of release back into circulation [82, 83]. SPR has been used to uncover some intriguing binding patterns of human and mouse FcRn across species. In work conducted by Ober et al., human FcRn was shown to have very selective binding to IgG from other species; only showing activity towards guinea pig and rabbit IgG [82]. In contrast, mouse FcRn was a highly promiscuous binder against human, rabbit, bovine, guinea pig, and sheep IgG. These findings were seminal toward understanding FcRn recycling and consequent mAb half-life, particularly in pre-clinical models. Although FcRn and FcγRs bind to distinct regions on IgGs [84], FcRn binding is a routine requirement for candidate mAbs when FcγR modifications are made to ensure no impacts on FcRn binding and ultimately half-life.

SPR is an ideal technology to study FcγR and FcRn binding in therapeutic mAbs. Depending on the questions being asked, experiments can be designed to simply report a yes/no answer regarding binding or more fully interrogate binding kinetics. The low sample requirements of SPR make it particularly well suited when limited supplies of FcγRs are available. In a detailed study of four IgG isotypes against the five human FcγRs using SPR, a wide range of binding affinities was demonstrated, consistent with findings from earlier studies using orthogonal techniques [85]. The authors further noted that in contrast to SPR, the ELISA format did not appear to have sufficient sensitivity to measure weaker binding interactions. Li et al. measured kinetic and steady-state equilibrium dissociation constants of two IgG isotypes against FcγRIIIa and found excellent comparability of SPR with a flow cytometry assay for the same interaction [86]. In another paper, effects of all known FcγR polymorphisms on IgG binding using steady-state fitting of equilibrium binding data was explored, demonstrating not only remarkable dependence of binding affinity on the type of polymorphism, but also good insight into how these polymorphisms may correlate with clinical observations of the mAbs [87]. Additionally it was also found that SPR could identify weak interactions between certain receptor and IgG combinations not detected using immunofluorescence analysis.

Further opportunities for SPR in studies of FcγRs and FcRn could likely center around designing assay formats capable of handling combinations of multiple IgG Fc variants and not only human receptors but also those of preclinical models. As additional in-vivo models of human physiology and pathology are identified it would be expected that upfront screening would be accomplished using much larger FcγR and FcRn receptor panels for rapid determination of desired binding profiles. Further expanding this notion, detailed kinetics or steady-state affinity analysis in a high-throughput manner for IgG variants against multispecies FcγR and FcRn would provide a wealth of information necessary to better engineer the IgG Fc domain of mAbs toward specific therapeutic applications.

5   Formulation and Stability

As a mAb drug candidate moves beyond discovery and approaches the development stage, detailed characterization including selectivity, specificity, and binding stability is required for regulatory approval. During this phase it is also of importance to ensure that the mAb is biophysically suited for manufacturing, long-term storage, and dosing requirements. In conjunction, it is crucial to find an appropriate formulation that satisfies these aspects.

SPR is one tool among many others, such as differential scanning calorimetry (DSC), thermal scanning fluorescence (TSF), light scattering, size-exclusion chromatography (SEC), capillary isoelectric focusing (cIEF), and mass spectrometry (MS) for evaluating the stability under stress conditions meant to reflect production, storage, and dosing scenarios. In this application, SPR can be used to identify changes in fractional activity and altered antigen or Fc receptor binding kinetics. Stress studies may include multiple buffer and excipient combinations stored at different temperatures under varied light conditions. Concentrations can also be varied to reflect conditions expected during manufacturing or dose formulation. Finally mechanical stresses can be introduced, for example, to study the stability of a mAb under different manufacturing paradigms or dose delivery strategies [88]. These stresses can induce conformational changes such as denaturation, formation of aggregates, chemical modifications such as oxidation, isomerization, deamidation, as well as clipping [89, 90]. Fincke et al. performed a study using SPR, among other biophysical techniques, to look at the three different biologic formats, including IgG1, exposed to temperature stress. The authors identified aggregates, fragments, and denaturation which, importantly, impacted fractional activity of both the IgG1 Fab and Fc domains [89]. Other studies have utilized SPR to monitor antigen binding activity based on observations of chemical modifications in complementarity-determining regions (CDRs) as a function of time and buffer conditions, providing a high level of detail around how these changes affect antigen binding kinetics [91, 92]. In addition to the Fab region, studies of IgG Fc stability have demonstrated that oxidation of select methionines can result in diminished FcRn binding in SPR consistent with destabilization of IgG1 FcRn binding domains [158].

6 Condition Scouting

In the course of designing a robust assay, SPR is commonly used to identify suitable conditions for binding an analyte to an antibody, as antibodies can be conformationally sensitive [93]. In general, SPR can be used to screen for optimal solubilization, purification, and crystallization conditions [33, 93]. Condition scouting is used to create either "(1) an experimental parameter to increase the fidelity of the affinity interaction or (2) a regeneration condition to improve the sensitivity and accuracy of sequential affinity-based analysis on a biosensor surface" [93]. More recently, several SPR sensors have been developed providing high-throughput mechanisms to screen a multitude of buffer conditions to determine appropriate conditions based on the necessary tertiary structure to facilitate ligand-analyte interactions, particularly in the context of the microenvironment created by the biosensor surface interaction [93].

G-protein coupled receptors (GPCRs) are membrane protein receptors that transmit signals from an extracellular stimulus to the interior of the cell by activation of GTP-binding proteins (G proteins). GPCRs mediate vital metabolic, sensorial, immunological, hormonal, and neurotransmission processes [94] and are triggered by a variety of extracellular stimuli including ions, hormones, light, lipids, glycoproteins, and ligand binding. Due to GPCRs involvement in a wide variety of physiological processes, including control of neuronal transmission and cardiac function, they are important targets for therapeutic intervention [95]. Up to half of the drugs on the market today modulate some form of GPCRs activity, and it is estimated that 25–50 % of the total drug targets are in the GPCR families [96, 97]. Elucidating GPCRs structure, function, and mechanism of interaction with different binding partners remains of critical importance to rational drug design [94, 95]. The great variety of receptor-stimulating ligands and high hydrophobicity of membrane proteins still poses significant challenges [94]. GPCRs are extremely hydrophobic as they are structurally characterized by seven transmembrane-spanning α-helices. They most often require a lipid environment to maintain the protein's native conformation. Compounding the situation further is the fact that GPCRs often are expressed at very low levels in the cell which has resulted in most GPCR studies being conducted using fluorescently labeled or radiolabeled ligands in cell-based assays [95]. Unfortunately, in order to overcome sensitivity limitations due to a low number of receptors, cell lines are often created that overexpress the GPCRs, which creates other problems. Many GPCRs are proving to be challenging targets for small molecule drugs, and as an alternative may be better approached with biologics, including mAbs (*see* Fig. 9) [98]. Significant to the challenges associated with GPCRs is finding conditions where the receptor is in a conformationally native state while still accessible for binding assays.

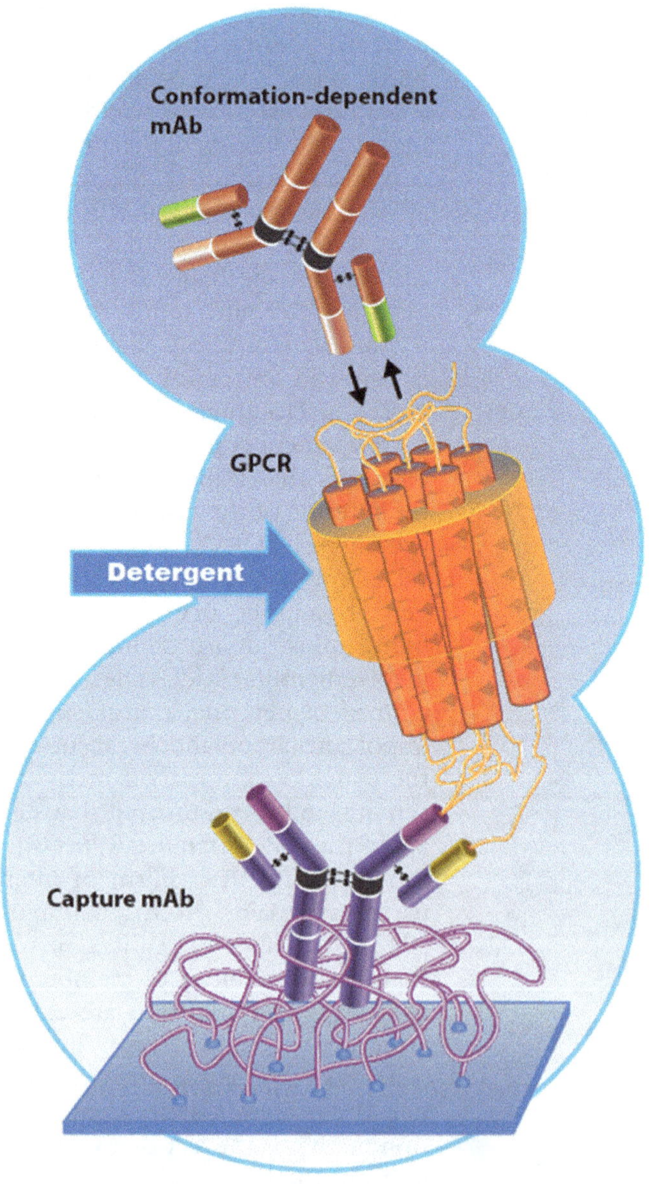

Fig. 9 GPCR schematic. Schematic showing how a GPCR can be captured for SPR analysis

SPR provides unique advantages when studying the binding activity of GPCRs including no labels, real-time information, and minimal sample preparation. Also, the conformational states of the receptors can be probed without labels in the presence and absence of a reconstituted bilayer. As Myszka et al. noted, "there are three advantages to using this receptor-capturing approach: (1) there is no need to purify the receptor prior to immobilization on the biosensor surface, (2) the receptors are homogeneously immobilized through the capturing step, and (3) the receptors can be captured at high enough densities to allow the study of relatively low-molecular-mass ligands (2,000–4,000 Da)" [95]. Multiple techniques have been described for characterizing GPCRs with SPR. Described here are some of the most prominent methods, including those from Karlsson and Löfås [99] and Myszka and Rich [95].

Karlsson and Löfås [99] used an SPR method with an L1 biosensor chip (a carboxymethyl dextran surface with additional hydrophobic alkane groups) to study GPCRs [100]. The L1 chip is used to capture lipids to form a synthetic membrane environment [101, 102]. The synthetic membrane is created by amine-coupling purified rhodopsin into a lipid bilayer environment around the receptors using lipid/detergent-mixed micelles [99]. This method, while encouraging, requires significant effort to purify the GPCR prior to analysis. Also, the GPCRs are not uniformly oriented on the biosensor surface due to the fact that the amine-coupling procedure is not site specific and may bind any amine group on the surface of rhodopsin [103].

The second method is described by Myszka and Rich [95, 104] and referred to as capture and reconstitution. In this method a specific capturing molecule is used to concentrate a GPCR from a crude cell preparation, and then reconstitute a lipid bilayer environment on a biosensor chip. This method requires the production of paramagnetic proteoliposomes containing pure, uniformly oriented native GPCRs [105, 106]. Successful experiments with conformationally sensitive monoclonal antibodies illustrate how to study membrane-associated receptors [95, 104]. Additional methods/techniques based on these two approaches are described in the following references [104, 107, 108].

Despite these advantages and a large demand for the capabilities of SPR sensing in GPCR applications, the ability to perform assays in a highly parallel fashion has historically been a major limiting factor in its application [12, 18, 19] and overall remains challenging even after decades of study [94]. GPCRs are the most studied of the major drug target classes, and yet the introduction of new drugs based upon GPCR targets into the market in the last decade has been limited. Binding assays have remained an important first step in understanding ligand-receptor specificity, binding dynamics, and in generating quantitative data. With ever increasing evidence as to the importance of GPCR heterodimerism, functional selectivity, and the exhibition of polypharmacology by drugs, the complexity of ligand-receptor activity is increasing and the need is evident for higher-throughput assay methods to cope with this complexity.

7   Immunogenicity of Therapeutic mAbs

While uncommon to small molecule pharmaceuticals, therapeutic mAbs have the potential to elicit unwanted immune responses in both preclinical and clinical settings. These responses can be humoral and/or cell-mediated in nature, resulting in the formation of anti-drug antibodies (ADAs) [109]. Presence of ADAs can neutralize the active concentration of therapeutic mAb, resulting in diminished pharmacokinetics/pharmacodynamics (PK/PD). Although the ADA response has been recognized for some time in the literature [110] there are still challenges with effectively de-immunizing mAbs. A number of in-silico prediction tools have being developed [111] along with traditional engineering strategies [112] to remove immunogenic "hot spots" from mAbs early in the drug discovery process. In the case of mAbs generated in mice or rabbits for example, efforts are put toward "humanizing" lead candidates [113]. Beyond primary sequence and structure, glycosylation patterns, chemical modifications, and formation of aggregates all have been found to increase incidence of immunogenicity [112].

Careful monitoring of immunogenicity, and in particular ADAs, is crucial for accurate interpretation of PK/PD parameters and overall improvement of safety outcomes in clinical trials. Traditionally ELISA have been the staple for ADA screening, composed of a bridging assay where mAb drug is coupled to the plate wells, followed by addition of serum or plasma, then washed and probed using the mAb drug with a reporter label. More recently, similar formats have been incorporated into newer technologies such as electrochemiluminescence (ECL) and donor/acceptor bead signaling (e.g. MSD and AlphaScreen, respectively) [114, 115]. The aforementioned assays are all endpoint in nature and to an extent face challenges in terms of clearly delineating ADAs as neutralizing versus nonneutralizing as well as identifying the isotype of the ADA which is often of interest toward better understanding the immune response and requires additional follow up analyses. *See* Fig. 8 for information on the different human isotypes and the corresponding immune response mechanisms.

Current SPR platforms are well suited to address these more detailed, structure-based questions and have been effectively utilized to these ends [116, 117]. SPR platforms can determine ADA nonspecific binding issues, semi-quantitate concentration, isotype, and affinity. SPR has the added benefit of being able to observe the primary binding of ADAs to a mAb drug surface followed by secondary binding of either mAb drug to confirm specificity, anti-isotype mAbs, or other reagents to better understand the ADA epitope(s). Several studies have reported good comparability of SPR to ECL or ELISA with respect to limits of detection, and in some instances found that for low affinity mAbs, SPR is actually superior. Reflective of the rich SPR kinetic information absent in the other techniques, discrepancies across these methods appear attributable to signal reporting not being matched to differences, in particular, to dissociation rates [118]. Weeraratne et al. also described a head-to-head comparison of ECL and SPR, finding that SPR was superior for both sensitivity and drug tolerance for a peptide-Fc fusion drug in clinical trial [119]. Currently the major hurdle for SPR as a key screening tool in immunogenicity as opposed to being second or third tier in the assay paradigm is achieving throughput on the scale of plate-based technologies such as ELISA and ECL. To some extent for preclinical studies and undoubtedly for clinical trials, sample numbers are likely to be substantial and require rapid processing. Additionally, array-based platforms such as the IBIS MX96 or Horiba EzPlex may allow for multiplexing of several different assay formats on a single surface, combining both detection as well as interrogation of isotype, binding mechanism, and so on.

8   SPR with Whole Cells

In whole cell SPR, living cells are brought to interact with the surface, similar to how antigen is coupled to an SPR surface with conventional assays. Cell adhesion results with the cell plasma membrane being approximately 10–100 nm away from the substrate surface. This means that optical biosensors of relatively short penetration depths are still able to sense the bottom portion of cells [98]. Sensing changes in the bottom portion of the cells as a result of changes in degree of cell adhesion or recruitment of intracellular proteins to activated receptors on the cell surface, for example, leads to a change in refractive index at the sensor surface which is detected using SPR. As opposed to conventional SPR that measures the amount of analyte binding to immobilized receptors, whole cell sensing is a result of the sum of all redistribution events within the sensing volume [98]. Researchers have explored the use of SPR to study the changes in the cell cytoskeleton, giving insight into changes in cell activity [99–102]. This includes work conducted by Fang et al. (2005) who used a biosensor similar to SPR to study the release of intracellular proteins from saponin-permeabilized Chinese hamster ovary (CHO) cells. Their work, combined with others [102, 103] led to the hypothesis that "most biomaterials are highly organized in cells primarily through direct binding or transient association with cytoskeletal filaments, and are not free to diffuse over a long distance," [98] which is a key component to understanding biomaterial-host interactions. Cleiren et al. explored the use of SPR to measure the interaction between hepatitis C virus NS5B polymerase and a small-molecule inhibitor. The kinetics and affinity of the enzyme-inhibitor interactions were measured, making it possible to select potent and promising lead candidates [104].

A fundamental limitation of the use of SPR biosensors for the study of whole cells is the limited distance that the plasmon wave can penetrate into the material above the sensor surface. An SPR biosensor can interrogate changes in refractive index up to 100 nm above the surface, giving knowledge of only the portion of the cell that is directly in contact with the surface. While this can be used to estimate the changes occurring over the entire membrane, the receptors, membrane proteins, and other cytoskeletal components may not be uniform around the cell. SPR analysis of whole cells remains a very challenging frontier. However, the potential of being able to interrogate cells in real-time with therapeutics, such as mAbs, means that new strategies will continue to be explored.

9   Nontraditional Antibody Formats

With around 30 monoclonal antibody (mAb) drugs on the market and more than 100 in clinical trials, engineered antibodies have become a mainstay in the pharmaceutical industry. By 2020, engineered antibodies, both full length and fragments, are predicted to account for a majority of all pharmaceutical revenues [120]. Antibody fragments (e.g. FAb and scFv) and engineered variants (diabodies, triabodies, minibodies, and single-domain antibodies) are leading the next generation of mAb-based biotherapeutics after the engineered mAb. Antibody fragments and engineered variants possess a highly tuned structure, smaller size, more efficient manufacturing, and properties which can be engineered (e.g. easier tissue penetration), as well as possess other unique and superior properties of diagnostic and therapeutic applications [121]. As a result they are being designed "into multivalent and multispecific reagents, linked to therapeutic payloads (such as radionuclides, toxins, enzymes, liposomes, and viruses) and engineered for enhanced therapeutic efficacy" [121]. Antibody fragments are becoming important engineering platforms for future drug candidates [122]. However, they often possess a shorter half-life and lack Fc mediated effector mechanisms that affect both efficacy of the drugs and the PK/PD [123]. These drawbacks seem to be outweighed by the advantages of fragment formats (*see* Fig. 8) [120].

Generally, techniques that work effectively for whole antibody characterization apply to antibody fragments and engineered variants. Although SPR is routinely used to generate both sensitive and reliable kinetic data from antibody/antigen interactions, several issues arise when using SPR for antibody fragments including the method of surface attachments (capture or couple) and the state of purification (purified or crude). With respect to the trade-offs for the method of surface attachment, two approaches to surface attachment are coupling the antibody fragment to the surface, which involves direct covalent attachment of the molecule to the surface (usually through amine or carboxy chemistries) and capture, which involves covalently attaching another capture molecule on the surface (usually an anti-FC antibody, NTA/His$_6$, biotin/avidin, or another ligand). The selection criteria include the type of antibody and the host where the protein is being produced. Capture options are usually more limited with antibody fragments and engineered variants because the molecules possess a smaller number of useable targets—most notably missing in most fragments is the FC region; however, that would not be the case if a tag was engineered into the protein. Researchers commonly select capture because protein orientation and paratope availability is more predictable [36]. Despite the disadvantages described here, antibody fragments are still often used for kinetic screening, such as the studies conducted with human Ab fragments against Tie-1 [124], human tissue kallikrein 1 [125], and PcrV protein [43].

Fragment selection, while commonly practiced, remains a time consuming process and commonly occurs through multiple rounds of binding studies [126]. Specific phages are characterized, then eluted, reinfected into the host, followed by numerous rounds of panning [127, 128]. While phage display is widely used in many pharmaceutical laboratories [129], the successful selection of specific antibodies remains a challenge [130]. Common problems include the optimization of selection conditions, preferential recovery of high avidity (i.e. highest display level on an individual phage particle) and a large number of biopanning rounds [131, 132].

Currently, endpoint assays are used most frequently to screen the large number of antibodies in a library. However, endpoint assays such as ELISAs are commonly unreliable due to differences in antibody valence and host expression levels [124]. Several techniques have been explored to screen antibody fragments and engineered variants in a more rapid fashion from crude matrices using optical biosensor platforms [63, 133]. Because the process is so time intensive, the ability to screen using an SPR system with high throughput (an order of magnitude greater than current machines) would be highly desirous. In addition, the ability to screen directly from crude sample using either capture or coupling techniques would also be highly desirable. Using epitope binning on the front end would also help, as it is important that a comprehensive number of individual clones, rather than a small representative subset, are analyzed [131]. High-throughput SPR has significant potential for removing long delays by providing relatively short testing times.

Phage display technologies can generate thousands of clones for screening against most antigens while the traditional immunized organism approach can generate hundreds if not thousands of clones as well. Current SPR systems lack the throughput to screen all of the clones as a primary screen [133]; moreover, many screening assays entail rigorous sample preparation and purification prior to SPR analysis. Besides vigorous sample prep, current SPR systems are limited in their throughput [133]. Greater throughput would be a boon to the label-free screening of antibody fragments.

10   Commercial SPR Platforms with Increased Throughput

Biacore has historically established the benchmark for SPR instrumentation, most commonly with lower-throughput platforms, such as the T200. The T200 is equipped with four flow cells that can be fluidically addressed either as individual cells, pairs of cells or all four cells. Currently the only commercially available higher-throughput platform offered by Biacore is the 4000, with four flow cells comprised of five monitored spots within each flow cell, yielding the ability to measure four analyte injections against five ligand surfaces in parallel. Including the needed reference surfaces in each flow cell, the 4000 can monitor up to 16 binding events simultaneously.

In terms of higher-throughput formats, several other instruments have taken a nonstandard approach to determining kinetics that will be briefly reviewed here including the BioRad Proteon, Sensiq Pioneer, Sierra Mass-1, Horiba Ez-Plex, and IBIS MX96. The ProteOn XPR36 is a parallel array imaging SPR biosensor utilizing a six channel microfluidic flow path that can be rotated 90° on the chip surface. By immobilizing ligands in one orientation and then delivering analytes in the corresponding perpendicular direction, up to 36 interactions can be monitored simultaneously, with surface referencing accomplished via "interspots" on the empty surface between the immobilized ligands [116]. Response data can be collected at six different concentrations of an analyte over six different ligands. This enables a "one-shot" kinetics approach that generates high-quality kinetic data on 6 mAbs at a time [134].

The SensíQ Pioneer utilizes dynamic injection SPR (diSPR™) in which buffer and sample streams are mixed immediately upstream of the reaction surface allowing for multiple analyte injections from a single loaded analyte concentration to be tested across up to three ligand surfaces. In doing so, the Pioneer generates a full concentration series while reducing time and workload [135].

The Sierra Sensors MASS-1 utilizes eight flow cells, each containing two individually addressable ligand surfaces. Depending on how reference surfaces are arranged, up to 16 spots can be monitored in real time [136]. The high sensitivity of the MASS-1 also enables monitoring of antibody fragment and small molecule binding.

The Horiba Ez-Plex utilizes SPR imaging (SPRi) to monitor an array of up several hundred ligand spots in real-time. Spots are generated either by contact or flow printing [137].

Lastly, the IBIS MX96 utilizes SPRi to scan up to 144 regions of interest (ROI) on the sensor surface. In a typical experiment, 96 ligands are flow printed as an array on the surface of the SPR sensor, followed by repeated injections of analytes across the entire surface, while utilizing interspots for reference surface correction. This array format significantly increases throughput for both kinetics as well as epitope binning studies with minimal sample consumption [138].

From the brief descriptions of the above platforms it is evident that multiple technological approaches are being taken to address SPR throughput requirements. Ultimately these efforts will be critical toward accelerating bottlenecks in therapeutic mAb development and open up possibilities for new SPR applications.

11   Alternative Techniques to SPR

While SPR detection is the most widely used label-free technology for the detection of biomolecular interactions, other techniques exist such as isothermal titration calorimetry (ITC), interferometry, diffraction, DNA levers, atomic force microscopy (AFM), and quartz crystal microbalance (QCM). All except ITC require surface coupling of at least one of the binding partners being interrogated.

Traditionally analyte/ligand interactions have been assessed by labeled, end-point detection mechanisms (ELISA, radio immunoprecipitation, high performance liquid chromatography (HPLC), etc.) [139], where the label is used to amplify the signal. However label-free biosensors (e.g., SPR, kinetic exclusion assay (KinExA), oblique-incidence reflectivity difference (OIRD), bio-layer interferometry, etc.) are becoming increasingly popular due to the potential for more physiologically relevant interactions in the absence of a label. Nevertheless, such techniques are not without their limitations. Experimental designs to assess analyte/ligand interactions should consider the sensitivity, specificity, complexity, and throughput of the technique chosen.

11.1 End-Point Detection

ELISA-based testing has become the clinical standard for many endpoint detection needs due to its simplicity, reproducibility, and cost effectiveness [140]. However, the ELISA may not be sensitive enough for certain applications (e.g., AHL small molecules which require the specificity [141] and sensitivity provided by SPR [140]), usually requiring antibodies with high affinity to minimize the amount of required reagents [142]. Radio immunoprecipitation may circumvent some of these pitfalls while providing for highly sensitive and specific solution phase interactions; however, radiolabelling may (1) interfere with interactions, (2) fail to detect rapid disassociations, and (3) present safety concerns [141, 143]. Ellipsometry, mass spectrometry, and HPLC could also be used to determine interactions between different molecules; however, limited kinetic data is often gleaned from these techniques and sample preprocessing is frequently required [144, 145]. Finally, AFM may offer an alternative end-point detection method that can combine both elements of a bioassay with an optical biosensor [146]; however, the throughput is limited as is the sensitivity of the technique.

11.2 Real-Time Detection Methods

11.2.1 Biosensors

There are two primary types of biosensors: electrochemical or impedance-based and optical. Electrochemical/impedance biosensors are not frequently used to assess analyte/ligand interactions, but are more often used to evaluate bacterial/antibiotic or cellular interactions [147–149]. Alternatively, a variety of optical biosensors are available to measure the kinetics of analyte/ligand binding.

11.2.2 Optical Biosensors for Surface-Bound Antigens

Although Biacore systems may be the most well-known optical biosensing instrument, there are several other commercially available systems, listed in Table 3. Despite widespread utilization, some of the upfront challenges with use of SPR, as highlighted previously in this chapter, include (1) immobilization of the ligand and surface chemistry that may impact binding kinetics due to altered conformation [141], (2) boundaries in resolution for particularly slow disassociation constants [26, 150], (3) multivalency and multiple modes of binding which are difficult to fit [59, 151], (4) restrictions in the resolution of small molecule interactions, and (5) surface regeneration conditions that are difficult to quality control. In addition to these conditions, which may constrain the utility of SPR, mass transport effects must also be considered [59, 151], although appropriate experimental design and flow conditions can minimize this effect. Localized SPR (LSPR), which is based on a nanoparticle-based detection, can overcome some of these disadvantages due to a much smaller working distance [152]. However, LSPR technology is relatively new and the utility remains to be proven.

Similar to SPR but with slightly different underlying physics, phase-based common path interferometry offers a real-time, label-free

Table 3
Commercially available biosensors

Manufacturer	Model(s)
BiaCore	4000 T200 X100 3000 SPR-MALDI Interface C
Bio-Rad	Proteon
BiOptix	404pi
Horiba	EzPlex OpenPlex
Ibis	MX96
SensiQ	Pioneer
Reichert	SR7500
Sierra	SPR-2
GWC	SPRimager

mechanism to determine antibody/antigen interactions with detection sensitivity as low as 14 fg [139, 153]. Bio-layer interferometry (BLI) also utilizes wavelength shifts as a measure of signal, though this signal is more related to changes in sensor surface optical thickness, rather than additive mass as in traditional SPR [154]. Despite this difference in detector signal, BLI shares substantial overlap in applications with SPR.

11.2.3 Optical Biosensors for Solution Phase Antigens

To address concerns regarding accuracy and fidelity of kinetic measurements from a surface-bound analyte, solution measurements can also be made. KinExA not only provides indirect solution phase association and disassociation kinetics over a wide range, including extremely slow disassociation rates, but it can also measure a percentage of active antibody [155]. This technology enables calculation of exceptionally high affinity binders that are typically beyond the range of SPR instruments [120]. SPR correlates well with the KinExA method derived kinetic constants [26]. Notably, however, the system is unable to measure the binding association constant when the analyte and antibody concentration needed for a measurable signal reach equilibrium within 2 s [155]. Similar to LSPR, KinExA analysis depends on analyte presentation on beads/hapten. This leads to more manually intensive procedures in order to prime and clean the system before and after a series of runs, a significant disadvantage when multiple samples must be processed.

Furthermore, although the system requires very little antibody to detect binding kinetics, reactants are only detectable at concentrations around or below their affinity for one another.

11.2.4 Isothermal Titration Calorimetry

ITC presents an alternative to surface-based detection methodologies by acquiring solution phase affinity, stoichiometry, and thermodynamic data; however, instrumentation can be challenging to use and often cost prohibitive [155–160]. Moreover, measurements require a large amount of sample due to their limited sensitivity and disassociation constant range [144]. This said, solution-based ITC measurements have been found to correlate well with those obtained using SPR [43]. Although efforts have been made to increase the automation of ITC, in comparison to SPR it remains a relatively low-throughput application best suited for confirmation of binding stoichiometry and thermodynamics, or in cases where surface immobilization of one of the binding components is not feasible.

11.3 Bioassays

Although both traditional SPR and solution phase kinetic measurements can provide data on analyte/ligand interactions, none of the techniques previously reviewed, including the end-point-labeled detection techniques, can provide functional validation of interaction. Only bioassays are able to provide a more systems biology approach to analyze an interaction. Resonant wavelength grating biosensors use living cells under physiological conditions [161]. Importantly, the resonant wavelength grating approach only measures reactions from the bottom layer of adherent cells. Unfortunately, as with any biological system approach, bioassays are costly, technically demanding, difficult to standardize, and labor intensive. Furthermore, data represent an integrated set of cellular responses, including off target effects.

12   Future Outlook for SPR

The ability to monitor biomolecular interactions in real time has enabled the development of a large number of applications for SPR biosensors in mAb drug development. Historically, an area that SPR has suffered from is limited throughput; however, higher-throughput approaches have emerged that allow for the analysis of many thousands of interactions. Currently, the trade-off for this is decreased sensitivity when compared to lower-throughput platforms that will necessitate improvements in SPR sensor and detection technologies.

Looking forward, increased throughput and sensitivity opens up a number of interesting possibilities for SPR applications. SPR has been a workhorse for generating kinetics and affinity data and as platforms incorporating more array-based detection systems emerge, the opportunity to screen even greater number of therapeutic candidates will continue to grow. This would likely also be the case for epitope profiling, which has historically been relegated to characterizing lead candidates as opposed to being a front-line ranking tool. Additionally, SPR may begin to supplant many of the current endpoint assays in mAb production platforms such as ELISA for affinity ranking, titer, and isotyping both in supernatants as well as small-scale purifications. One could envision combinatorial assays being developed that encompass antigen binding/kinetics, isotyping, FcγR-, and FcRn binding into one sample injection. Furthermore, the more recent successful application of SPR as a tool in characterizing ADAs might enable additional routine applications in the clinical space with systems that can array a large number of binding interactions, while meeting or exceeding sensitivity limits found on lower-throughput SPR platforms. The push toward biosimilars will continue to rely heavily on the use of SPR to confirm comparability to innovator mAbs, in many cases being the first-line in demonstrating equivalence. Overall the utility of SPR as a critical tool in therapeutic mAb discovery and development will continue to grow.

References

1. Boozer C, Kim G, Cong S et al (2006) Looking towards label-free biomolecular interaction analysis in a high-throughput format: a review of new surface plasmon resonance technologies. Curr Opin Biotechnol 17:400–405. doi:10.1016/j.copbio.2006.06.012

2. Evans JB, Syed BA (2014) From the analyst's couch: next-generation antibodies. Nat Rev Drug Discov 13(6):413–414

3. Epstein MS, Ehrenpreis ED, Kulkarni PM (2014) Biosimilars: the need, the challenge, the future: the FDA perspective. Am J Gastroenterol 109:1856–1859. doi:10.1038/ajg.2014.151

4. Sitte HH, Freissmuth M (2013) Biosimilars versus generics: scientific basics and clinical implications. Mag Eur Med Oncol 6(3): 202–206

5. Walsh G (2014) Biopharmaceutical benchmarks. Nat Biotechnol 32:992–1000. doi:10.1038/nbt.3040

6. Arnum PV (2013) Tracking growth in biologics. Pharm Technol 37:16

7. Rich RL, Myszka DG (2004) Why you should be using more SPR biosensor technology. Drug Discov Today Technol 1:301–308

8. Myszka DG, Rich RL (2003) SPR's high impact on drug discovery: resolution, throughput and versatility. Drug Discov World 49(1):49–55

9. Homola J, Yee SS, Gauglitz G (1999) Surface plasmon resonance sensors: review. Sens Actuators B Chem 54:3–15. doi:10.1016/S0925-4005(98)00321-9

10. Homola J, Piliarik M (2006) Surface plasmon resonance (SPR) sensors. In: Surface plasmon resonance sensors. Springer, p 45–67

11. Weingart CL, Broitman-Maduro G, Dean G et al (1999) Fluorescent labels influence phagocytosis of Bordetella pertussis by human neutrophils. Infect Immun 67:4264–4267

12. Altschuh D, Dubs MC, Weiss E, Zeder-Lutz G, Van Regenmortel MHV (1992) Determination of kinetic constants for the interaction between a monoclonal antibody and peptides using surface plasmon resonance. Biochemistry 31(27):6298–6304

13. Wammes AEM, Fischer MJE, de Mol NJ et al (2013) Site-specific peptide and protein immobilization on surface plasmon resonance chips via strain-promoted cycloaddition. Lab Chip 13:1863–1867. doi:10.1039/c3lc41338a

14. Kooyman RPH, Corn RM, Frazier RA et al (2008) Handbook of surface plasmon resonance: RSC, 1st edn. Royal Society of Chemistry, Cambridge, UK

15. Rich RL, Myszka DG (2008) Survey of the year 2007 commercial optical biosensor literature. J Mol Recognit 21:355–400

16. Haab BB, Dunham MJ, Brown PO (2001) Protein microarrays for highly parallel detection and quantitation of specific proteins and antibodies in complex solutions. Genome Biol 2(2)

17. MacBeath G, Schreiber SL (2000) Printing proteins as microarrays for high-throughput function determination. Science 289:1760–1763

18. Houseman BT, Mrksich M (2002) Towards quantitative assays with peptide chips: a surface engineering approach. Trends Biotechnol 20:279–281. doi:10.1016/S0167-7799(02)01984-4

19. Vijayendran RA, Leckband DE (2001) A quantitative assessment of heterogeneity for surface-immobilized proteins. Anal Chem 73:471–480. doi:10.1021/ac000523p

20. Firestone MA, Shank ML, Sligar SG, Bohn PW (1996) Film architecture in biomolecular assemblies. Effect of linker on the orientation of genetically engineered surface-bound proteins. J Am Chem Soc 118:9033–9041. doi:10.1021/ja961046o

21. Canziani GA, Klakamp S, Myszka DG (2004) Kinetic screening of antibodies from crude hybridoma samples using Biacore. Anal Biochem 325:301–307. doi:10.1016/j.ab.2003.11.004

22. Natarajan S, Katsamba PS, Miles A et al (2008) Continuous-flow microfluidic printing of proteins for array-based applications including surface plasmon resonance imaging. Anal Biochem 373:141–146. doi:10.1016/j.ab.2007.07.035

23. Leckband D (2000) Measuring the forces that control protein interactions. Annu Rev Biophys Biomol Struct 29:1–26. doi:10.1146/annurev.biophys.29.1.1

24. Holmberg A, Blomstergren A, Nord O, Lukacs M, Lundeberg J, Uhlén M (2005) The biotin-streptavidin interaction can be reversibly broken using water at elevated temperatures. Electrophoresis 26(3):501–510

25. Schuck P, Zhao H (2010) The role of mass transport limitation and surface heterogeneity in the biophysical characterization of macromolecular binding processes by SPR biosensing. Methods Mol Biol 627:15–54. doi:10.1007/978-1-60761-670-2_2

26. Drake AW, Myszka DG, Klakamp SL (2004) Characterizing high-affinity antigen/antibody complexes by kinetic- and equilibrium-based methods. Anal Biochem 328:35–43. doi:10.1016/j.ab.2003.12.025

27. Myszka DG (1997) Kinetic analysis of macromolecular interactions using surface plasmon resonance biosensors. Curr Opin Biotechnol 8:50–57

28. Karlsson R, Michaelsson A, Mattsson L (1991) Kinetic analysis of monoclonal antibody-antigen interactions with a new biosensor based analytical system. J Immunol Methods 145:229–240. doi:10.1016/0022-1759(91)90331-9

29. Christensen LLH (1997) Theoretical analysis of protein concentration determination using biosensor technology under conditions of partial mass transport limitation. Anal Biochem 249:153–164. doi:10.1006/abio.1997.2182

30. Van Regenmortel MH, Altschuh D, Chatellier J et al (1998) Measurement of antigen-antibody interactions with biosensors. J Mol Recognit 11:163–167

31. Myszka DG, He X, Dembo M et al (1998) Extending the range of rate constants available from BIACORE: interpreting mass transport-influenced binding data. Biophys J 75:583–594

32. Myszka DG (1999) Improving biosensor analysis. J Mol Recognit 12:279–284

33. Drake AW, Papalia GA (2012) Biophysical considerations for development of antibody-based therapeutics. In: Bornstein GG, Klakamp SL, Tabrizi MA (eds) Developments in antibody-based therapies. Springer, New York, NY, pp 95–139

34. Wijaya E, Lenaerts C, Maricot S et al (2011) Surface plasmon resonance-based biosensors: from the development of different SPR structures to novel surface functionalization strategies. Curr Opin Solid State Mater Sci 15:208–224. doi:10.1016/j.cossms.2011.05.001

35. Buenger D, Topuz F, Groll J (2012) Hydrogels in sensing applications. Prog Polym Sci 37:1678–1719. doi:10.1016/j.progpolymsci.2012.09.001

36. Van Der Merwe PA (2001) Surface plasmon resonance. Oxford University Press, New York, NY

37. Andersson DI, Hughes D (2012) Evolution of antibiotic resistance at non-lethal drug concentrations. Drug Resist Updat 15:162–172. doi:10.1016/j.drup.2012.03.005

38. Murphy M, Jason-Moller L, Bruno J (2001) Using Biacore to measure the binding kinetics

of an antibody-antigen interaction. Curr Protoc Protein Sci. Chapter 19:Unit 19.14. doi: 10.1002/0471142301.ps1914s45

39. Drake AW, Klakamp SL (2011) A strategic and systematic approach for the determination of biosensor regeneration conditions. J Immunol Methods 371:165–169. doi:10.1016/j.jim.2011.06.003

40. Rich RL, Myszka DG (2000) Advances in surface plasmon resonance biosensor analysis. Curr Opin Biotechnol 11:54–61

41. Karlsson R, Fält A (1997) Experimental design for kinetic analysis of protein-protein interactions with surface plasmon resonance biosensors. J Immunol Methods 200:121–133. doi:10.1016/S0022-1759(96)00195-0

42. Katsamba PS, Navratilova I, Calderon-Cacia M et al (2006) Kinetic analysis of a high-affinity antibody/antigen interaction performed by multiple Biacore users. Anal Biochem 352:208–221. doi:10.1016/j.ab.2006.01.034

43. Papalia GA, Baer M, Luehrsen K et al (2006) High-resolution characterization of antibody fragment/antigen interactions using Biacore T100. Anal Biochem 359:112–119. doi:10.1016/j.ab.2006.08.032

44. Säfsten P, Klakamp SL, Drake AW et al (2006) Screening antibody–antigen interactions in parallel using Biacore A100. Anal Biochem 353:181–190. doi:10.1016/j.ab.2006.01.041

45. Jason-Moller L, Murphy M, Bruno J (2006) Overview of Biacore systems and their applications. Curr Protoc Protein Sci. Chapter 19: Unit 19.13.doi:10.1002/0471140864.ps1913s45

46. Morton TA, Myszka DG, Chaiken IM (1995) Interpreting complex binding kinetics from optical biosensors: a comparison of analysis by linearization, the integrated rate equation, and numerical integration. Anal Biochem 227:176–185. doi:10.1006/abio.1995.1268

47. Mol NJ, Fischer MJE (2010) Surface plasmon resonance: a general introduction. In: Fischer MJE, Mol NJ (eds) Surface plasmon resonance. Humana, New York, NY, pp 1–14

48. O'Shannessy DJ (1994) Determination of kinetic rate and equilibrium binding constants for macromolecular interactions: a critique of the surface plasmon resonance literature. Curr Opin Biotechnol 5:65–71. doi:10.1016/S0958-1669(05)80072-2

49. Cheskis B, Freedman LP (1996) Modulation of nuclear receptor interactions by ligands: kinetic analysis using surface plasmon resonance. Biochemistry (Mosc) 35:3309–3318. doi:10.1021/bi952283r

50. Heding A, Gill R, Ogawa Y et al (1996) Biosensor measurement of the binding of insulin-like growth factors i and ii and their analogues to the insulin-like growth factor-binding protein-3. J Biol Chem 271:13948–13952. doi:10.1074/jbc.271.24.13948

51. Persson E, Ezban M, Shymko RM (1995) Kinetics of the interaction between the human factor VIIIa subunits: effects of pH, ionic strength, Ca2+ concentration, heparin, and activated protein C-catalyzed proteolysis. Biochemistry (Mosc) 34:12775–12781. doi:10.1021/bi00039a038

52. Gertler A, Grosclaude J, Strasburger CJ et al (1996) Real-time kinetic measurements of the interactions between lactogenic hormones and prolactin-receptor extracellular domains from several species support the model of hormone-induced transient receptor dimerization. J Biol Chem 271:24482–24491. doi:10.1074/jbc.271.40.24482

53. Masson L, Lu Y, Mazza A et al (1995) The CryIA(c) receptor purified from Manduca sexta displays multiple specificities. J Biol Chem 270:20309–20315. doi:10.1074/jbc.270.35.20309

54. Edlund M, Blikstad I, Öbrink B (1996) Calmodulin binds to specific sequences in the cytoplasmic domain of c-cam and down-regulates c-cam self-association. J Biol Chem 271:1393–1399. doi:10.1074/jbc.271.3.1393

55. Raghavan M, Wang Y, Bjorkman PJ (1995) Effects of receptor dimerization on the interaction between the class I major histocompatibility complex-related Fc receptor and IgG. Proc Natl Acad Sci U S A 92: 11200–11204

56. Raghavan M, Bonagura VR, Morrison SL, Bjorkman PJ (1995) Analysis of the pH dependence of the neonatal Fc receptor/immunoglobulin G interaction using antibody and receptor variants. Biochemistry (Mosc) 34:14649–14657

57. Sasaki T, Göhring W, Pan T et al (1995) Binding of mouse and human fibulin-2 to extracellular matrix ligands. J Mol Biol 254:892–899. doi:10.1006/jmbi.1995.0664

58. Sundberg F (2009) Kinetics from SPR. Drug Discov Dev 12(2):22–24

59. Myszka DG, Morton TA, Doyle ML, Chaiken IM (1997) Kinetic analysis of a protein antigen-antibody interaction limited by mass transport on an optical biosensor. Biophys Chem 64:127–137. doi:10.1016/S0301-4622(96)02230-2

60. Keighley W (2011) The need for high throughput kinetics early in the drug discovery process. Drug Discov World 12:39–45

61. Brooks BD (2014) The importance of epitope binning for biological drug discovery. Curr Drug Discov Technol 11(2):109–112

62. Brooks BD, Miles A, Abdiche Y (2014) High-throughput epitope binning of therapeutic monoclonal antibodies: why you need to bin the fridge. Drug Discov Today 19(8):1040–1044. doi:10.1016/j.drudis.2014.05.011

63. Abdiche Y, Malashock D, Pinkerton A, Pons J (2008) Determining kinetics and affinities of protein interactions using a parallel real-time label-free biosensor, the Octet. Anal Biochem 377:209–217. doi:10.1016/j.ab.2008.03.035

64. Abdiche YN, Lindquist KC, Stone DM et al (2012) Label-free epitope binning assays of monoclonal antibodies enable the identification of antigen heterogeneity. J Immunol Methods 382:101–116. doi:10.1016/j.jim.2012.05.010

65. Abdiche YN, Malashock DS, Pinkerton A, Pons J (2009) Exploring blocking assays using Octet, ProteOn, and Biacore biosensors. Anal Biochem 386:172–180. doi:10.1016/j.ab.2008.11.038

66. Brooks BD, Albertson AE, Jones JA et al (2008) Efficient screening of high-signal and low-background antibody pairs in the bio-bar code assay using prion protein as the target. Anal Biochem 382:60–62. doi:10.1016/j.ab.2008.07.009

67. Miller PL, Wolfert RL, Diedrich G (2011) Epitope binning of murine monoclonal antibodies by a multiplexed pairing assay. J Immunol Methods 365:118–125. doi:10.1016/j.jim.2010.12.021

68. Lobo ED, Hansen RJ, Balthasar JP (2004) Antibody pharmacokinetics and pharmacodynamics. J Pharm Sci 93:2645–2668. doi:10.1002/jps.20178

69. Carter PJ (2011) Introduction to current and future protein therapeutics: a protein engineering perspective. Exp Cell Res 317:1261–1269. doi:10.1016/j.yexcr.2011.02.013

70. Luzzago A, Felici F, Tramontano A et al (1993) Mimicking of discontinuous epitopes by phage-displayed peptides, I. Epitope mapping of human H ferritin using a phage library of constrained peptides. Gene 128:51–57. doi:10.1016/0378-1119(93)90152-S

71. Stephen CW, Lane DP (1992) Mutant conformation of p53: precise epitope mapping using a filamentous phage epitope library. J Mol Biol 225:577–583. doi:10.1016/0022-2836(92)90386-X

72. Zuiderweg ERP (2002) Mapping protein–protein interactions in solution by NMR spectroscopy†. Biochemistry (Mosc) 41:1–7. doi:10.1021/bi011870b

73. Marciano DP, Dharmarajan V, Griffin PR (2014) HDX-MS guided drug discovery: small molecules and biopharmaceuticals. Curr Opin Struct Biol 28:105–111. doi:10.1016/j.sbi.2014.08.007

74. Mihai S, Nimmerjahn F (2013) The role of Fc receptors and complement in autoimmunity. Autoimmun Rev 12:657–660. doi:10.1016/j.autrev.2012.10.008

75. Rosales C, Uribe-Querol E (2013) Fc receptors: cell activators of antibody functions. Adv Biosci Biotechnol 4:21

76. Mellor JD, Brown MP, Irving HR et al (2013) A critical review of the role of Fc gamma receptor polymorphisms in the response to monoclonal antibodies in cancer. J Hematol Oncol 6:8722–8726

77. Clynes R (2006) Antitumor antibodies in the treatment of cancer: fc receptors link opsonic antibody with cellular immunity. Hematol Oncol Clin North Am 20:585–612. doi:10.1016/j.hoc.2006.02.010

78. Nimmerjahn F, Ravetch JV (2012) Translating basic mechanisms of IgG effector activity into next generation cancer therapies. Cancer Immun 12:13

79. Lazar GA, Dang W, Karki S et al (2006) Engineered antibody Fc variants with enhanced effector function. Proc Natl Acad Sci U S A 103:4005–4010. doi:10.1073/pnas.0508123103

80. Strohl WR (2009) Optimization of Fc-mediated effector functions of monoclonal antibodies. Curr Opin Biotechnol 20:685–691

81. Roopenian DC, Akilesh S (2007) FcRn: the neonatal Fc receptor comes of age. Nat Rev Immunol 7:715–725

82. Ober RJ, Radu CG, Ghetie V, Ward ES (2001) Differences in promiscuity for antibody–FcRn interactions across species: implications for therapeutic antibodies. Int Immunol 13:1551–1559

83. Chen Y, Balthasar JP (2012) Evaluation of a catenary PBPK model for predicting the in vivo disposition of mAbs engineered for high-affinity binding to FcRn. AAPS J 14:850–859

84. Carter PJ (2006) Potent antibody therapeutics by design. Nat Rev Immunol 6:343–357. doi:10.1038/nri1837

85. Patel R, Johnson KK, Andrien BA, Tamburini PP (2013) IGg subclass variation of a monoclonal antibody binding to human fc-gamma receptors. Am J Biochem Biotechnol 9:206

86. Li P, Jiang N, Nagarajan S et al (2007) Affinity and kinetic analysis of Fcgamma receptor IIIa (CD16a) binding to IgG ligands. J Biol Chem 282:6210–6221. doi:10.1074/jbc.M609064200

87. Bruhns P, Iannascoli B, England P et al (2009) Specificity and affinity of human Fcγ receptors and their polymorphic variants for human IgG subclasses. Blood 113: 3716–3725

88. Kiese S, Papppenberger A, Friess W, Mahler H-C (2008) Shaken, not stirred: mechanical stress testing of an IgG1 antibody. J Pharm Sci 97:4347–4366. doi:10.1002/jps.21328

89. Fincke A, Winter J, Bunte T, Olbrich C (2014) Thermally induced degradation pathways of three different antibody-based drug development candidates. Eur J Pharm Sci 62:148–160. doi:10.1016/j.ejps.2014.05.014

90. Bhatnagar BS, Bogner RH, Pikal MJ (2007) Protein stability during freezing: separation of stresses and mechanisms of protein stabilization. Pharm Dev Technol 12:505–523

91. Haberger M, Bomans K, Diepold K, et al. (2014) Assessment of chemical modifications of sites in the CDRs of recombinant antibodies: Susceptibility vs. functionality of critical quality attributes. *mAbs.* Landes Bioscience, p 327

92. Chumsae C, Gaza-Bulseco G, Sun J, Liu H (2007) Comparison of methionine oxidation in thermal stability and chemically stressed samples of a fully human monoclonal antibody. J Chromatogr B 850:285–294

93. Rich RL, Miles AR, Gale BK, Myszka DG (2009) Detergent screening of a G-protein-coupled receptor using serial and array biosensor technologies. Anal Biochem 386:98–104. doi:10.1016/j.ab.2008.12.011

94. Locatelli-Hoops S, Yeliseev AA, Gawrisch K, Gorshkova I (2013) Surface plasmon resonance applied to G protein-coupled receptors. Biomed Spectrosc Imaging 2:155–181. doi:10.3233/BSI-130045

95. Stenlund P, Babcock GJ, Sodroski J, Myszka DG (2003) Capture and reconstitution of G protein-coupled receptors on a biosensor surface. Anal Biochem 316:243–250

96. Parrill AL (2008) Crystal structures of a second g protein-coupled receptor: triumphs and implications. ChemMedChem 3:1021–1023. doi:10.1002/cmdc.200800070

97. Overington JP, Al-Lazikani B, Hopkins AL (2006) How many drug targets are there? Nat Rev Drug Discov 5:993–996. doi:10.1038/nrd2199

98. Hutchings CJ, Koglin M, Marshall FH (2010) Therapeutic antibodies directed at G protein-coupled receptors. mAbs 2:594–606. doi:10.4161/mabs.2.6.13420

99. Karlsson OP, Löfås S (2002) Flow-mediated on-surface reconstitution of g-protein coupled receptors for applications in surface plasmon resonance biosensors. Anal Biochem 300:132–138. doi:10.1006/abio.2001.5428

100. Hodnik V, Anderluh G (2010) Capture of intact liposomes on biacore sensor chips for protein–membrane interaction studies. In: Fischer MJE, Mol NJ (eds) Surface plasmon reson. Humana, New York, NY, pp 201–211

101. Cooper MA (2002) Optical biosensors in drug discovery. Nat Rev Drug Discov 1: 515–528

102. Cooper MA, Hansson A, Löfås S, Williams DH (2000) A vesicle capture sensor chip for kinetic analysis of interactions with membrane-bound receptors. Anal Biochem 277:196–205. doi:10.1006/abio.1999.4389

103. Johnsson B, Löfås S, Lindquist G (1991) Immobilization of proteins to a carboxymethyldextran-modified gold surface for biospecific interaction analysis in surface plasmon resonance sensors. Anal Biochem 198:268–277. doi:10.1016/0003-2697(91)90424-R

104. Navratilova I, Dioszegi M, Myszka DG (2006) Analyzing ligand and small molecule binding activity of solubilized GPCRs using biosensor technology. Anal Biochem 355:132–139

105. Mirzabekov T, Kontos H, Farzan M et al (2000) Paramagnetic proteoliposomes containing a pure, native, and oriented seven-transmembrane segment protein, CCR5. Nat Biotechnol 18:649–654. doi:10.1038/76501

106. Babcock GJ, Mirzabekov T, Wojtowicz W, Sodroski J (2001) ligand binding characteristics of cxcr4 incorporated into paramagnetic proteoliposomes. J Biol Chem 276:38433–38440. doi:10.1074/jbc.M106229200

107. Chen L, Jin L, Zhou N (2012) An update of novel screening methods for GPCR in drug discovery. Expert Opin Drug Discov 7:791–806. doi:10.1517/17460441.2012.699036

108. Harding PJ, Hadingham TC, McDonnell JM, Watts A (2006) Direct analysis of a GPCR-agonist interaction by surface plasmon resonance. Eur Biophys J 35:709–712. doi:10.1007/s00249-006-0070-x

109. Hwang WYK, Foote J (2005) Immunogenicity of engineered antibodies. Methods 36:3–10

110. Wright A, Shin S-U, Morrison SL (1991) Genetically engineered antibodies: progress and prospects. Crit Rev Immunol 12: 125–168

111. De Groot AS et al (2008) Prediction of immunogenicity: in silico paradigms, ex vivo and in vivo correlates. Curr Opin Pharmacol 8:620–626. doi:10.1016/j.coph.2008.08.002

112. Harding FA, Stickler MM, Razo J, Du Bridge RB (2010) The immunogenicity of humanized and fully human antibodies: residual immunogenicity resides in the CDR regions. mAbs 2:256–265

113. Cheung NK, Guo H, Hu J et al (2012) Humanizing murine IgG3 anti-GD2 antibody m3F8 substantially improves antibody-dependent cell-mediated cytotoxicity while retaining targeting in vivo. Oncoimmunology 1:477–486

114. Kaliyaperumal A, Pennucci J, Nagatani J et al (2014) A method to quantitate the neutralizing capacity of anti-therapeutic protein antibodies in serum and their correlation to clinical impact. J Pharm Biomed Anal 102C:176–183. doi:10.1016/j.jpba.2014.09.009

115. Mikulskis A, Yeung D, Subramanyam M, Amaravadi L (2011) Solution ELISA as a platform of choice for development of robust, drug tolerant immunogenicity assays in support of drug development. J Immunol Methods 365:38–49

116. Nechansky A (2010) HAHA–nothing to laugh about. Measuring the immunogenicity (human anti-human antibody response) induced by humanized monoclonal antibodies applying ELISA and SPR technology. J Pharm Biomed Anal 51:252–254

117. Barbosa MD, Gokemeijer J, Martin AD, Bush A (2013) Altering drug tolerance of surface plasmon resonance assays for the detection of anti-drug antibodies. Anal Biochem 441:174–179

118. Lofgren JA, Dhandapani S, Pennucci JJ et al (2007) Comparing ELISA and surface plasmon resonance for assessing clinical immunogenicity of panitumumab. J Immunol 178:7467–7472

119. Weeraratne DK, Lofgren J, Dinnogen S et al (2013) Development of a biosensor-based immunogenicity assay capable of blocking soluble drug target interference. J Immunol Methods 396:44–55

120. Elvin JG, Couston RG, van der Walle CF (2013) Therapeutic antibodies: market considerations, disease targets and bioprocessing. Int J Pharm 440:83–98. doi:10.1016/j.ijpharm.2011.12.039

121. Holliger P, Hudson PJ (2005) Engineered antibody fragments and the rise of single domains. Nat Biotechnol 23:1126–1136. doi:10.1038/nbt1142

122. Beck A, Wurch T, Bailly C, Corvaia N (2010) Strategies and challenges for the next generation of therapeutic antibodies. Nat Rev Immunol 10:345–352. doi:10.1038/nri2747

123. Nelson AL, Reichert JM (2009) Development trends for therapeutic antibody fragments. Nat Biotechnol 27:331–337

124. Steukers M, Schaus J-M, van Gool R et al (2006) Rapid kinetic-based screening of human Fab fragments. J Immunol Methods 310:126–135. doi:10.1016/j.jim.2006.01.002

125. Wassaf D, Kuang G, Kopacz K et al (2006) High-throughput affinity ranking of antibodies using surface plasmon resonance microarrays. Anal Biochem 351:241–253. doi:10.1016/j.ab.2006.01.043

126. Hoogenboom HR, de Bruïne AP, Hufton SE et al (1998) Antibody phage display technology and its applications. Immunotechnology 4:1–20. doi:10.1016/S1380-2933(98)00007-4

127. Kehoe JW, Kay BK (2005) Filamentous phage display in the new millennium. Chem Rev 105:4056–4072. doi:10.1021/cr000261r

128. Azzazy HME, Highsmith WE Jr (2002) Phage display technology: clinical applications and recent innovations. Clin Biochem 35:425–445. doi:10.1016/S0009-9120(02)00343-0

129. Hoogenboom HR (2005) Selecting and screening recombinant antibody libraries. Nat Biotechnol 23:1105–1116. doi:10.1038/nbt1126

130. Mondon P (2008) Human antibody libraries: a race to engineer and explore a larger diversity. Front Biosci 13:1117. doi:10.2741/2749

131. Conroy PJ, Hearty S, Leonard P, O'Kennedy RJ (2009) Antibody production, design and use for biosensor-based applications. Semin Cell Dev Biol 20:10–26. doi:10.1016/j.semcdb.2009.01.010

132. Bradbury AR, Marks JD (2004) Antibodies from phage antibody libraries. J Immunol Methods 290:29–49

133. Leonard P, Säfsten P, Hearty S et al (2007) High throughput ranking of recombinant avian scFv antibody fragments from crude lysates using the Biacore A100. J Immunol Methods 323:172–179. doi:10.1016/j.jim.2007.04.010

134. Bravman T, Bronner V, Lavie K et al (2006) Exploring "one-shot" kinetics and small molecule analysis using the ProteOn XPR36 array

biosensor. Anal Biochem 358:281–288. doi:10.1016/j.ab.2006.08.005

135. Rich RL, Quinn JG, Morton T et al (2010) Biosensor-based fragment screening using FastStep injections. Anal Biochem 407: 270–277

136. Shepherd CA, Hopkins AL, Navratilova I (2014) Fragment screening by SPR and advanced application to GPCRs. Prog Biophys Mol Biol 116:113–123. doi:10.1016/j.pbiomolbio.2014.09.008, pii: S0079-6107(14)00110-2

137. Chardin H et al (2014) Surface Plasmon Resonance imaging: a method to measure the affinity of the antibodies in allergy diagnosis. J Immunol Methods 405:23–28. doi:10.1016/j.jim.2013.12.010

138. Schasfoort R, de Lau W, van der Kooi A et al (2012) Method for estimating the single molecular affinity. Anal Biochem 421: 794–796

139. Liu S, Zhu JH, He LP et al (2014) Label-free, real-time detection of the dynamic processes of protein degradation using oblique-incidence reflectivity difference method. Appl Phys Lett 104:163701. doi:10.1063/1.4873676

140. Wöllner K, Chen X, Kremmer E, Krämer PM (2010) Comparative surface plasmon resonance and enzyme-linked immunosorbent assay characterisation of a monoclonal antibody with N-acyl homoserine lactones. Anal Chim Acta 683:113–118. doi:10.1016/j.aca.2010.10.015

141. Thorpe R, Swanson SJ (2005) Assays for detecting and diagnosing antibody-mediated pure red cell aplasia (PRCA): an assessment of available procedures. Nephrol Dial Transplant 20:16–22. doi:10.1093/ndt/gfh1086

142. Heinrich L, Tissot N, Hartmann DJ, Cohen R (2010) Comparison of the results obtained by ELISA and surface plasmon resonance for the determination of antibody affinity. J Immunol Methods 352:13–22. doi:10.1016/j.jim.2009.10.002

143. Tacey R, Greway A, Smiell J et al (2003) The detection of anti-erythropoietin antibodies in human serum and plasma. Part I. Validation of the protocol for a radioimmunoprecipitation assay. J Immunol Methods 283: 317–329

144. Jecklin MC, Schauer S, Dumelin CE, Zenobi R (2009) Label-free determination of protein-ligand binding constants using mass spectrometry and validation using surface plasmon resonance and isothermal titration calorimetry. J Mol Recognit 22:319–329. doi:10.1002/jmr.951

145. Azzam RMA, Rigby PG, Krueger JA (1977) Kinetics of protein adsorption and immunological reactions at a liquid/solid interface by ellipsometry. Phys Med Biol 22:422. doi:10.1088/0031-9155/22/3/002

146. Ndieyira JW, Watari M, Barrera AD et al (2008) Nanomechanical detection of antibiotic-mucopeptide binding in a model for superbug drug resistance. Nat Nanotechnol 3:691–696. doi:10.1038/nnano.2008.275

147. Ciambrone GJ, Liu VF, Lin DC et al (2004) Cellular dielectric spectroscopy: a powerful new approach to label-free cellular analysis. J Biomol Screen 9:467–480. doi:10.1177/1087057104267788

148. Peters MF, Vaillancourt F, Heroux M et al (2010) Comparing label-free biosensors for pharmacological screening with cell-based functional assays. Assay Drug Dev Technol 8:219–227. doi:10.1089/adt.2009.0232

149. Chua JH, Chee R-E, Agarwal A et al (2009) Label-free electrical detection of cardiac biomarker with complementary metal-oxide semiconductor-compatible silicon nanowire sensor arrays. Anal Chem 81:6266–6271. doi:10.1021/ac901157x

150. Navratilova I (2005) Measuring long association phases using Biacore. Anal Biochem 344:295–297. doi:10.1016/j.ab.2005.05.025

151. Abdiche YN, Malashock DS, Pons J (2008) Probing the binding mechanism and affinity of tanezumab, a recombinant humanized anti-NGF monoclonal antibody, using a repertoire of biosensors. Protein Sci 17:1326–1335. doi:10.1110/ps.035402.108

152. Mayer KM, Hafner JH (2011) Localized surface plasmon resonance sensors. Chem Rev 111:3828–3857. doi:10.1021/cr100313v

153. Sun Y-S, Landry JP, Fei Y, Zhu X (2013) An oblique-incidence reflectivity difference study of the dependence of probe-target reaction constants on surface target density using streptavidin-biotin reactions as a model. Instrum Sci Technol 41:535–544. doi:10.108 0/10739149.2013.775590

154. Concepcion J, Witte K, Wartchow C et al (2009) Label-free detection of biomolecular interactions using biolayer interferometry for kinetic characterization. Comb Chem High Throughput Screen 12:791–800

155. Chiu Y-W, Li QX, Karu AE (2001) Selective binding of polychlorinated biphenyl congeners by a monoclonal antibody: analysis by kinetic exclusion fluorescence immunoassay. Anal Chem 73:5477–5484. doi:10.1021/ac0102462

156. Murphy KP, Freire E, Paterson Y (1995) Configurational effects in antibody–antigen interactions studied by microcalorimetry. Proteins Struct Funct Bioinforma 21:83–90. doi:10.1002/prot.340210202

157. Leder L, Berger C, Bornhauser S et al (1995) Spectroscopic, calorimetric, and kinetic demonstration of conformational adaptation in peptide-antibody recognition. Biochemistry (Mosc) 34:16509–16518

158. Kreimann M, Brandt S, Krauel K et al (2014) Interaction between platelet factor 4 and heparins: thermodynamics determines conformational changes required for binding of anti-platelet factor 4/heparin antibodies. Blood. doi: 10.1182/blood-2014-03-559518

159. Ciulli A (2013) Biophysical screening for the discovery of small-molecule ligands. Methods Mol Biol 1008:357–388. doi:10.1007/978-1-62703-398-5_13

160. Gell DA, Grant RP, Mackay JP (2012) The detection and quantitation of protein oligomerization. Adv Exp Med Biol 747:19–41. doi:10.1007/978-1-4614-3229-6_2

161. Fleming MR, Shamah SM, Kaczmarek LK (2014) Use of label-free optical biosensors to detect modulation of potassium channels by G-protein coupled receptors. J Vis Exp 84:e51307. doi:10.3791/51307

Chapter 4

Label-Free Cell-Based Biosensor Methods in Drug Toxicology Analysis

Jie Zhou, Xianxin Qiu, and Ping Wang

Abstract

Cell-based biosensors are one kind of devices that employ immobilized living cells as sensing elements combined with sensors or transducers to detect the intracellular and extracellular microenvironment conditions, physiological parameters and responses of cells upon stimulation. Because of their advantages associated with long-term recording in a noninvasive way, fast response time, and label-free experimentation, these biosensors have been widely utilized in many fields such as cellular physiological analysis, pharmaceutical evaluation, environmental monitoring, and medical diagnosis. Drug toxicology analysis is a vital step in drug discovery and development. This chapter discusses the principles and applications of cell-based biosensors including microelectrode arrays, electrical cell–substrate impedance sensing, field effect transistors, light-addressable potentiometric sensors, patch-clamp chips, quartz crystal microbalance in drug toxicology analysis.

Key words Cell-based biosensor, Drug toxicity, Electrical cell–substrate impedance sensing, Field effect transistors, Light-addressable potentiometric sensors, Microelectrode arrays, Patch-clamp chips, Quartz crystal microbalance

1   Introduction

Cell-based biosensors are one kind of devices that employ immobilized living cells as sensing elements combined with sensors or transducers to detect the intracellular and extracellular microenvironment conditions, physiological parameters and responses of cells upon stimulation. A typical cell-based biosensor consists of two parts: one is living cells or neural network cultured on the surface of a transducer and another is the transducer including potential and chemical sensing (Fig. 1). Stimulus elements may also be included. The living cells serve as the sensing element or primary transducer to respond to external stimuli such as electric and chemical stimulus, antiviral drugs and various receptor ligands, leading to corresponding output responses, such as changes of intracellular molecules and ions, action potential, and cellular

Ye Fang (ed.), *Label-Free Biosensor Methods in Drug Discovery*, Methods in Pharmacology and Toxicology,
DOI 10.1007/978-1-4939-2617-6_4, © Springer Science+Business Media New York 2015

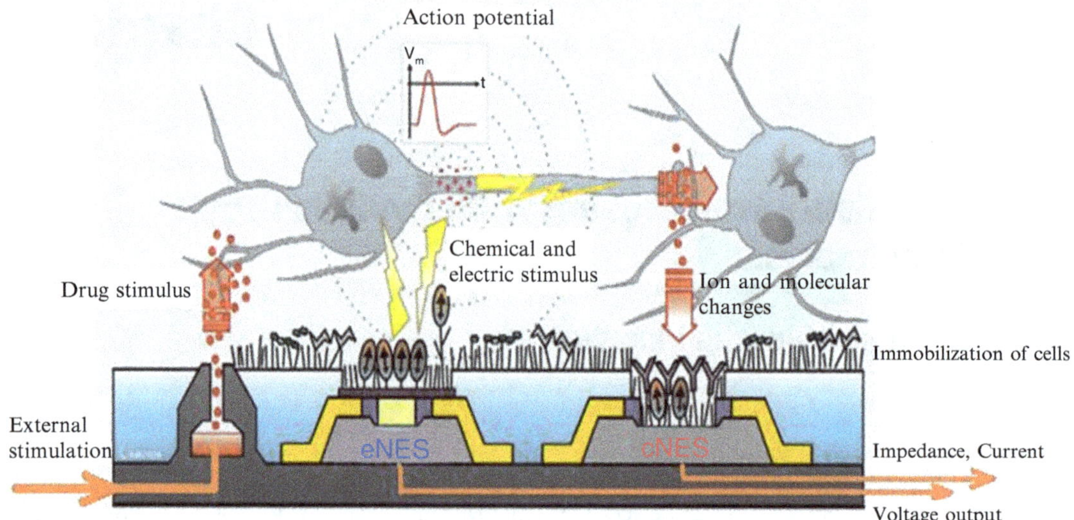

Fig. 1 Basic schematic diagram of cell-based biosensors. Cell-based biosensors combine living cells and sensors or transducers for cellular physiological parameter detection. When external stimulation, such as drugs, chemical and electric stimulus are added into cell-based biosensors, cells cultured on chip would produce action potential or extracellular ion and molecular changes which can be detected by devices through a thin layer of electrolyte. The potential and current changes coupled with the transducers, inducing the changes of extracellular potential or cellular impedance which were monitored by cell-based biosensors

impedance. The transducer or secondary transducer can detect these output responses and convert them into biosensor signals. The commonly used transducers include microelectrodes array (MEA), field-effect transistor (FET), light addressable potentiometric sensor (LAPS), electric cell–substrate impedance sensor (ECIS), patch-clamp chip, quartz crystal microbalance (QCM), and surface plasmon resonance (SPR).

By using living cells as sensitive elements, cell-based biosensors are able to respond to many chemical and biological analytes and obtain functional information. Compared with traditional biological assays, cell-based biosensors have the advantages of label-free, long-term recording in a noninvasive way, fast response time, high throughput, and high sensitivity. These biosensors have been widely utilized in many fields including drug discovery and toxicology analysis.

This chapter discusses several cell-based biosensors and their applications in drug toxicology analysis.

2   Microelectrode Array Sensors

2.1   Principle of MEA Sensors

With the development of microfabrication techniques, MEA sensors were developed for stimulation and recording of electrical activity of electrogenic cells and tissue cultures with high resolution. MEA sensors were pioneered by Thomas [1], in which multiple metallic film sites with diameter of several micrometers are fabricated on a

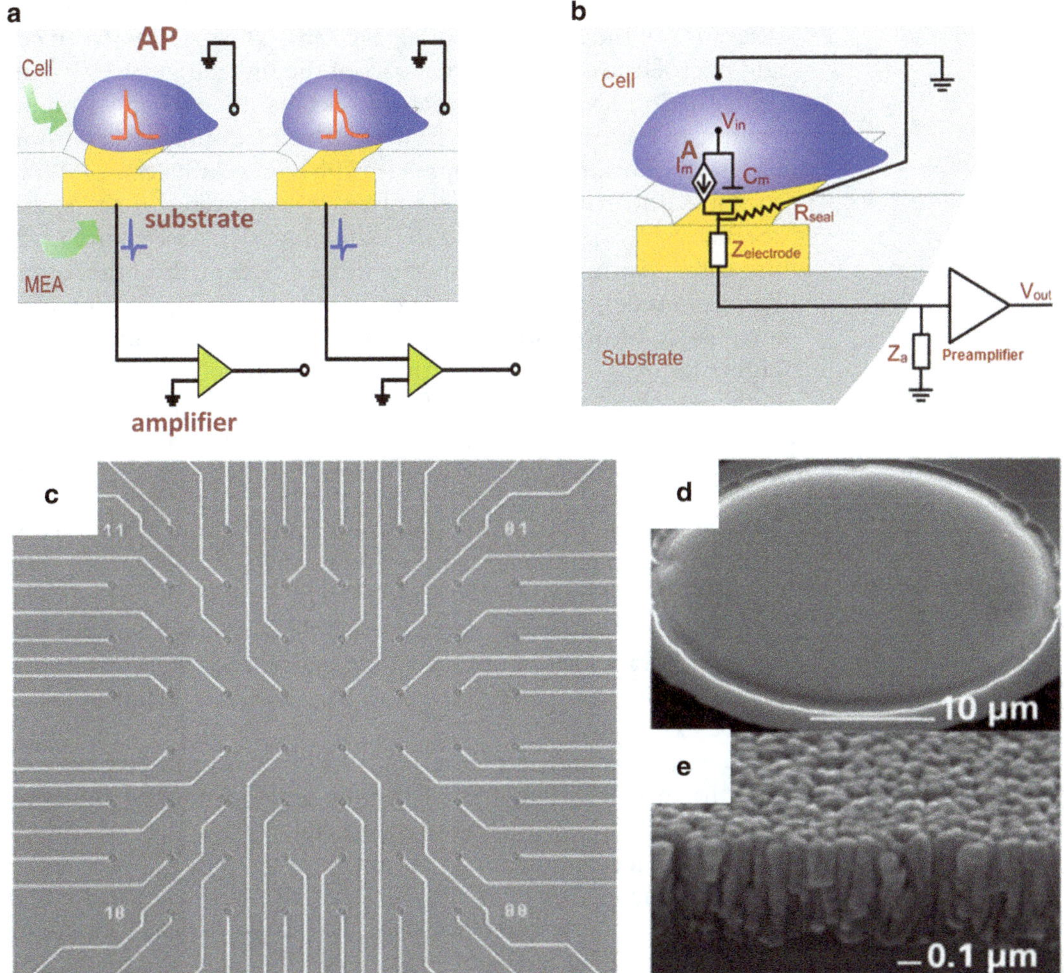

Fig. 2 Microelectrode array sensors for cell electrophysiology studies. (**a**) Schematic setup of a traditional MEA sensor; (**b**) The Randles model; (**c–e**) a typical MEA chip from commercial MultiChannel Systems: (**c**) the chip layout of the 8 × 8 MEA; (**d**) the electronic microscopic image of a TiN-coated electrode; (**e**) the surface morphology of the electrode as revealed using electronic microscopy

glass substrate (Fig. 2a). Cells are cultured in the chamber, adhering to the substrate and microelectrodes. The intracellular action potential originating at cell itself is created by ions passing through gated protein channels on the cell membranes, while the movement of ions in the extracellular solution creates potentials that can be detected at different sites.

Alternatively, the H-H model with capacitance and resistance of the cell membrane in parallel is used to describe the cellular electrophysiology. The current flowing through the basal membrane is the sum of ionic and capacitive current which is given by:

$$I_{\text{total}} = K \frac{\mathrm{d}^2 V_{\text{M}}}{\mathrm{d}t} = C_{\text{M}} \frac{\mathrm{d} V_{\text{M}}}{\mathrm{d}t} + I_{\text{ionic}} \tag{1}$$

So the voltage developed at the node A is proportional to the second derivative of the action potential (Fig. 2b). The space between cells and microelectrodes is the vital part of the signaling process. When cell adhesion to the microelectrode occurs, there is still a minute volume of electrolyte which forms an electric double layer with the electrode. This minute volume electrolyte also induces a side track for ionic flow to the bulk electrolyte. It is expressed as the sealing resistance (R_{seal}) in parallel to the cellular model. As seen in Fig. 2a, the total transmembrane current flows through the branch with Randles model, the impedance of the electrode $Z_{electrode}$, the input impedance of preamplifier Z_{in} in series and the R_{seal} branch. The bigger the R_{seal} is, the smaller the leaked current is, thus inducing a higher recorded extracellular field potential V_{EP}.

$$V_{EP} = \left(I_{total} - I_{leakage} \right) \times R_{in} \tag{2}$$

Both extracellular and transmembrane action potentials are useful for characterizing drug pharmacology, although they differ greatly in amplitude, shape, and kinetics. The amplitude of extracellular action potential detected by MEA is much smaller than transmembrane action potential. By analyzing some characteristic parameters of the recorded signal, the effects of drug molecules can be examined.

The layout and structure of MEA have been optimized over time to meet the demand of specific and operational biological problems. The essential design principle obeys the "sandwich" structure since Thomas et al. pioneered it in 1972 [1]. The metallic film is deposited between the insulative substrate and passivation layer. Only the electrode sites and pad are exposed for electric sensing and signal output, respectively. Generally, the diameter of electrodes is 10–100 μm. For improving the performance, a TiN layer with regular "column" morphology is deposited on the electrodes [2]. However, the developments of MEA designs are mainly in the aspects of layout, structures of electrodes, and functional expansion.

With nearly 40-year development, MEA has been commercialized and its products are mainly from companies of MultiChannel Systems (Germany), Ayanda Biosystems (USA), and Panasonic (Japan). To date, MEA sensors are generally used for low-throughput cell analysis.

2.2 MEA Sensors for Drug-Induced Cardiotoxicity Assessment

Drug-induced cardiotoxicity is one of the major side-effects of drugs that cause damages on the normal function of the heart. In the past couple decades, at least a dozen top-selling drugs were withdrawn from the market due to undesired cardiotoxicity, resulting in huge economic losses for the related companies. Assessment of drug-induced cardiotoxicity is mandated by drug regulatory agencies.

MEA provides a convenient and versatile system solution for in vitro recordings of cardiomyocytes. The multisite design enables the recording of electrical activity of cardiomyocytes in different locations, so the spatiotemporal behaviors of the culture including the generation of extracellular action potential and the propagation pathway can studied [3]. The characteristics of electrophysiological mapping of cardiomyocytes on MEAs are sensitive to various stimuli, ranging from mechanical stress to electrical pulse to drug molecules.

Ion channels, primarily sodium, potassium, and calcium channels, are indispensable elements in determining the action potential generation of cardiomyocytes, thus are important targets for drugs that affect cardiomyocytes. A variety of cardiac system disorders are caused by the dysfunction of ion channels. For instance, the fast inward Na^+ current can drive the depolarization. When treated with Na^+ channel blockers, the amplitude of extracellular field potential recorded by MEA is greatly decreased and conduction delay increased [4, 5]. Ca^{2+} is closely related with the cardiac contractility. The drugs like quinidine and nifedipine could cause changes on the shape of extracellular field potentials and beating behavior [6, 7]. MEAs also have been used to assess the cardiotoxicity of different molecules, such as potassium channel openers, pesticide, angiotensin II [8–10].

The abnormal prolongation of the QT interval in electrocardiogram (ECG) is known to be associated with cardiac arrhythmia. Studies have found that many drugs can cause the prolongation of the QT interval, suggesting the necessity of assessing the drug effects on QT interval prolongation. QT interval prolongation directly corresponds to the prolonged ventricular action potential, which is also correlated with the duration of field potentials measured by the MEA. To achieve high-throughput pharmacological screening of QT prolongation, a six-well multichannel electrode chip was used, where each of the wells contained ten microelectrodes. To validate the system, the QT-prolonging effect of some compounds with known effects, such as antiarrhythmic agents such as quinidine and E-4031, and noncardiac agents such as cisapride, sparfloxacin, were tested. Figure 3 shows an example of the field potential for human embryonic stem cell-derived cardiomyocytes (hESC-CMs) measured by a QT screen system in the presence of increasing amounts of E-4031, indicating the prolongation of field potential duration in response to E-4031. Compared with conventional cell-based assays, such as human ether-a-go-go-related gene (hERG) assays, MEAs can detect cardiomyocyte action potential regulation with full mechanisms.

2.3 MEA Sensors for Neuronal Pharmacology Profiling

The electrophysiology of neuronal networks underlies the memory storage, learning ability, and signal processing in human brain. Based on the synaptic connections, most of the neuronal networks develop spontaneous bursting activities and reach synchronous

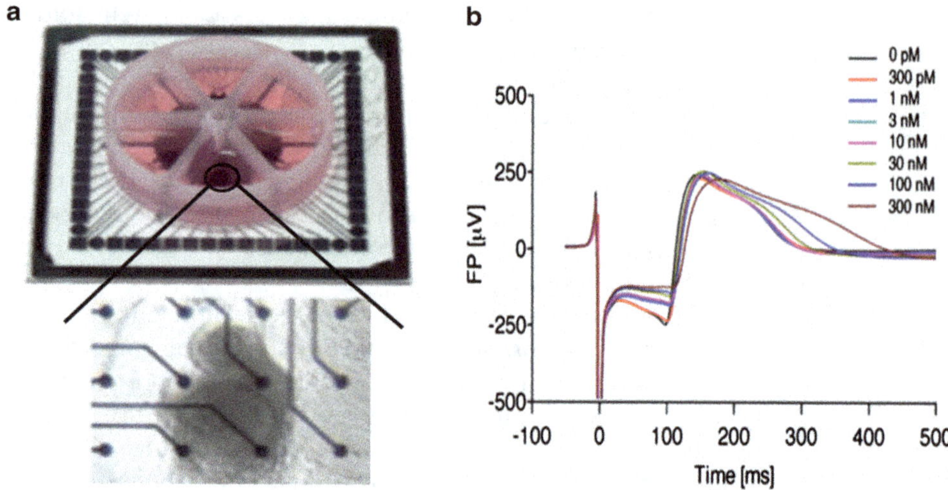

Fig. 3 (**a**) Six-well multichannel electrode chip for the QT-Screen and the micrograph of electrodes in one well with hESC-CMs attached and cultured on them. (**b**) Field potential for hESC-CMs in the presence of increasing amounts of E-4031. Reprinted with permission from ref. 11. Copyright 2010 Elsevier

when culture matures [12, 13]. Thus, even without the homeostatic control of the central nervous system, the dissociated neural networks cultured on MEAs are still a promising model for a variety of applications, including the study of neuronal topology, the development, mechanisms, and drug pharmacology of various neuronal networks. The neuronal activity deviation in physiological level could be mapped out when the neuronal networks are exposed to a wide variety of chemical compounds such as drugs and environmental toxins. Based on inherent electrophysiological mechanisms of neural network, their influences are classified as direct metabolic effects, specific synaptic effects, transmission effects, and generic membrane effects [14]. In the past decades, a lot of substances with effects of excitation or inhibition have been studied using MEA sensors, such as neurotransmitters (GABA, dopamine, serotonin) [15–18], glycine receptor antagonist (strychnine) [19, 20], 5-HT receptor antagonist (fluoxetine) [21], NMDA receptor antagonists (APV, NBQX) [22], GABA receptor antagonists (gabazine, bicuculline, TMPP) [23], cannabinoid receptor-mediated apoptosis (anandamide and methanandamide) [24], NMDA receptors blocker (ethanol), Na-K-ATPase inhibitor (ouabain) [25], Gp120 protein of the AIDS virus [14], and even heavy metals (Mn, Hg, Zn) [26, 27] (Table 1). These studies demonstrated that neuronal networks from different brain regions gave rise to different pharmacological responses [28]. Through MEA platform, it can generate a database of well-characterized profiles of different drugs, so the unknown neuronal active substances could be recognized by comparisons of the induced changes on spike patterns.

Table 1
The pharmacology on various neuronal networks based on MEA

Cellular component	Stimulus and concentration	Description
Frontal cortical neurons	Chloroquine (0–30 μM)	Chloroquine dose-dependently depressed the spike rate and inhibited whole-cell calcium current [29]
Cortex networks	Domoic acid (0–2 μM)	Domoic acid of 50 nM increased the basal spontaneous electrical activity [30]
Cortex networks	Borna disease virus	The virus blocked the activity-dependent enhancement of neuronal network activity [31].
Cortex networks	Botulinum toxin (10 ng/mL)	Botulinum toxin increased duration and number of spikes and unique oscillatory behavior with each burst [32]
Auditory cortex network	Fluoxetine (1–25 μM)	Excitation, initial inhibition and activity cessation were caused at 1–20 μM, 15 μM and 20–25 μM, respectively [21]
Auditory cortex networks	Quinine (1–40 μM)	Response of auditory cortex networks to quinine was with an excitatory phase followed by inhibition [29]
Spinal cord networks	Glutamate (0–100 μM)	A concentration-dependent increase of spike rate was caused at elevated levels [33]
Spinal cord networks	Strychnine (0 nM to 20 μM)	Bursting was increased at 5–20 nM and coordinated above 5 μM [19]
Hippocampal neuronal networks	Gabazine (10 μM) Bicuculline (10 μM)	Gabazine increased the firing. Bicuculline exhibited heterogeneity of action on firing rate [18]
Retinal ganglion slice	AP-4 (100 μM)	Activated with AP-4, cells are hyperpolarized in presence of light and in darkness [34]
Olfactory epithelium	Acetic acid (25 μM) Butanedione (25 μM)	Different firing patterns are generated after treatment of these two different odorants [35]
Olfactory bulb slice	Glutamic acid (10 μM to 5 mM)	Glutamic acid increased the amplitude and the firing rate of signals [36]
Olfactory placode neurons	GABA (10 μM) Bicuculline (10 μM)	GABA almost immediately inhibited firing activities. Bicuculline has the facilitatory effect or lack of effect [37]

The profiles of the neuroactive substances are usually expressed by the spike rate, burst rate, waveform shape and the attributes like synchronicity, regularity of oscillation, burst structure, connectivity. Of note, the neuronal networks mainly include those dissociated from central nervous system and peripheral nervous system. Until now, the dissociated and cultured neuronal networks, tissues, and slices all have been widely used as the pharmacological models.

3 Electric Cell–Substrate Impedance Sensor

3.1 Principle of ECIS

Cell adhesion to a substrate to grow and propagate is always the first step in a cell-based experiment. Electrical cell–substrate impedance sensing (ECIS) is one of the electrochemical techniques that can be applied to monitor cell adhesion, spreading, and motility in real time [38]. Figure 4 shows a schematic overview of the measurement setup pioneered by Giaever and Keese [39]. Microelectrodes are constructed beneath the cell attachment platform. An alternating current is applied and the voltage is monitored using a lock-in amplifier. When no cells are attached, electric current in the form of ions can flow freely from the surface to the electrodes. Cells growing on the electrode "impede" the flow of current and thus will increase the resistance of the system as cell membranes act as insulators. Electrodes without any cells will produce minimal "baseline" resistance. The addition of analytes that either rupture the cell monolayer or cause disturbances will lead to impedance changes.

ECIS has emerged as one of the most important and interesting label-free technologies for in vitro cell-based assays, due to its advantages of giving real-time and dynamic information of cellular responses, easy to construct and miniaturization. Applications of ECIS in biochemistry and biomedicine up to now are listed in Table 2.

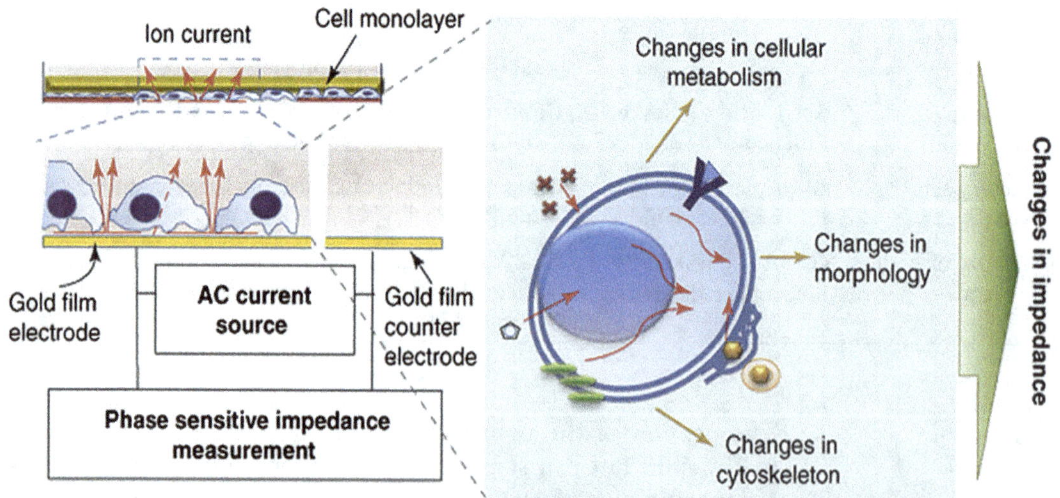

Fig. 4 An ECIS sensor for monitoring cell–substrate impedance. The phase sensitive impedance measurement unit contains a lock-in amplifier with a phase sensitive detector and computer interface for collecting data. A constant current source used to make the in-phase and out-of-phase potentials, proportional to the real and imaginary component of impedance, respectively, are measured in parallel. Certain cell responses such as changes in cellular metabolism, morphology, and cytoskeletal structure cause impedance changes

Table 2
ECIS for biochemistry and biomedicine applications

Application	Description	Cell types (references)
Cell adhesion and proliferation	Biochemicals alter adhesion and proliferation by interfering with cell–ECM interaction, cell-signaling pathways, or cytoskeletal architecture	Fibroblast cells: lung [38, 40–42], kidney [43], liver [44–52], muscle [53–56] Carcinoma cells: hepatoma [57], pancreatic [58]
Cell migration and invasion	Migration causes changes in local area impedance with temporal and spatial resolution	Fibroblast cells: kidney [59, 60] Endothelial cells: umbilical vein [61], renal microvascular[62] Carcinoma cells: hela [60], ovarian [61], hepatoma [63], lung [64], breast [65, 66], prostate [67]
Barrier function	Biochemicals induce barrier dysfunction by perturbing extracellular matrix and cytoskeleton	Epithelial cells: bronchial [68], laryngeal [69], choroid plexus [70], corneal [71] Endothelial cells: pulmonary microvessel [72], brain microvascular [73], brain capillary [74–76], umbilical vein [77], lung microvascular [78, 79], corneal [71, 80]
Cytotoxicity assays and drug discovery	Cytotoxicity and drugs influence cell adhesion and morphology, which induces change of cell–substrate or intercellular impedance in an acute or chronic way	Fibroblast cells: lung [41, 81, 82], orbital [83] Epithelial cells: ovarian [84] Adenocarcinoma cells: colon [85, 86], cervix [87, 88] Carcinoma cells: hepatoma [89, 90], epithelial [91], hepatoma [89], lymphoma [87], lung [57], ovarian [92] Sarcoma cells: fibrosarcoma [93], osteosarcoma [92]

3.2 ECIS for Cytotoxicity Assessment and Drugs Discovery

Cells respond to cytoxins in the forms of loss of adhesion, cell rounding, membrane protrusions or blebbing, formation of apoptotic bodies and ultimately engulfment of apoptotic bodies by phagocytosis. These apopototic responses change cell adhesion and morphology, which ultimately will induce decline of cell–substrate impedance. Such nonlinear dynamic changes depend largely on cell types, compound properties and concentration, and compound exposure duration. Some recommended reference chemicals for evaluating a cytotoxicity test such as antipyrine, trichlorfon, dimethyl formamide, and sodium dichromate, as well as some familiar toxins such as sodium arsenite, mercury chloride, enzalkonium chloride, Triton X-100, sodium lauryl sulfate, cadmium chloride, 1,3,5-trinitrobenzene, cycloheximide, and neutral red solution have been tested using an impedance-based, real-time cell electronic sensing (RT-CES™)

system with various types of cells [82, 94, 95]. In our laboratory, we applied ECIS for rapid and real-time detection of environmental pollutants such as heavy metals, marine toxins with high sensitivity [96, 97].

In the case of drug discovery, cell-based assays using ECIS for investigation of pharmacodynamics can provide a more physiological approach when compared to biochemical assays. For instance, ECIS serves as a valuable approach for studying the effect of biomarkers or therapeutic target on cancer metastasis [98]. Tumor cell invasion and angiogenesis are foundations to tumor development and have been investigated by numerous assays. The typical cell-based assay by ECIS for cancer metastasis was first presented by Keese et al. [99] and is based on previous microscopic observations in which metastatic cells attached to and invaded a cell layer. The metastatic potential of tumor cells was indicated with impedance drop. Using similar assay, ECIS has been used to investigate the function of factors related to the tumor invasion process, such as proteases, cytoskeletal proteins, and adhesion molecules [61, 63–66], and to screen inhibitors that effectively block invasion and metastasis [67, 100, 101]. Here, compared to other chemotaxis assays including Boyden chamber assays, ECIS serves as a valuable tool for biomarkers or therapeutic targets exploration with better mimic of in vivo events, high sensitivity and real-time monitoring. In addition, compared with ex tissue and animal model assays, ECIS is especially suitable for cell-based high-throughput drug screening. ACEA Biosciences (USA) in partnership with Roche and Applied Biophysics (USA) has developed RT-CES products for in vitro monitoring of cells under drug challenge. Hu et al. designed an human induced pluripotent stem cell-derived cardiomyocytes (iPSC-CM)-based biosensor array with the human iPSC-CMs and impedance sensor array [102]. Compound profiling showed that the beating patterns of non-hERG inhibition compounds (isoproterenol, quinidine, and norepinephrine) were similar to the native mature beating patterns in control groups with slight differences in duration (Fig. 5a–c). However, all hERG inhibitors (sertindole, cisapride, and droperidol) tested gave rise to arrhythmic beating pattern (Fig. 5d–f). These known hERG blockers have been withdrawn from the market due to their hERG inhibition function, leading to prolongation of QT interval, even TdP. This rapid impedance assay is useful for drug safety assessment in the early stage of drug development.

Furthermore, the trend in screening applications is to measure an increasing number of cellular parameters in parallel to obtain a comprehensive view on the investigated cellular process [103–107]. Bionas (Germany) and Molecular Devices (USA) have developed products based on multiparametric microsensor chips.

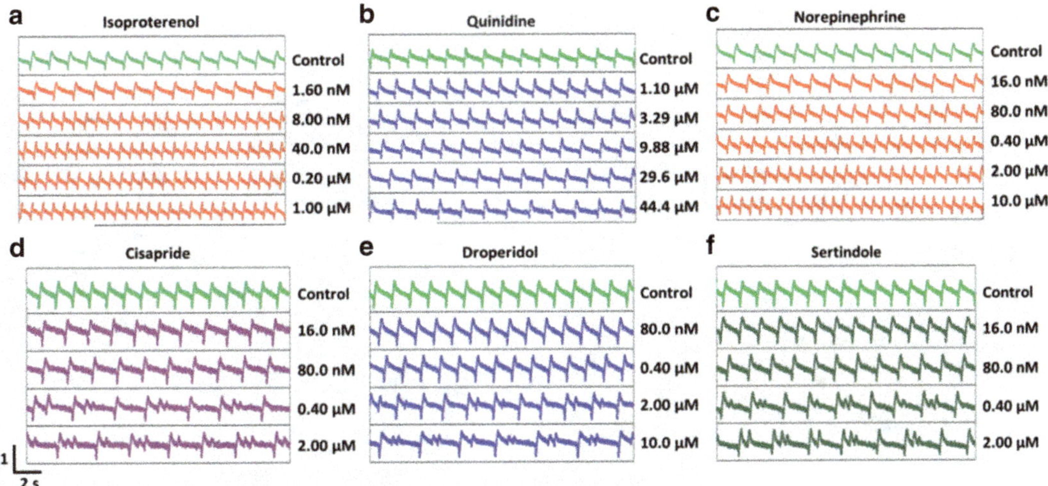

Fig. 5 An iPSC-CM-based biosensor for tracking the beating patterns of cultured cardiomyocytes under the non-hERG inhibition compounds isoproterenol (**a**), quinidine (**b**), norepinephrine (**c**) and hERG inhibitor sertindole (**d**), droperidol (**e**), and cisapride (**f**). Reprinted with permission from ref. 102. Copyright 2014 Elsevier

4 Light Addressable Potentiometric Sensors

4.1 Principle of LAPS

LAPS was first proposed by Hafeman in 1988, as a semiconductor device for biochemical system. In the past two decades, LAPS has been widely studied in biological analysis, and is commonly used as ion-sensitive FET (ISFET) [108–110]. Different LAPS systems have been designed to obtain better sensitivity, stability and compatibility with bioassay. The Cytosensor™ Microphysiometer for extracellular acidification and the Threshold Unit for immunoassays were commercialized by Molecular Devices Corp. (Sunnyvale, CA) [111], while the Potentiometric Alternating Biosensor system was commercialized by Technobiochip (Marciana (LI), Italy) [112].

LAPS is typically structured as conventional electrolyte/insulator/semiconductor (EIS) sensor [113]. By applying a DC bias voltage and modulated light stimulus, the photocurrent is generated. This photocurrent mainly depends on the localized surface potential, which is determined by the solid-liquid interface. Therefore, biological events that modify the electrochemical parameters of the interface could induce fluctuations in the photocurrent output. For example, cell metabolism in a micro-volume chamber results in proton accumulation (pH drop), thus resulting in a photocurrent [109]. Acidic products of energy metabolism acidify cellular environments and the microphysiometer measures the rate of proton excretion from cells (Fig. 6a, b). Many studies showed that the agonist-induced activation of certain receptors increases the rate of extracellular acidification (ECAR), which can be used as an indicator to estimate the effect of chemotherapy [114].

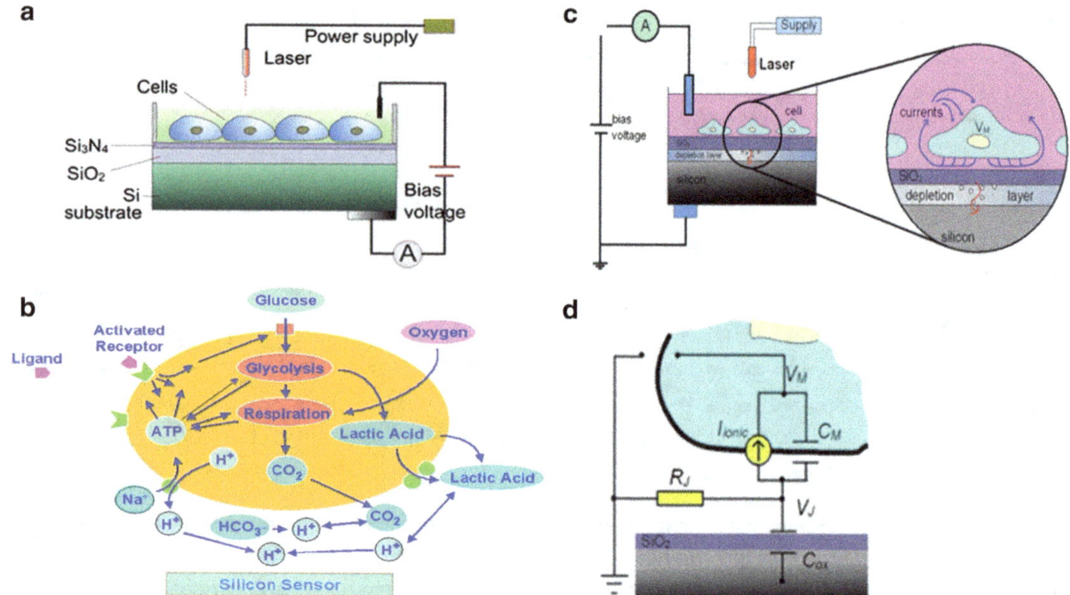

Fig. 6 (**a**, **b**) LAPS as microphysiometer. (**a**) Principle and structure of LAPS. (**b**) Proton release of cell metabolism. (**c**, **d**) Extracellular potential detection using LAPS. (**c**) Simplified cell–semiconductor interface. (**d**) Schematic circuit of the cell–LAPS hybrid system. Reprinted with permission from ref. 119. Copyright 2006 Elsevier

This microphysiometer is useful to evaluate and screen drugs and even suborganelle, against G protein-coupled receptors, receptors with intrinsic catalytic activity, ligand-gated ion channels, receptor tyrosine kinases [109, 115].

While constructing cell-based biosensors for extracellular microenvironment monitoring, LAPS is preferred to ISFET for its compatibility to MEMS fabrication, easier and less critical encapsulation, and satisfactory incorporation into micro volume chamber for bioassays. With cells cultured on silicon surface, extracellular action potential coupled to the sensor surface can also generate spikes in the photocurrent output [116]. Electrophysiology study with LAPS can overcome the geometric restrict of MEA and FET.

Recently, in some experiments the extracellular potentials of excitable cells have been monitored by LAPS [117, 118]. Here, when excitable cells were cultured on LAPS and the light pointer was focused onto the desired cell, the ionic currents (sodium, potassium, and calcium) produced by the cells would result in fluctuation of the photocurrent on LAPS.

The surface of LAPS is laterally unstructured. Cells can adhere on it without any spatial restrictions (Fig. 6c, d). When cells produces potential changes by the ionic currents related to Na^+ and K^+, which was equal to the change of bias voltage, its photocurrent fluctuates (Fig. 6c). When excitable cells are cultured on the oxidized silicon surface of the LAPS (Fig. 6d), it is possible to record changes of the extracellular potential by measuring the local surface potential at the illuminated region by focusing the light pointer on the LAPS surface underlying a target cell [119]. Most LAPS recordings were performed with self-excitable cells such as neurons and cardiomyocytes [116, 117, 120, 121].

4.2 LAPS for Drug Analysis

The functional measure of cellular physiology makes microphysiometer a valuable tool in drug research by allowing screening of pharmacologically active agents, characterization of dose responses and structure–activity relationships, and investigation of the mechanisms of action of drugs.

LAPS microphysiometer permits drug pharmacology testing. For instance, Rabinowitz et al. applied the microphysiometer to investigate the effects of cation channel blockers on the metabolism of a variety of human and murine cell lines [122]. At concentrations sufficient for cation channel blockade, most of these drugs tested have little or no effect on cellular metabolism as measured by acid release. In contrast, the potassium channel blocker clofilium triggers sustained increases in acid release at low concentration, and acid release persists in media containing high extracellular potassium. Fischer et al. measured the potency of four new drug molecules to inhibit the activity of the isoform 1 of the Na^+/H^+ exchanger [123]. The CHO K1 cells were enriched in the NHE-1 isoform of the Na^+/H^+ antiporter. The IC_{50} values obtained were in good agreement with traditional biological assays.

LAPS also enables in vitro toxicology testing. Cao et al. continuously monitored perturbations in metabolic rates of the human liver cell line ATCC-CCL-13 after individually exposed to ten different drugs (Fig. 7) [124]. All drugs produced concentration- and time-dependent reduction in acidification rate following 24 h exposure. Recovery after drug removal is compared. Excellent correlation ($r = 0.958$) was gained between IC_{50} value of 24 h exposure obtained from the cytosensor with the ten drugs and their published human lethal blood concentrations. One advantage of this methodology over other in vitro assays is that the microphysiometer allows for the determination of time points at which reversible change becomes irreversible.

Getting more information about the multifunctional cellular processing is essential to basic research and drug discovery. The concentrations of the extracellular ions, such as Na^+, K^+, and Ca^{2+}, may change along with the alteration of cell physiology. In order to analyze simultaneously the relations among the extracellular environmental H^+, Na^+, K^+, Ca^{2+} under the effects of drugs, our laboratory has developed a novel microphysiometer based on multi-LAPS (Fig. 8a) [125, 126]. The surface of the LAPS is deposited with different sensitive membranes by silicon microfabrication technique

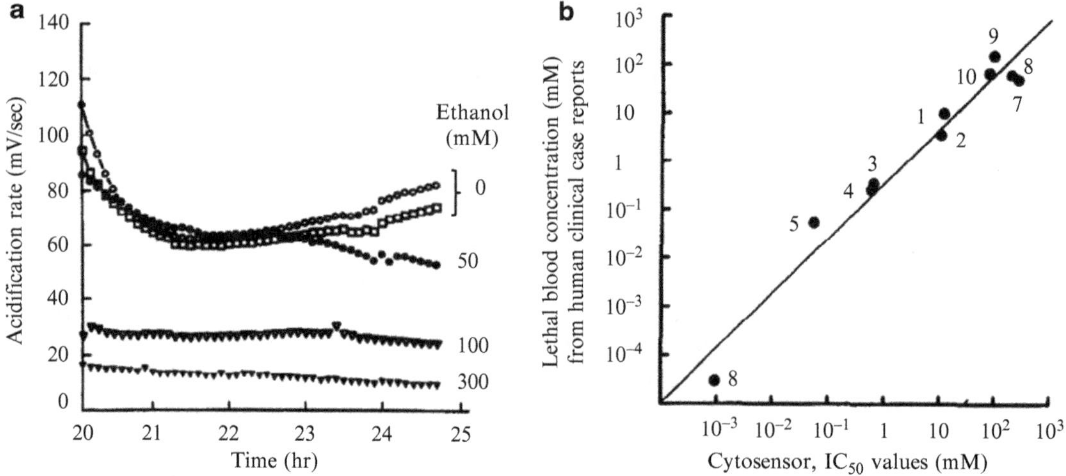

Fig. 7 LAPS microphysiometer for assessing drug-induced liver cell toxicity. (**a**) Effect of 24 h exposure to different concentrations of ethanol (50, 100, 300 mM) on human liver cells. (**b**) Correlation of in vitro cytotoxicity of the ten MEIC chemicals with their in vivo toxicity to humans. The *r* value is 0.958 for 24 h exposure. Each numeral identifies the test drug used: 1, acetaminophen; 2, acetylsalicylic acid; 3, ferrous sulfate; 4, diazepam; 5, amitriptyline; 6, digoxin; 7, ethylene glycol; 8, methanol; 9, ethanol; 10, isopropanol. Data of lethal blood concentrations were collected by the Swedish Poison Information Centre from clinical reports and autopsies. Reprinted with permission from ref. 126. Copyright 1997 Elsevier

and PVC membrane technique. The amplitude of each frequency component is measured online by software FFT analysis (Fig. 8b). Dilantin (phenytoin sodium) is an anti-epilepsy drug and has significant effects of tranquilizing, hypnotic, and anti-seizure. Dilantin is also one of the anti-arrhythmia drugs. Our multi-LAPS confirmed that dilantin has membrane stabilizing action on neural cells, as evidenced by its ability to reduce pericellular membrane ions (Na^+, Ca^{2+}) permeability, to inhibit Na^+ and Ca^{2+} influx, to stave K^+ efflux, thus prolonging refractory period, stabilizing pericellular membrane, and decreasing excitability (Fig. 8c).

LAPS also allows for multiparameter analysis of drug-induced effects on cultured cardiomyocytes [127]. As an agent of β-adrenoceptor agonist that contributes to cardio-activity, isoproterenol (ISO) enhances the L-type calcium channel activity, which causes an increase in Ca^{2+} signal. ISO administration was found to cause a dose-dependently and marked increase in beating frequency, amplitude, and duration of cardiomyocytes (Fig. 9). The cardiomyocyte contractibility all recovered after drugs washout. In contrast, carbamylcholine had opposite effect to ISO. In another study, the effects of heavy metal ions on cardiomyocyte function were also evaluated using LAPS [128].

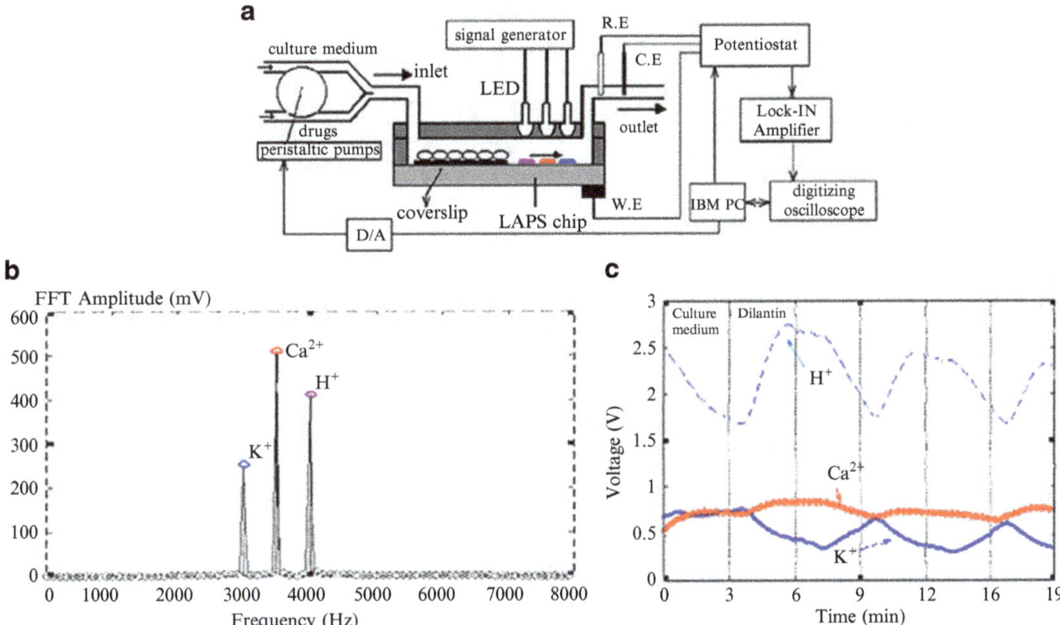

Fig. 8 Multi-LAPS as a novel microphysiometer. (**a**) The schematic drawing of the multi-LAPS system for monitoring three different extracellular ions (H⁺, K⁺, and Ca²⁺). (**b**) Illuminate simultaneously at the three sensitive membranes with three light sources at the three modulation frequencies. (**c**) H⁺, K⁺, Ca²⁺ analyze simultaneously by multi-LAPS. Reprinted with permission from refs. 127, 128. Copyright 2001 Elsevier

5　Field Effect Transistor Sensors

5.1　Principle of FET

FET sensors without gate metallization was originally applied for measuring ion concentration, thus termed ion sensitive FET (ISFET) in 1970 [129]. The measurement of ionic effluxes around neurons, together with oxygen consumption and other metabolic parameters, has wide implications in drug discovery. Over the past decades, FET and its derivatives have been developed and used for measuring the extracellular potential of muscle from locust leg [130], and living cells [131], and extended to cell micro-environmental monitoring and cell electrophysiological detection [132–136].

FET sensors use a transistor consisting of a single crystal substrate with two heavily doped regions, the source and drain regions, which are diffused into the top surface of the crystal. The current that flows from one to another of these two regions must flow through the narrow channel in the substrate between them. An extremely thin layer of silicon dioxide, a near-perfect insulator, is deposited upon the surface of the substrate between the two regions, which forms gate area. The biological or chemical reaction that results in electrical change can be measured by FET.

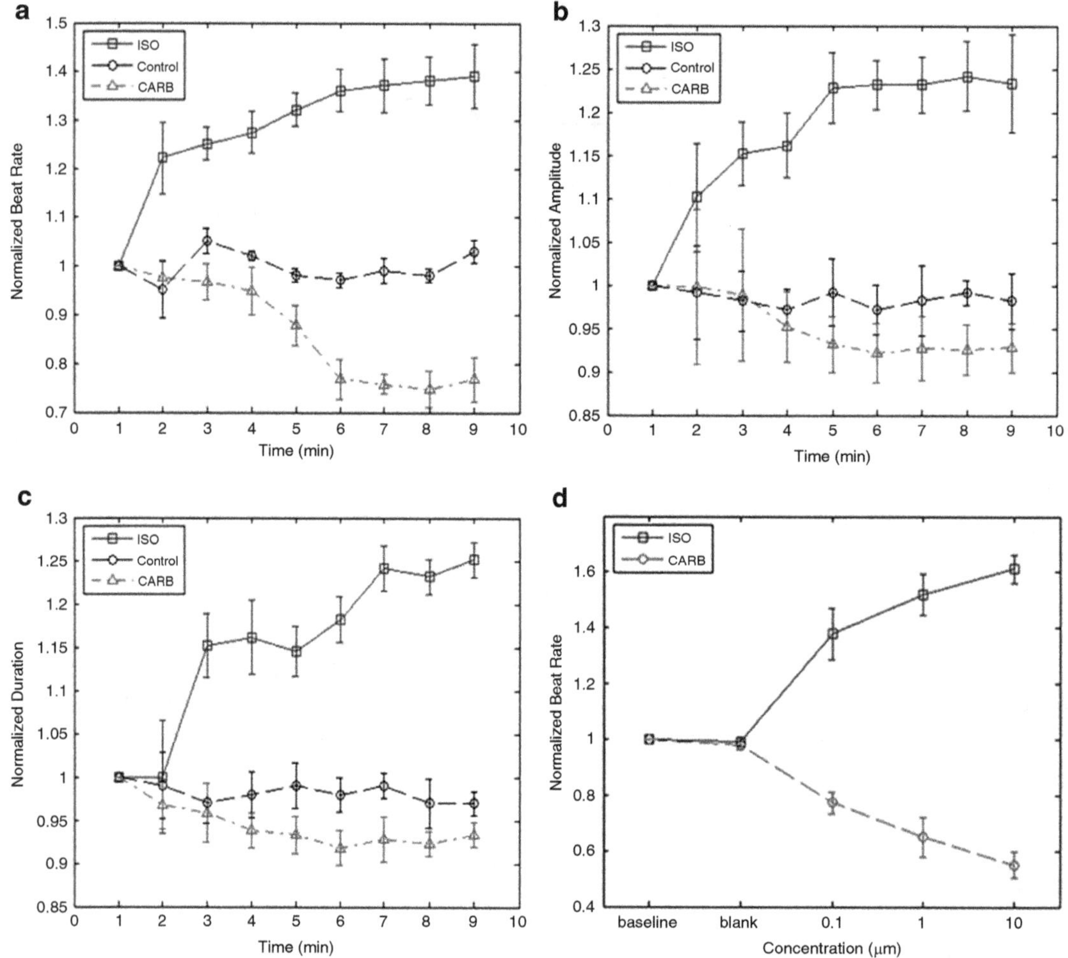

Fig. 9 Plots comparing the response of cardiomyocytes to the carbamylcholine (CARB), isoproterenol (ISO) and physiological solution as control. The concentration of drugs are all 1 μM. Drugs effect on the beat rate (**a**), amplitude (**b**) and duration (**c**) of the each extracellular potential. Effect of different drug concentration to beat rate (**d**). Each data point represents an average over 50 s. The experimental data is the average value of six times of repetition. Reprinted with permission from ref. 128. Copyright 2009 Elsevier

The most representative ISFET sensor is the proton-sensitive sensor. It consists of a pH-sensitive metal oxide, such as Al_2O_3, SiO_2 or TaO_2, as pH recognition element [137–139]. The detection of other ion types is achieved by depositing electrochemically sensitive layers, solid or polymeric materials onto the metal oxide gate of ISFET. The ISFET operational mechanism is identical to MOSFET with additional possibility to chemically modify the threshold voltage via the interfacial potential at the electrolyte-oxide interface. The basic model of electrolyte/insulator/silicon (EIS) structures was adopted by Bousse et al. [140]. Currently, the site-dissociation model is commonly accepted for describing the performance of the ISFET [141, 142].

Cell-based FET sensors usually adopt enhancement-type n-channel MOSFET. Under applied positive gate bias, the positive charges on the gate will attract minority carriers and form a channel that links the source and drain together. When bias voltage is applied between the source and the drain, the modulation of the drain-source current is determined by the gate voltage change. For the purpose of detecting cells or neuronal networks activities, the source, drain and bulk voltages are set at constant values when the transconductance dI_{SD}/dV_S reaches maximum. The selected point from the curves of I_{SD}–V_S characteristics is determined as working point. Cells are directly cultured on the dielectric material like SiO_2 or Si_3N_4. As soon as an action potential occurs, the surface potential of the dielectric layer will be lifted, resulting in a change in the density of mobile defect electrons. The neuron-silicon interaction causes a modulation of the current along the inversion layer driven by a voltage between source and drain. Finally, the changes in current convert into the junction voltage changes to represent cellular activities.

5.2 FET Sensors for Toxicity Assessment

The cell–transistor hybrid system can be used for many applications such as drug screening, neurophysiology, toxicology, and environmental measurements. This system is highly sensitive to minute changes of chemicals within the cellular environment.

Recording electrical signals of excitable cells or tissues by FET sensors were first reported in the middle of the 1970s to early 1980s [143]. Similar to MEA sensors, the excitation of cells or tissues coupled on the FET chip drives ionic and capacitive current through the membrane to the chip. The voltage is defined as Transductive Extracellular Potential $V_J(t)$, which can be detected by the FET. By monitoring the extracellular potential changes of electrogenic cells or tissues due to the influence of chemical stimuli on cellular activities, the drug discovery or toxicity assay can be achieved.

In the early phases of heart drug development, cardiomyocytes is a suitable in vitro model for the efficacy test. FET can perform long-term recording of the extracellular potentials of cardiomyocytes, which is a vital indicator of the cells' states. Ingebrandt developed an extracellular recording system for the detection of electrical cell signals using FET arrays [144]. Dissociated cardiac myocytes were cultured in high density on FET devices. Under the stimulation of cardiac stimulants (isoproterenol, norepinephrine) and relaxants (verapamil, carbamylcholine), the extracellular signal shapes of cardiomyocytes changes differently, confirming the characteristic effects of different agents on the heart cells.

FET arrays have potential for large scale multiplexing, enabling recording of both individual neurons and networks. Real-time recording and stimulating of neural cell's bioelectrical activity offers an unprecedented insight in understanding the functions of the nervous system and an efficient method for drug screening and neurotoxicity assay. Benfenati introduced a transparent organic cell stimulating and sensing FET (O-CST) providing simultaneous stimulation and recording of primary neurons [145]. With similar neuronal preparation procedures, the maximal amplitude-to-noise ratio of the extracellular recording achieved by the O-CST device is 16 times that of a microelectrode array system. They had applied the system for studying the effect of TetrodoToxin (TTX, a well-known Nav blocker) on neurons. After application of TTX, the number of positive spikes dramatically decreased, while some TTX resistant spikes were still recorded (Fig. 10), possible due to the fact that the action potential is mediated by both TTX-sensitive and TTX-insensitive Nav channels.

ISFET is mainly focused on monitoring the extracellular acidification rate (EAR) of a cell culture which is an important parameter reflecting the metabolism of cells. The EAR of cells is often altered by the external chemical stimulus such as toxins and drugs, making ISFET sensor a favorable platform for drug screening and toxicology analysis. For instance, Lehmann et al. fabricated a four-ISFET-array to measure the pH of adherent tumor cells in vitro [146].

Living cells are often involved in complex biochemical and biophysical processes to maintain their physiological functions. Only monitoring extracellular ionic concentration is not sufficient

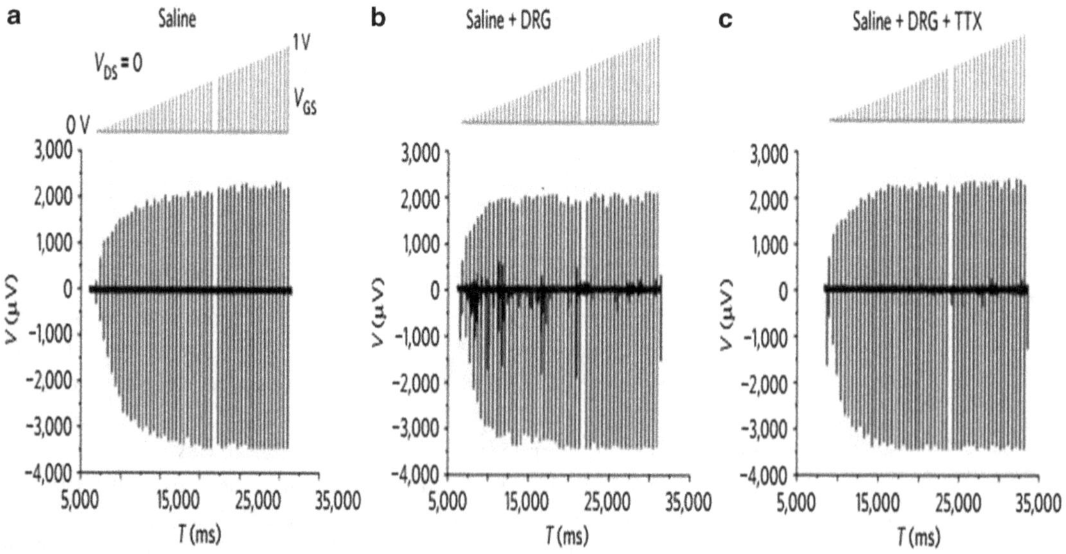

Fig. 10 Extracellular signals recorded by the O-CST upon biasing the device with the pulsed stimulation protocol (*top inset* in each panel: VDS = 0 V, VGS from 0 to 1 V with linearly increasing steps of 20 mV, pulse duration 200 μs, frequency rate 2 Hz) in different experimental conditions: when only saline is interfaced to the device (**a**), when neuronal cells are plated on top of the device (**b**) and when the same cells of (**b**) are exposed to the TTX neurotoxin (**c**). Reprinted with permission from ref. 145. Copyright 2013 Nature publishing system

to fully comprehend cell physiology. Therefore, integration of ISFET-based cell sensor with other sensors, such as temperature, conductivity, and oxygen sensors is useful [146, 147]. This technology enables the integration of these sensors located on the same silicon wafer at the bottom of a cell culturing chamber. Seeland developed an in vitro toxicological assay based on monitoring cellular oxygen consumption, acidification and impedance of HepG2 cells by using a multiparametric cytosensor system [148]. This system integrated ISFET, Clark-type sensors, and interdigital electrodes. Changes of the three cellular parameters under the treatment of eight marketed drugs were monitored, which revealed distinct patterns of drug-induced responses. Based on the analysis of these parameters, drugs can be classified as nontoxic (d-sorbitol), intrinsically toxic (antineoplastic drugs), or potentially toxic under conditions of exaggerated exposure.

6 Automated Patch-Clamp Chips

6.1 Principle of Automated Patch-Clamp Chips

Patch clamp has proven to be a powerful laboratory technique for the study of single or multiple ion channels in cells. Traditional patch-clamp recording uses a fire-polished glass pipette with an open tip diameter of about 1 μm to isolate a small membrane patch. The micropipette tip produces a smooth surface that assists in forming a giga-ohm resistance seal with the cell membrane, which is the key step of patch-clamp technique. The high resistance seal makes it possible to electronically isolate the currents measured across the membrane patch which often contains just one or a few ion channels (Fig. 11). Patch clamp allows the research of the single channel behaviors on a small membrane patch or the macroscopic current from the whole cellular membrane, which play crucial roles in cellular signal transduction, impulse conduction, cellular microenvironment balance, and so on. On the other hand, ion channels are important drug targets because about 8 % of all clinically used drugs are the agonists or antagonists of ion channels. However, patch clamp suffers from some of its intrinsic drawbacks, such as low throughput, precision micromanipulation under high power visual magnification, vibration damping, and the requirement of an experienced and skillful experimenter [149].

The first improvement of the conventional microelectrode was achieved by Flyion who put forward a technology called flip-tip and developed a novel automatic patch-clamp instrument, which is known as the Flyscreen 8500 system [150]. The interface between cell and electrode was inverted, which make it possible to place the cells inside the microelectrode. By this way, cells can reach the tip of the pipette and form a seal from the inside. However, this single microelectrode-based system cannot realize

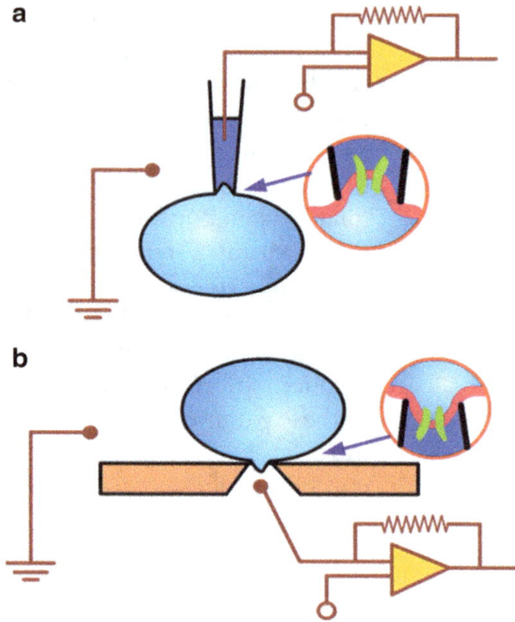

Fig. 11 The configuration of the conventional patch clamp (**a**) and the planar patch-clamp chip (**b**)

the high-throughput measurements. Another improvement was the development of patch-clamp chip that started in the late 1990s. These automated patch-clamp chip replaces the glass microelectrode with a planar structure (Fig. 11b) [149]. In these patch-clamp chips, cells were guided onto the aperture by a negative pressure or static electricity field. The high seal resistance between cell and chip is obtained by the application of another negative pressure. Patch-clamp chip holds many advantages over conventional patch clamp. First, more convenient and rapid operation can be carried out on patch-clamp chip, which can be easily combined with optical measurements and micromanipulator, such as atomic force microscopy and fluorescent microscopy. Second, the patch-clamp chip configured with microelectrodes could record multiple cells simultaneously, which make it suitable for high-throughput measurements. Third, due to its planar structure, its capacitance (about 1 pF) should be less than that of a glass pipette (several pF) and the resistance is reduced resulting in a lower distributed RC noise and a higher resolution.

6.2 Planar Patch-Clamp Chip for High-Throughput Drug Screening

The significant advantages of patch-clamp chip make it suitable for high-throughput screening of drugs targeting ionic channels [151, 152]. Ion channels are drug targets for numerous therapeutic agents aimed at treating a variety of disorders, including hypertension, arrhythmias, seizures, pain, stroke and diabetes. With the development of human genome and protein, more and more drug targets will be discovered and demonstrated. It is estimated that ionic channels may account for 15 % in around 5,000 druggable targets. However, the measurements of ionic channels are complicated by their properties of variety and complexity indicated by genomics and proteomics [153]. The expression of ionic channels also differs greatly, consequently, leading to the inconsistency of the measurement data.

The parallel, automated, and high-throughput patch-clamp chip system can greatly improve the work efficiency during drug screening. Lau et al. presented a novel open-access patch-clamp chip with raised cell trapping microfluidic channels to better resemble traditional glass micropipette openings [154]. The main fluidic chamber was open to the air, providing an easy-to-use platform for fluidic exchange. The smooth surface of open-access patch-clamp sites accomplished by the microscale hole punching method and seal resistances are characterized. Extensive whole-cell patch-clamp experiments are then performed on CHO cells expressing Kv2.1 ion channels, including ion channel I–V characterizations, drug dose–response characterizations, and also dynamic drug activity characterizations. This open-access platform was suitable for high-throughput screening of ion channel electrophysiology, since it provides easier handling and a shorter data turnaround time compared to the traditional patch-clamp set-up.

In order to make multi-cell recording simultaneously, Molecular Devices launched a novel product of Ionworks Quattro system by adopting the population patch-clamp technology, which is suitable for the fast analysis of the structure and function of massive mutant ionic channel [155]. In this system, multiple cells can be voltage clamped by multiple micro apertures in multiple wells, each of which approximately 7,000–10,000 cells are added. This system was used to record the non-inactivated channels hKv1.5 expressed in CHO cells in a whole-cell recording mode [153].

Another patch-clamp chip system that can be used in high-throughput screening of ionic channels is the 16-channel planar patch-clamp system, known as PatchXpress (Axon Instruments, Mol. Devices, USA). In the case of ionic channels screening for the investigation of the effects of small molecules on hERG channels, it can obtain 2,000 reliable data points per day, which is improved by fourfold in throughput [156]. Qpatch 16 (Sophion Bioscience, Denmark) is also a 16-channel automated planar patch-clamp screening system. Its throughput can reach 250–1,200 data points in the case of whole-cell recordings on hERG channels expressed in CHO cells. When it was used to screen the hERG and KCNQ4 channels expressed in CHO and HEK cells, respectively, the successful rate of giga-ohm seal is 40–90 % and about 67 % of cells can sustain whole-cell recordings for more than 20 min [157]. Similarly, as compared with those of conventional patch clamps, the IonWorks HT planar patch-clamp (Molecular Devices, USA) system can also achieve reliable and comparable data when it was used to screen hERG channels expressed in CHO cells using quinidine [151].

It is evident that patch-clamp chip technology has become an effective approach in the basic scientific research of ion channels as well as drug discovery. In the future, some improvements, such as higher throughput, higher successful rate, and primary cell recordings, are necessary for patch-clamp chip to satisfy the applications in basic research and drug discovery as well as to explore new domains and applications.

7　Quartz Crystal Microbalance (QCM) Biosensor

7.1　Principle of QCM

The resonant device is sensitive to mass and viscosity changes, which makes it a promising and powerful tool to study biological molecular interactions, especially for affinity cell-based biosensors. The typical resonant device is QCM, which detects tiny mass changes by monitoring the oscillation frequency shifts of the crystal resulting from pressure changes on the crystal surface by mass-loading. An increase of mass loading to the sensitive surface causes a decrease of oscillation frequency. Consequently, the mass-sensing sensors can respond to the mass changes of coated material on the sensitive area. The oscillation frequency decrease is proportional to the mass changes [158].

QCM was discovered by the Curie brothers [159]. The linear relationship between the mass changes and the oscillation frequency changes in quartz crystal was revealed by Sauerbrey [160]. In the 1980s, Nomura and Okuhara designed oscillator circuits that allow this sensor to be used not only in a vacuum or air, but also in liquids [161], making the QCM an attractive and promising analytical tool in the field of biosensors. In the case of cell-based biosensors, the living cells do not behave as elastic masses on the QCM surface, which makes QCM can not only provide mass changes on the crystal surface but also more valuable information about reactions and conditions at the liquid-solid interface. The resonant resistance (R) of quartz crystal combined with the oscillation frequency (f) is used to characterize the viscoelastic properties of deposited inelastic masses on the surface of the crystal, whose values are affected by the medium density and viscosity. The f decrease is due to both mass binding and viscoelastic energy dissipation behavior while R increases. When solution and crystal surface contact tightly without relative sliding, the oscillation frequency shift can be calculated by the Kanazawa equation [162]. The resonant resistance change can be calculated by the Muramatsu equation [163]. When QCM operates in solution, the total f changes may result from a bound mass as well as the solution contributions. The viscoelastic properties and the energy-dissipating

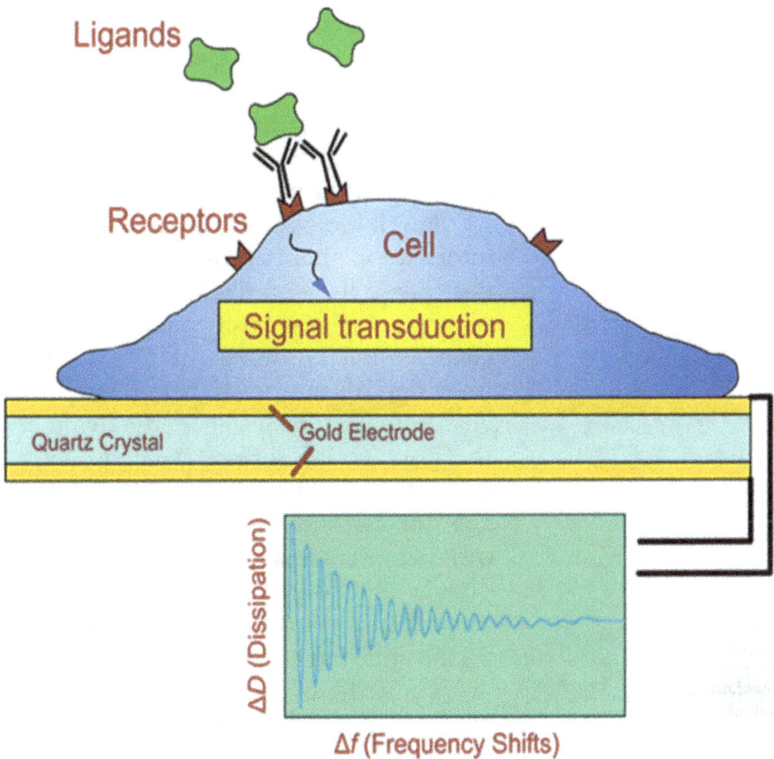

Fig. 12 The principle of QCM sensors for whole-cell sensing

properties of surface with masses attached, such as living cells, can be evaluated relative to density-viscosity changes of a liquid solution. According to these equations, QCM technique has the sensitive and quantitative capability to investigate the behavior of adherent cells in response to chemical, biological, or physical changes in the environment. In addition, QCM has a wide detection range from a monolayer of small molecules to much greater masses—even complex arrays of cells. Some properties of cultured cells had been successfully monitored with QCM, such as the cell attachment, proliferation, and cell–substrate interaction under different conditions (Fig. 12). QCM can also measure the exocytosis, vesicle retrieval of cell populations, and cell–microparticle interactions in real time.

7.2 QCM Biosensor for Drug Discovery

The process of drug discovery and drug analysis is a long, complex, and multistage process. The successful odds of this process are very low with high cost. The main reason may be due to the lack of powerful tools for high-throughput and information-rich content screening of candidate drugs. This is also the major driving force for enterprise within pharmaceutical industry to find novel measurement techniques to evaluate the effect of drug compounds on specific pharmaceutical targets and ultimately improve the overall efficiency of the drug discovery and development.

QCM biosensor integrating with living cells as sensitive elements have been used in a number of studies for drug discovery and drug analysis. The whole-cell-based biosensors are suitable for drug detection because it detects the magnitude and kinetics of a whole-cell biological response, which is much closer to the type of information pharmaceutical companies require as drug testing output. The cell-based QCM biosensors can also provide information on changes in viscosity properties of cells in addition to mass changes. Furthermore, the QCM technique holds the advantage over optical sensor of being less sensitive to changes in fluid environment. For instance, the living endothelial cells adhering to the gold QCM surface were used for detecting the actions of nocodazole, which is a known microtubule-binding drug that can alter the cytoskeletal properties of living cells [164]. By simultaneous measurements of the shift values in the QCM steady state frequency and motional resistance, the cell-based QCM biosensor can effectively monitor the process of cell microtubules disruption by the addition of nocodazole.

The cell-based QCM biosensors have also been applied in the prediction of drug resistance of tumor cells. A cell-based QCM biosensor was developed for the real-time screening of cell lines and their sensitivity to anticancer drugs, which can predict tumor responses to drugs prior to therapy or before resistance or hypersensitivity develops [165].

The underlying mechanisms that determine the QCM signal for a particular cell type were explored by the using of AC impedance analysis in a frequency range [166], indicating that many subcellular compartments contribute to the resonators' fundamental frequency such as extracellular matrix, the actin cytoskeleton, the medium that overlays the cell layer, as well as the liquid compartment that is known to exist between the basal plasma membrane and the culture substrate. Recently, the adhesion and growth of rat epithelial cells and lung melanoma cells on the QCM has been monitored in real time by continuous measuring the changes in the oscillation frequency and resistance values of the piezoelectric resonators [167]. The behavior of human patellar tendon fibroblasts was also monitored by QCM coated with indium-tin oxide (ITO). On the other hand, the real-time monitoring of MCF-7 cell growth and assessment of chemical cytotoxicity was achieved by a QCM with polyporphyrin film modified gold electrode surface [168]. The responses of human oral epithelial cells to microspheres were monitored by a cell-based QCM biosensor in real time [169]. In addition, QCM combined with impedance analysis can be a completely new approach for determining electrical and viscoelastic properties of the epithelial and endothelial cell monolayers that form controlled barriers in vivo [170].

QCM with dissipation (QCM-D) is a novel and attractive technique for in vitro real-time characterization of cell attachment and spreading. The cell adhesion and spreading can be monitored more accurately and allows in situ real-time measurements. It has been successfully applied in the characterization of initial adhesion and spreading of fibroblasts in contact with protein pre-coated biocompatible surfaces [171]. The QCM-D technique can also be applied in the measurements of complex dynamic processes relating to dense-core vesicle release and retrieval. The mass change and rigidity of populations of excitable cells during exocytosis and subsequent retrieval of dense-core vesicles can be simultaneously monitored. In the case of two cell lines, NG 108-15 and PC 12, it was demonstrated that their differences in release and retrieval with cells of different morphology, sizes, and numbers of dense-core vesicles by being cultured on piezoelectric quartz crystals can be effectively monitored [172].

8 Summary

The most important reason for developing cell-based biosensors is that by using living cells components capable of a direct response to incoming information of an external physical or chemical stimulus. This functional information with additional qualitative and/or quantitative analytical information can be very important with respect to clinical diagnostics, pharmacology and drug screening, cell biology, toxicology and environmental monitoring. By means of such biosensors, it could be possible to study the effects of pharmaceutical compounds, toxic substances, pollutants, etc., on a physiological system and in particular on cellular metabolism.

The model of the cell–silicon, cell–metal electrode interface and the detection models of MEA, FET, LAPS, and ECIS are very important for improving the property of cell-based biosensors. For example, the characteristic of transmembrane ionic current are given based on the conductance and permeability of cellular membrane. With the development of microelectronic mechanical system (MEMS) and cell biology, the research on cell-based biosensor has reached on the cellular and molecular level. Cells provide and express a series of elements such as naturally evolved receptor, ion channels, and enzymes that can be the targets of biological active analytes. When stimulated, the living cell responds and takes actions: induce electronic activity, excrete something, or absorb something. Cell-based biosensors that treat cells as biological sensing elements have the capacity to respond to analytes in a physiologically relevant manner. However, cell-based biosensors still suffer from some intrinsic shortcomings. The common problems faced by the optimization of cell-based biosensors include how to achieve satisfactory stability, how to analyze the selectivity of a special sensor design, and how to enhance the cells' lifetime. Fortunately, cellular mimicking and sensing are expected to be exploited in the near future, with the development of biotechniques such as nanotechnology, microfluidics, and high-content screening.

References

1. Thomas C Jr, Springer P, Loeb G et al (1972) A miniature microelectrode array to monitor the bioelectric activity of cultured cells. Exp Cell Res 74(1):61–66

2. Metz S, Bartlett R, Jenkins J, et al (1996) Controller design for extracorporeal life support. in Engineering in Medicine and Biology Society, 1996. Bridging disciplines for biomedicine. Proceedings of the 18th annual international conference of the IEEE. IEEE

3. Egert U (2006) Network on chips. In: BioMEMS. Springer. pp. 309–349

4. Borkholder DA (1998) Cell-based biosensors using microelectrodes. Ph.D. thesis, Standford University, CA.

5. Halbach MD, Egert U, Hescheler J et al (2003) Estimation of action potential changes from field potential recordings in multicellular mouse cardiac myocyte cultures. Cell Physiol Biochem 13(5):271–284

6. Reppel M (2007) Effect of cardioactive drugs on action potential generation and propagation in embryonic stem cell-derived cardiomyocytes. Cell Physiol Biochem 19(5/6):12

7. Gilchrist KH (2003) Characterization and validation of cell-based biosensors. Ph.D. thesis, Stanford University, CA.

8. Natarajan A, Molnar P, Sieverdes K et al (2006) Microelectrode array recordings of cardiac action potentials as a high throughput method to evaluate pesticide toxicity. Toxicol in Vitro 20(3):375–381

9. Tsai CT, Chiang FT, Chen WP et al (2011) Angiotensin II induces complex fractionated electrogram in a cultured atrial myocyte monolayer mediated by calcium and sodium-calcium exchanger. Cell Calcium 49(1):1–11

10. Yeung C, Sommerhage F, Wrobel G et al (2007) Drug profiling using planar microelectrode arrays. Anal Bioanal Chem 387(8): 2673–2680

11. Braam SR, Tertoolen L, van de Stolpe A et al (2010) Prediction of drug-induced cardiotoxicity using human embryonic stem cell-derived cardiomyocytes. Stem Cell Res 4(2): 107–116

12. Gross G, Kowalski JM (1991) Experimental and theoretical analysis of random nerve cell networks dynamics. In: Antognetti P, Miltunovic E (eds) Neural networks: concepts, applications and implementations. Prentice Hall, New Jersey, pp 47–110

13. Kamioka H, Maeda E, Jimbo Y et al (1996) Spontaneous periodic synchronized bursting during formation of mature patterns of connections in cortical cultures. Neurosci Lett 206(2–3):109–112

14. Gross GW, Harsch A, Rhoades BK et al (1997) Odor, drug and toxin analysis with neuronal networks in vitro: extracellular array recording of network responses. Biosens Bioelectron 12(5):373–393

15. Eytan D, Minerbi A, Ziv N et al (2004) Dopamine-induced dispersion of correlations between action potentials in networks of cortical neurons. J Neurophysiol 92(3): 1817–1824

16. Moss BL, Fuller AD, Sahley CL et al (2005) Serotonin modulates axo-axonal coupling between neurons critical for learning in the leech. J Neurophysiol 94(4):2575–2589

17. Otto F, Görtz P, Fleischer W et al (2003) Cryopreserved rat cortical cells develop functional neuronal networks on microelectrode arrays. J Neurosci Methods 128(1–2): 173–181

18. Sokal DM, Mason R, Parker TL (2000) Multi-neuronal recordings reveal a differential effect of thapsigargin on bicuculline- or gabazine-induced epileptiform excitability in rat hippocampal neuronal networks. Neuropharmacology 39(12):2408–2417

19. Harsch A, Ziegler C, Göpel W (1997) Strychnine analysis with neuronal networks in vitro: extracellular array recording of network responses. Biosens Bioelectron 12(8): 827–835

20. Krause G, Lehmann S, Lehmann M et al (2006) Measurement of electrical activity of long-term mammalian neuronal networks on semiconductor neurosensor chips and comparison with conventional microelectrode arrays. Biosens Bioelectron 21(7):1272–1282

21. Xia Y, Gopal KV, Gross GW (2003) Differential acute effects of fluoxetine on frontal and auditory cortex networks in vitro. Brain Res 973(2):151–160

22. Mistry SK, Keefer EW, Cunningham BA et al (2002) Cultured rat hippocampal neural progenitors generate spontaneously active neural networks. Proc Natl Acad Sci U S A 99(3): 1621–1626

23. Rijal SO, Gross GW (2008) Dissociation constants for GABAA receptor antagonists determined with neuronal networks on microelectrode arrays. J Neurosci Methods 173(2):183–192

24. Morefield SI, Keefer EW, Chapman KD et al (2000) Drug evaluations using neuronal networks cultured on microelectrode arrays. Biosens Bioelectron 15(7–8):383–396

25. Xia Y, Gross GW (2003) Histiotypic electrophysiological responses of cultured neuronal networks to ethanol. Alcohol 30(3):167–174

26. Dasari S, Yuan Y (2010) In vivo methylmercury exposure induced long-lasting epileptiform activity in layer II/III neurons in cortical slices from the rat. Toxicol Lett 193(2):138–143

27. Parviz M, Gross GW (2007) Quantification of zinc toxicity using neuronal networks on microelectrode arrays. Neurotoxicology 28(3): 520–531

28. Gopal KV, Gross GW (2004) Unique responses of auditory cortex networks in vitro to low concentrations of quinine. Hear Res 192(1–2):10–22

29. O'Shaughnessy TJ, Zim B, Ma W et al (2003) Acute neuropharmacologic action of chloroquine on cortical neurons in vitro. Brain Res 959(2):280–286

30. Hogberg HT, Sobanski T, Novellino A et al (2011) Application of micro-electrode arrays (MEAs) as an emerging technology for developmental neurotoxicity: evaluation of domoic acid-induced effects in primary cultures of rat cortical neurons. Neurotoxicology 32(1):158–168

31. Volmer R, Prat CMA, Le Masson G et al (2007) Borna disease virus infection impairs synaptic plasticity. J Virol 81(16):8833–8837

32. Scarlatos A, Cadotte AJ, DeMarse TB, Welt BA (2008) Cortical networks grown on microelectrode arrays as a biosensor for botulinum toxin. J Food Sci 73(3):129–136

33. Manos P, Pancrazio JJ, Coulombe MG et al (1999) Characterization of rat spinal cord neurons cultured in defined media on microelectrode arrays. Neurosci Lett 271(3): 179–182

34. Guenther E, Herrmann T, Stett A (2006) The retinasensor: an in vitro tool to study drug effects on retinal signaling. In: Taketani M, Baudry M (eds) Advances in network electrophysiology. Springer, USA, pp 321–331

35. Liu Q, Ye W, Xiao L et al (2010) Extracellular potentials recording in intact olfactory epithelium by microelectrode array for a bioelectronic nose. Biosens Bioelectron 25(10): 2212–2217

36. Chen Q, Xiao L, Liu Q et al (2011) An olfactory bulb slice-based biosensor for multi-site extracellular recording of neural networks. Biosens Bioelectron 26(7):3313–3319

37. Suyama K, Daikoku S, Funabashi T et al (2004) Effects of GABA and bicuculline on the electrical activity of rat olfactory placode neurons derived at e13.5 and cultured for 1 week on multi-electrode dishes. Endocr J 51(2):171–176

38. Wegener J, Keese CR, Giaever I (2000) Electric cell-substrate impedance sensing (ecis) as a noninvasive means to monitor the kinetics of cell spreading to artificial surfaces. Exp Cell Res 259(1):158–166

39. Giaever I, Keese CR (1986) Use of electric fields to monitor the dynamical aspect of cell behavior in tissue culture. Biomed Eng IEEE T Biomed Eng 33(2):242–247

40. Mitra P, Keese CR, Giaever I (1991) Electric measurements can be used to monitor the attachment and spreading of cells in tissue culture. Biotechniques 11(4):504–510

41. Xiao C, Lachance B, Sunahara G et al (2002) An in-depth analysis of electric cell-substrate impedance sensing to study the attachment and spreading of mammalian cells. Anal Chem 74:1333–1339

42. Mayer M, Brunner P, Merwa R et al (2005) Monitoring of lung edema using focused impedance spectroscopy: a feasibility study. Physiol Meas 26(3):185–192

43. Lo CM, Keese CR, Giaever I (1995) Impedance analysis of MDCK cells measured by electric cell-substrate impedance sensing. Biophys J 69(6):2800–2807

44. Cascales-Sanchez P, Fernandez-Cornejo V, Tomas-Gomez A et al (2007) Electrical impedance of the liver during experimental long-term liver preservation. Transplant Proc 39(7):2118–2119

45. Parramon D, Erill I, Guimera A et al (2007) In vivo detection of liver steatosis in rats based on impedance spectroscopy. Physiol Meas 28(8):813–828

46. Parsonnet V, Marak MJ, Panken E et al (2007) Detection of early renal transplant rejection by minimally-invasive monitoring of

impedance variability. Biosens Bioelectron 22(11):2749–2753

47. Antaki F, French MM, Moonka DK et al (2008) Bioelectrical impedance analysis for the evaluation of hepatic fibrosis in patients with chronic hepatitis C infection. Dig Dis Sci 53(7):1957–1960

48. Spottorno J, Multigner M, Rivero G et al (2008) Time dependence of electrical bio-impedance on porcine liver and kidney under a 50 Hz ac current. Phys Med Biol 53(6): 1701–1713

49. Bhati CS, Silva MA, Wigmore SJ et al (2009) Use of bioelectrical impedance analysis to assess liver steatosis. Transplant Proc 41(5): 1677–1681

50. Hessheimer AJ, Parramon D, Guimera A et al (2009) A rapid and reliable means of assessing hepatic steatosis in vivo via electrical bio-impedance. Transplantation 88(5):716–722

51. Hwang S, Yu YD, Park GC et al (2010) Bioelectrical impedance analysis for evaluation of donor hepatic steatosis in living-donor liver transplantation. Transplant Proc 42(5): 1492–1496

52. Park JY, Lee YS, Chang BY et al (2010) Label-free impedimetric sensor for a ribonucleic acid oligomer specific to hepatitis C virus at a self-assembled monolayer-covered electrode. Anal Chem 82(19):8342–8348

53. Tarulli AW, Chin AB, Partida RA et al (2006) Electrical impedance in bovine skeletal muscle as a model for the study of neuromuscular disease. Physiol Meas 27(12):1269–1279

54. Yang M, Lim CC, Liao R et al (2007) A novel microfluidic impedance assay for monitoring endothelin-induced cardiomyocyte hypertrophy. Biosens Bioelectron 22(8):1688–1693

55. Balasubramanian L, Yip K-P, Hsu T-H et al (2008) Impedance analysis of renal vascular smooth muscle cells. Am J Physiol Cell Physiol 295(4):954–965

56. Haas S, Jahnke HG, Glass M et al (2010) Real-time monitoring of relaxation and contractility of smooth muscle cells on a novel biohybrid chip. Lab Chip 10(21):2965–2971

57. Kirstein SL, Atienza JM, Xi B et al (2006) Live cell quality control and utility of real-time cell electronic sensing for assay development. Assay Drug Dev Technol 4(5):545–553

58. Atienza JM, Zhu J, Wang X et al (2005) Dynamic monitoring of cell adhesion and spreading on microelectronic sensor arrays. J Biomol Screen 10(8):795–805

59. Keese CR, Wegener J, Walker SR et al (2004) Electrical wound-healing assay for cells in vitro. Proc Natl Acad Sci U S A 101(6):1554–1559

60. Wang L, Zhu J, Deng C et al (2008) An automatic and quantitative on-chip cell migration assay using self-assembled monolayers combined with real-time cellular impedance sensing. Lab Chip 8(6):872–878

61. Ren J, Y-j X, Singh LS et al (2006) Lysophosphatidic acid is constitutively produced by human peritoneal mesothelial cells and enhances adhesion, migration, and invasion of ovarian cancer cells. Cancer Res 66(6): 3006–3014

62. Noiri E, Hu Y, Bahou WF et al (1997) Permissive role of nitric oxide in endothelin-induced migration of endothelial cells. J Biol Chem 272(3):1747–1752

63. Saxena NK, Sharma D, Ding X et al (2007) Concomitant activation of the jak/stat, pi3k/akt, and erk signaling is involved in leptin-mediated promotion of invasion and migration of hepatocellular carcinoma cells. Cancer Res 67(6):2497–2507

64. Chen J, Ye L, Zhang L et al (2008) Placenta growth factor, PLGF, influences the motility of lung cancer cells, the role of Rho associated kinase, Rock1. J Cell Biochem 105(1): 313–320

65. Earley S, Plopper GE (2008) Phosphorylation of focal adhesion kinase promotes extravasation of breast cancer cells. Biochem Biophys Res Commun 366(2):476–482

66. Saxena NK, Taliaferro-Smith L, Knight BB et al (2008) Bidirectional crosstalk between leptin and insulin-like growth factor-i signaling promotes invasion and migration of breast cancer cells via transactivation of epidermal growth factor receptor. Cancer Res 68(23): 9712–9722

67. Sgambato A, De Paola B, Migaldi M et al (2007) Dystroglycan expression is reduced during prostate tumorigenesis and is regulated by androgens in prostate cancer cells. J Cell Physiol 213(2):528–539

68. Sun T, Swindle EJ, Collins JE et al (2010) On-chip epithelial barrier function assays using electrical impedance spectroscopy. Lab Chip 10:1611–1617

69. Ko KSC, Lo CM, Ferrier J et al (1998) Cell-substrate impedance analysis of epithelial cell shape and micromotion upon challenge with bacterial proteins that perturb extracellular matrix and cytoskeleton. J Microbiol Methods 34(2):125–132

70. Wegener J, Hakvoort A, Galla HJ (2000) Barrier function of porcine choroid plexus epithelial cells is modulated by cAMP-dependent pathways in vitro. Brain Res 853(1):115–124

71. Yin F, Watsky MA (2005) LPA and S1P increase corneal epithelial and endothelial cell transcellular resistance. Invest Ophthalmol Vis Sci 46(6):1927–1933

72. Tiruppathi C, Malik AB, Del Vecchio PJ et al (1992) Electrical method for detection of endothelial cell shape change in real time: assessment of endothelial barrier function. Proc Natl Acad Sci U S A 89(17):7919–7923

73. Chang YC, Stins MF, McCaffery MJ et al (2004) Cryptococcal yeast cells invade the central nervous system via transcellular penetration of the blood-brain barrier. Infect Immun 72(9):4985

74. Treeratanapiboon L, Psathaki K, Wegener J et al (2005) In vitro study of malaria parasite induced disruption of blood-brain barrier. Biochem Biophys Res Commun 335(3): 810–818

75. Weidenfeller C, Schrot S, Zozulya A et al (2005) Murine brain capillary endothelial cells exhibit improved barrier properties under the influence of hydrocortisone. Brain Res 1053(1–2):162–174

76. Hartmann C, Zozulya A, Wegener J et al (2007) The impact of glia-derived extracellular matrices on the barrier function of cerebral endothelial cells: an in vitro study. Exp Cell Res 313(7):1318–1325

77. Moy AB, Van Engelenhoven J, Bodmer J et al (1996) Histamine and thrombin modulate endothelial focal adhesion through centripetal and centrifugal forces. J Clin Invest 97(4): 1020–1027

78. Usatyuk PV, Vepa S, Watkins T et al (2003) Redox regulation of reactive oxygen species-induced p38 MAP kinase activation and barrier dysfunction in lung microvascular endothelial cells. Antioxid Redox Signal 5(6):723–730

79. Usatyuk PV, Parinandi NL, Natarajan V (2006) Redox regulation of 4-hydroxy-2-nonenal-mediated endothelial barrier dysfunction by focal adhesion, adherens, and tight junction proteins. J Biol Chem 281(46): 35554–35566

80. Shivanna M, Rajashekhar G, Srinivas SP (2010) Barrier dysfunction of the corneal endothelium in response to TNF-α: role of p38 MAP kinase. Invest Ophthalmol Vis Sci 51(3):1575–1582

81. Boyd JM, Huang L, Xie L et al (2008) A cell-microelectronic sensing technique for profiling cytotoxicity of chemicals. Anal Chim Acta 615(1):80–87

82. Xiao C, Luong JHT (2003) On-line monitoring of cell growth and cytotoxicity using electric cell-substrate impedance sensing (ECIS). Biotechnol Prog 19(3):1000–1005

83. Wang H, Keese CR, Giaever I et al (1995) Prostaglandin E2 alters human orbital fibroblast shape through a mechanism involving the generation of cyclic adenosine monophosphate. J Clin Endocrinol Metab 80(12): 3553–3558

84. Litkouhi B, Kwong J, Lo CM et al (2007) Claudin-4 overexpression in epithelial ovarian cancer is associated with hypomethylation and is a potential target for modulation of tight junction barrier function using a C-terminal fragment of Clostridium perfringens enterotoxin. Neoplasia 9(4):304–314

85. Ehret R, Baumann W, Brischwein M et al (1997) Monitoring of cellular behaviour by impedance measurements on interdigitated electrode structures. Biosens Bioelectron 12(1):29–41

86. Ehret R, Baumann W, Brischwein M et al (2001) Multiparametric microsensor chips for screening applications. Fresenius J Anal Chem 369(1):30–35

87. Ciambrone GJ, Liu VF, Lin DC et al (2004) Cellular dielectric spectroscopy: a powerful new approach to label-free cellular analysis. J Biomol Screen 9(6):467–480

88. Verdonk E, Johnson K, McGuinness R et al (2006) Cellular dielectric spectroscopy: a label-free comprehensive platform for functional evaluation of endogenous receptors. Assay Drug Dev Technol 4(5):609–619

89. Yeon JH, Park JK (2005) Cytotoxicity test based on electrochemical impedance measurement of HepG2 cultured in microfabricated cell chip. Anal Biochem 341(2):308–315

90. Guo M, Chen J, Yun X et al (2006) Monitoring of cell growth and assessment of cytotoxicity using electrochemical impedance spectroscopy. Biochim Biophys Acta 1760(3): 432–439

91. Glamann J, Hansen AJ (2006) Dynamic detection of natural killer cell-mediated cytotoxicity and cell adhesion by electrical impedance measurements. Assay Drug Dev Technol 4(5):555–563

92. Solly K, Wang X, Xu X et al (2004) Application of real-time cell electronic sensing (rt-ces) technology to cell-based assays. Assay Drug Dev Technol 2(4):363–372

93. Zhu J, Wang X, Xu X et al (2006) Dynamic and label-free monitoring of natural killer cell cytotoxic activity using electronic cell sensor arrays. J Immunol Methods 309(1–2):25–33

94. Xing JZ, Zhu L, Jackson JA et al (2005) Dynamic monitoring of cytotoxicity on

microelectronic sensors. Chem Res Toxicol 18(2):154–161

95. Xing JZ, Zhu L, Gabos S et al (2006) Microelectronic cell sensor assay for detection of cytotoxicity and prediction of acute toxicity. Toxicol In Vitro 20(6):995–1004

96. Zhou J, Wu C, Tu J et al (2013) Assessment of cadmium-induced hepatotoxicity and protective effects of zinc against it using an improved cell-based biosensor. Sens Actuators A-Phys 199:156–164

97. Zou L, Hu N, Zhou J et al (2014) A novel electrical cell-substrate impedance biosensor for rapid detection of marine toxins. Sensor Lett 12(6–7):1041–1045

98. Shaw LM (2005) Tumor cell invasion assays. In: Guan J-L (ed) Cell migration. Humana, Totowa, pp 97–105

99. Keese CR, Bhave K, Wegener J, Giaever I (2002) Real-time impedance assay to follow the invasive activities of metastatic cells in culture. Biotechniques 33(4):842–850

100. Taliaferro-Smith L, Nagalingam A, Zhong D et al (2009) LKB1 is required for adiponectin-mediated modulation of AMPK-S6K axis and inhibition of migration and invasion of breast cancer cells. Oncogene 28(29):2621–2633

101. Patani N, Douglas-Jones A, Mansel R et al (2010) Tumour suppressor function of MDA-7/IL-24 in human breast cancer. Cancer Cell Int 10(1):29–32

102. Hu N, Wang T, Wang Q et al (2014) High-performance beating pattern function of human induced pluripotent stem cell-derived cardiomyocyte-based biosensors for hERG inhibition recognition. Biosens Bioelectron 67:146–153

103. Otto AM, Brischwein M, Niendorf A et al (2003) Microphysiological testing for chemo-sensitivity of living tumor cells with multiparametric microsensor chips. Cancer Detect Prev 27(4):291–296

104. Brischwein M, Motrescu ER, Cabala E et al (2003) Functional cellular assays with multiparametric silicon sensor chips. Lab Chip 3(4):234–240

105. Geisler T, Ressler J, Harz H et al (2006) Automated multiparametric platform for high-content and high-throughput Analytical screening on living cells. IEEE Trans Autom Sci Eng 3(2):169–176

106. Ceriotti L, Kob A, Drechsler S et al (2007) Online monitoring of BALB/3T3 metabolism and adhesion with multiparametric chip-based system. Anal Biochem 371(1):92–104

107. Becker B, Lob V, Janzen N, et al (2008) Automated multi-parametric label free 24 channel real-time screening system. In: 14th Nordic-Baltic conference on biomedical engineering and medical physics. pp 186–189

108. Hafeman DG, Parce JW, McConnell HM (1988) Light-addressable potentiometric sensor for biochemical systems. Science 240:1182–1185

109. Hafner F (2000) Cytosensor((R)) microphysiometer: technology and recent applications. Biosens Bioelectron 15(3–4):149–158

110. McConnell HM, Owicki JC, Parce JW et al (1992) The cytosensor microphysiometer: biological applications of silicon technology. Science 257:1906–1912

111. Owicki JC, Bousse LJ, Hafeman DG et al (1994) The light-addressable potentiometric sensor: principles and biological applications. Annu Rev Biophys Biomol Struct 23:87–114

112. Adami M, Sartore M, Nicolini C (1995) PAB: a newly designed potentiometric alternating biosensor system. Biosens Bioelectron 10(1–2):155–167

113. Wagner T, Werner CF, K-i M et al (2012) Development and characterisation of a compact light-addressable potentiometric sensor (LAPS) based on the digital light processing (DLP) technology for flexible chemical imaging. Sens Actuators B 170(31):34–39

114. Miller DL, Olson JC, Parce JW et al (1993) Cholinergic stimulation of the Na+/K+ adenosine-triphosphatase as revealed by microphysiometry. Biophys J 64(3):813–823

115. Wang P, Xu GX, Qin LF et al (2005) Cell-based biosensors and its application in biomedicine. Sens Actuators B-Chem 108(1–2):576–584

116. Xu G, Ye X, Qin L et al (2005) Cell-based biosensors based on light-addressable potentiometric sensors for single cell monitoring. Biosens Bioelectron 20(9):1757–1763

117. Ismail ABM, Yoshinobu T, Iwasaki H et al (2003) Investigation on light-addressable potentiometric sensor as a possible cell-semiconductor hybrid. Biosens Bioelectron 18(12):1509–1514

118. Stein B, George M, Gaub HE et al (2004) Extracellular measurements of averaged ionic currents with the light-addressable potentiometric sensor (LAPS). Sens Actuators B-Chem 98(2–3):299–304

119. Liu QJ, Cai H, Xu Y et al (2006) Olfactory cell-based biosensor: a first step towards a neurochip of bioelectronic nose. Biosens Bioelectron 22(2):318–322

120. Parak WJ, George M, Domke J et al (2000) Can the light-addressable potentiometric sensor (LAPS) detect extracellular potentials of

cardiac myocytes? IEEE Trans Biomed Eng 47(8):1106–1113

121. Zhang W, Li Y, Liu Q et al (2008) A novel experimental research based on taste cell chips for taste transduction mechanism. Sens Actuators B 131(1):24–28

122. Rabinowitz JD, Rigler P, Carswell-Crumpton C et al (1997) Screening for novel drug effects with a microphysiometer: a potent effect of clofilium unrelated to potassium channel blockade. Life Sci 61(7):87–94

123. Fischer H, Seelig A, Beier N et al (1999) New drugs for the Na+/H+ exchanger. Influence of Na+ concentration and determination of inhibition constants with a microphysiometer. J Membr Biol 168(1):39–45

124. Cao C, Mioduszewski R, Menking D et al (1997) Validation of the cytosensor for in vitro cytotoxicity studies. Toxicol In Vitro 11(3):285–293

125. Yicong W, Ping W, Xuesong Y et al (2001) Drug evaluations using a novel microphysiometer based on cell-based biosensors. Sens Actuators B 80(3):215–221

126. Wu Y, Wang P, Ye X et al (2001) A novel microphysiometer based on MLAPS for drugs screening. Biosens Bioelectron 16(4): 277–286

127. Yu H, Cai H, Zhang W et al (2009) A novel design of multifunctional integrated cell-based biosensors for simultaneously detecting cell acidification and extracellular potential. Biosens Bioelectron 24(5):1462–1468

128. Liu Q, Cai H, Xu Y et al (2007) Detection of heavy metal toxicity using cardiac cell-based biosensor. Biosens Bioelectron 22(12): 3224–3229

129. Bergveld P (1970) Development of an ion-sensitive solid-state device for neurophysiological measurements. IEEE Trans Biomed Eng 17(1):70–71

130. Bergveld P, Wiersma J, Meertens H (1976) Extracellular potential recordings by means of a field-effect transistor without gate metal, called osfet. IEEE Trans Biomed Eng 23(2): 136–144

131. Fromherz P, Offenhausser A, Vetter T et al (1991) A neuron-silicon junction: a Retzius cell of the leech on an insulated-gate field-effect transistor. Science 252(5010):1290–1293

132. Bergveld P (2003) Thirty years of ISFETOLOGY: What happened in the past 30 years and what may happen in the next 30 years. Sens Actuators B 88(1):1–20

133. Lee CS, Kim SK, Kim M (2009) Ion-sensitive field-effect transistor for biological sensing. Sensors 9(9):7111–7131

134. Dzyadevych SV, Soldatkin AP, EI'skaya AV et al (2006) Enzyme biosensors based on ion-selective field-effect transistors. Anal Chim Acta 568(1–2):248–258

135. Fromherz P (2003) Semiconductor chips with ion channels, nerve cells and brain. Physica E 16(1):24–34

136. Schoning MJ (2005) "Playing around" with field-effect sensors on the basis of EIS structures, LAPS and ISFETs. Sens Actuators B 5:126–138

137. Kurzweil P (2009) Metal oxides and ion-exchanging surfaces as ph sensors in liquids: state-of-the-art and outlook. Sensors 9: 4955–4985

138. Niu M-N, Ding X-F, Tong Q-Y (1996) Effect of two types of surface sites on the characteristics of Si_3N_4-gate pH-ISFETs. Sens Actuators B 37:13–17

139. Ujihira Y, Okabe Y, Suggano T et al (1982) IEEE Trans Electron Dev 29:1936

140. Bousse L, Derooij NF, Bergveld P (1983) operation of chemically sensitive field-effect sensors as a function of the insulator-electrolyte interface. IEEE T Electron Dev 30(10):1263–1270

141. Van Hal REG, Eijkel JCT, Bergveld P (1996) A general model to describe the electrostatic potential at electrolyte oxide interfaces. Adv Colloid Interface Sci 69(1–3):31–62

142. Raiteri R, Margesin B, Grattarola M (1998) An atomic force microscope estimation of the point of zero charge of silicon insulators. Sens Actuators B 46(2):126–132

143. Jobling DT, Smith JG, Wheal HV (1981) Active microelectrode array to record from the mammalian central nervous-system in vitro. Med Biol Eng Comput 19(5): 553–560

144. Ingebrandt S, Yeung C-K, Krause M et al (2001) Cardiomyocyte-transistor-hybrids for sensor application. Biosens Bioelectron 16(7): 565–570

145. Benfenati V, Toffanin S, Bonetti S et al (2013) A transparent organic transistor structure for bidirectional stimulation and recording of primary neurons. Nat Mater 12(7):672–680

146. Baumann W, Lehmann M, Schwinde A et al (1999) Microelectronic sensor system for microphysiological application on living cells. Sens Actuators B 55(1):77–89

147. Otto AM, Brischwein M, Motrescu E et al (2004) Analysis of drug action on tumor cell metabolism using electronic sensor chips. Arch Pharm 337(12):682–686

148. Seeland S, Török M, Kettiger H et al (2013) A cell-based, multiparametric sensor approach

characterises drug-induced cytotoxicity in human liver HepG2 cells. Toxicol in Vitro 27(3):1109–1120

149. Chen PH, Zhang W, Zhou J et al (2009) Development of planar patch clamp technology and its application in the analysis of cellular electrophysiology. Proc Natl Acad Sci U S A 19(2):153–160

150. Lepple-Wienhues A, Ferlinz K, Seeger A et al (2003) Flip the tip: an automated, high quality, cost-effective patch clamp screen. Receptors Channel 9(1):13–17

151. Kiss L, Bennett PB, Uebele VN et al (2003) High throughput ion-channel pharmacology: Planar-array-based voltage clamp. Assay Drug Dev Techn 1(1):127–135

152. Dunlop J, Bowlby M, Peri R et al (2008) High-throughput electrophysiology: an emerging paradigm for ion-channel screening and physiology. Nat Rev Drug Discov 7(4): 358–368

153. Schroeder K, Neagle B, Trezise DJ et al (2003) IonWorks (TM) HT: a new high-throughput electrophysiology measurement platform. J Biomol Screen 8(1):50–64

154. Lau AY, Hung PJ, Wu AR et al (2006) Open-access microfluidic patch-clamp array with raised lateral cell trapping sites. Lab Chip 6(12):1510–1515

155. Finkel A, Wittel A, Yang N et al (2006) Population patch clamp improves data consistency and success rates in the measurement of ionic currents. J Biomol Screen 11(5): 488–496

156. Tao HM, Ana DS, Guia A et al (2004) Automated tight seal electrophysiology for assessing the potential hERG liability of pharmaceutical compounds. Assay Drug Dev Techn 2(5):497–506

157. Kutchinsky J, Friis S, Asmild M et al (2003) Characterization of potassium channel modulators with QPatch (TM) automated patch-clamp technology: system characteristics and performance. Assay Drug Dev Techn 1(5):685–693

158. Sauerbrey G (1959) Use of quartz vibrator for weighing thin films on a microbalance. Z Phys 155(2):206–210

159. Curie J, Curie P (1880) Piezoelectric and allied phenomena in Rochelle salt. Comput Rend Acad Sci Paris 91:294–297

160. Sauerbrey G (1959) Use of quartz crystal vibrator for weighting thin films on a microbalance. Z Phys 155:206–222

161. Nomura T, Okuhara M (1982) Frequency shifts of piezoelectric quartz crystals immersed in organic liquids. Anal Chim Acta 142:281–284

162. Keiji Kanazawa K, Gordon JG (1985) The oscillation frequency of a quartz resonator in contact with liquid. Anal Chim Acta 175: 99–105

163. Muramatsu H, Tamiya E, Karube I (1988) Computation of equivalent circuit parameters of quartz crystals in contact with liquids and study of liquid properties. Anal Chem 60(19): 2142–2146

164. Marx KA, Zhou T, Montrone A et al (2007) A comparative study of the cytoskeleton binding drugs nocodazole and taxol with a mammalian cell quartz crystal microbalance biosensor: different dynamic responses and energy dissipation effects. Anal Biochem 361(1):77–92

165. Braunhut SJ, McIntosh D, Vorotnikova E et al (2005) Detection of apoptosis and drug resistance of human breast cancer cells to taxane treatments using quartz crystal microbalance biosensor technology. Assay Drug Dev Techn 3(1):77–88

166. Wegener J, Seebach J, Janshoff A et al (2000) Analysis of the composite response of shear wave resonators to the attachment of mammalian cells. Biophys J 78(6):2821–2833

167. Fohlerová Z, Skládal P, Turanek J (2007) Adhesion of eukaryotic cell lines on the gold surface modified with extracellular matrix proteins monitored by the piezoelectric sensor. Biosens Bioelectron 22(9–10): 1896–1901

168. Guo M, Chen J, Zhang Y et al (2008) Enhanced adhesion/spreading and proliferation of mammalian cells on electropolymerized porphyrin film for biosensing applications. Biosens Bioelectron 23(6):865–871

169. Elsom J, Lethem MI, Rees GD et al (2008) Novel quartz crystal microbalance based biosensor for detection of oral epithelial cell-microparticle interaction in real-time. Biosens Bioelectron 23(8):1259–1265

170. Steinem C, Janshoff A, Wegener J (1997) Impedance and shear wave resonance analysis of ligand-receptor interactions at functionalized surfaces and of cell monolayers. Biosens Bioelectron 12(8):787–808

171. Lord MS, Modin C, Foss M et al (2006) Monitoring cell adhesion on tantalum and oxidised polystyrene using a quartz crystal microbalance with dissipation. Biomaterials 27(26):4529–4537

172. Cans AS, Höök F, Shupliakov O et al (2001) Measurement of the dynamics of exocytosis and vesicle retrieval at cell populations using a quartz crystal microbalance. Anal Chem 73(24):5805–5811

Part II

Biochemical Profiling and Screening

Chapter 5

Kinetics Characterization of Ligand–Receptor Interactions Using Oblique-Incidence Reflectivity Difference Method

Shuang Liu, Guozhen Yang, Huibin Lu, and Heng Zhu

Abstract

The oblique-incidence reflectivity difference (OIRD) method is a novel optical biosensor which has recently been applied to label-free, real-time detection of molecular interactions in microarray format using a functionalized glass substrate. The capability of the OIRD to independently monitor association and dissociation kinetics enables real-time profiling of ligand–receptor interactions. The microarray format of the OIRD method makes it a practical platform for high-throughput, system-wide affinity profiling of the interactions of proteins, DNA, or whole cells with a diverse set of biomolecules.

Key words Binding kinetics, Biomolecular interactions, High-throughput, Label-free, Oblique-incidence reflectivity difference (OIRD)

1 Introduction

Microarrays are created by immobilizing biomolecules on a solid substrate to generate a high-content, large-scale platform for simultaneous analysis of hundreds to thousands of biochemical interactions. This technology has been applied to gene expression profiling and analyzing protein–protein, protein–small molecule interactions [1–3]. A variety of detection methods, such as fluorescence, Surface Plasmon Resonance (SPR), and OCTET (ForteBio, Inc.), have emerged as tools for monitoring these interactions [4–6]. Fluorescence is a highly sensitive and widely used label method, which requires labeling with fluorescent molecules, but is rarely applied for binding kinetics measurements, whereas label-free, real-time methods, such as SPR and OCTET, for profiling of ligand–receptor kinetics are inherently low-throughput or require an expensive sensor surface.

Oblique-incidence reflectivity difference (OIRD) as a recently developed biosensor compatible with microarray technology can enable monitoring the kinetics of biomolecular interactions in a label-free and high-throughput manner [7–12]. OIRD method was previously used to monitor the process of growing of oxide thin

Ye Fang (ed.), *Label-Free Biosensor Methods in Drug Discovery*, Methods in Pharmacology and Toxicology, DOI 10.1007/978-1-4939-2617-6_5, © Springer Science+Business Media New York 2015

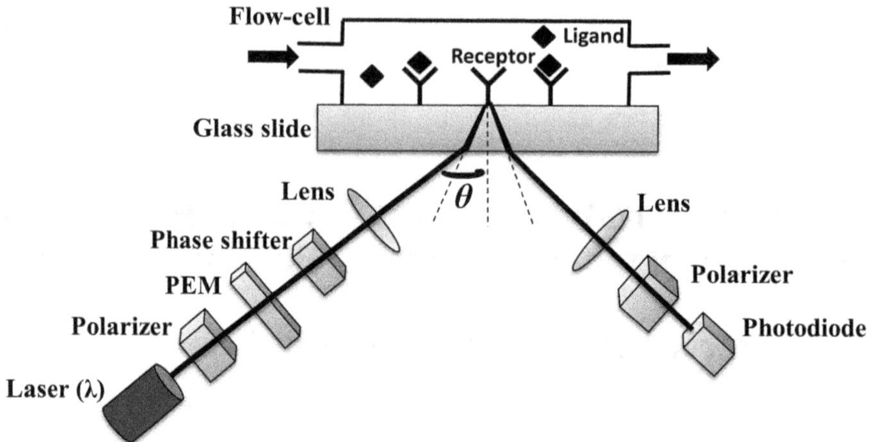

Fig. 1 Sketch of the OIRD system for microarray detection, where a flow-cell is mounted on the top of the system. *PEM* photoelastic modulator for polarization modulation

films and surface modifications in real-time [13–15]. In principle, OIRD method measures the fractional difference between the reflectivity of the p- and s-polarized lights from a surface at oblique incidence, termed as "$\Delta_p - \Delta_s$," and can acquire two signals consisting of an imaginary part $Im\{\Delta_p - \Delta_s\}$ and a real part $Re\{\Delta_p - \Delta_s\}$, which provide us with phase and amplitude information of the "$\Delta_p - \Delta_s$". Based on the common functional slide, the $Im\{\Delta_p - \Delta_s\}$ signal is applied for detection in our experiment because of its higher sensitivity than $Re\{\Delta_p - \Delta_s\}$. A small change in thickness or mass density of the molecular layer leads to changes of reflectivity of the p- and s-polarized lights which enables OIRD method a high sensitivity optical biosensor [16].

The basic layout of the OIRD system is sketched in Fig. 1. A 632.8 nm wavelength, p-polarized He-Ne laser beam passes through a photo-elastic modulator (PEM), which modulates the probe beam to oscillate between p- and s-polarization at a constant frequency $\Omega = 50$ kHz. After that a phase shifter introduces a variable phase between p- and s-polarization, the beam is then focused on the glass surface at a 60° incident angle. The reflected beam, following a polarization analyzer, is detected by a silicon photodiode. Finally, the first harmonic $I(\Omega)$ and second harmonic $I(2\Omega)$ of the AC components are simultaneously monitored by two digital lock-in amplifiers.

Here, we will introduce the specific binding of antigen–monoclonal antibody and methylated DNA motif–protein interactions as the ligand–receptor models applied by OIRD method.

2 Materials

2.1 Antigen–
Monoclonal
Antibody Model

Antigen protein is printed onto the microarray and is assembled into the flow-cell containing multiple chambers allowing for multiple reactions on a single slide. Monoclonal antibody is then pumped through the flow-cell assembled on the OIRD system in Fig. 1. Antigen and monoclonal antibody are purified and suspended in 1× PBS.

Buffer: 1× PBS (phosphate-buffered saline), 1× PBST (0.1 % Tween 20 in 1× PBS), 1 % BSA (w/v, BSA: Albumin from bovine serum). These buffers are stored at room temperature with the exception of the 1 % BSA which is stored at 4 °C.

(a) Reagent: Glycerol, Triton, and Tween 20.

(b) The functionalized substrate: The surface of proteins often contain reactive functional groups in the side chains (Table 1, from ref. 17) which can be used for immobilizing these biomolecules on microarrays [17]. For OIRD method, the common used surface of functionalized standards glass slide

Table 1
Various methods of coupling proteins on a microarray platform

Functional side group on peptide	Available surface for derivatization	Type of binding
Natural		
–COOH (carboxylic acid)	Amino	Electrostatic
Asp		Covalent amide (after carboxy activation)
–NH$_2$ (amino)	Carboxylic acid, active ester, epoxy, aldehyde	Electrostatic
Lys, Gln, Arg		Covalent amide
–SH (thiol)	Maleimide	Covalent thio ether
Cys		
–OH	Epoxy	Covalent ether
Ser, Thr		
Synthetic		
His-Tag	Ni-NTA complex	Coordination complex
Strep-Tag	Strep-Tactin	Supramolecular complex
Biotin	Streptavidin	Supramolecular complex

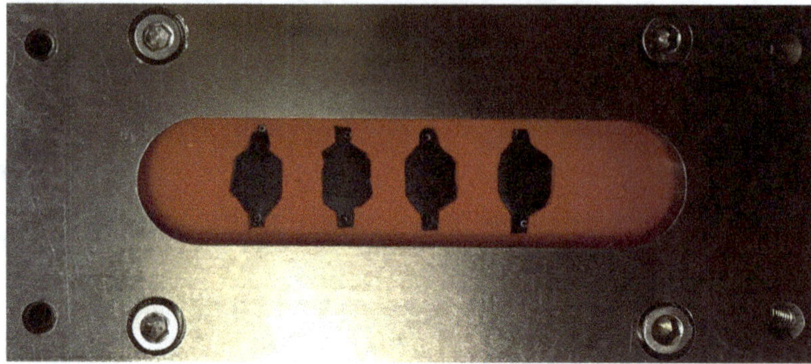

Fig. 2 The flow-cell: a rubber pad (*orange color*) with four rectangular holes is mounted onto a glass slide to generate four chambers that each contained an identical sub-array. Each chamber is 8 mm × 10 mm × 1 mm

($25 \times 76 \times 0.94$ mm or $25 \times 75 \times 0.94$ mm) is coated with epoxides or aldehydes to create a functionalized surface for protein immobilization.

(c) The printing machine: the microarrays are generated using a contact printing machine that uses pins [18].

(d) The flow-cell chamber: the flow-cell as shown in Fig. 2 is designed for the OIRD system and allows four concentrations of ligand to interact with the receptors isolated in different chambers. Each chamber is $8 \times 10 \times 1$ mm and manipulated by a peristaltic pump which controls the flow rate and direction in the chamber.

2.2 Methylated DNA Motif–Protein Model

DNA motifs suspended in 50 % DMSO are printed on an amine surface (*see* **Note 1**) of a functionalized glass slide. Proteins of interest are pumped into the flow-cells assembled on the OIRD system.

Buffer: DMSO (Dimethyl Sulfoxide), EMSA (1 base buffer in ref. 19), they are stored in room temperature.

3 Methods

3.1 Antigen–Monoclonal Antibody Model

3.1.1 Printing

The antigen proteins and negative control BSA are suspended in 1× PBS, 30 % Glycerol, 0.03 % Triton in 96 or 384 wells and then printed by a contact-printing machine at concentration 0.5 mg/mL on epoxy or aldehyde glass slide (*see* **Note 2**).

After printing, the antigen microarray is incubated at 4 °C overnight to ensure that the antigen or BSA bind to the glass surface completely.

3.1.2 OIRD Detection

1. Assemble the microarray into the flow-cell and scan with OIRD program compiled in LabVIEW (NI, USA) to create a first 2D image of OIRD intensity after printing (*see* **Note 3**).

2. Block the mounted antigen slide by incubating with 1 mg/mL BSA in 1× PBS for 1 h at RT.

3. Sequentially pump 1× PBS and 1× PBST buffer into the flow-cell to wash the antigen slide for 10 min at a flow rate of 1 mL/min and obtain a second 2D image OIRD image after the washing is complete.

4. Scan across the centerlines of the printing spots on the antigen microarray using the 632.8 nm laser beam to confirm the coordinate of the starting point and to give the real-time scanning program a 5 min baseline scan (*see* **Note 4**).

5. Pump multiple dilutions of monoclonal antibody into their respective reaction chambers in the flow cell while the scanning program records binding event to generate on-curves (*see* **Note 5**).

6. After the OIRD signals reach saturation, pump 1× PBS into the flow-cell at a flow rate of 200 μL/min (*see* **Note 6**) and generate the off-curves simultaneously. To obtain a better off-curve, a two times of on-curve scanning time is taken.

7. Obtain a final OIRD 2D image by the third 2D scanning program after the off-curve measurement.

3.1.3 Analysis of OIRD Data

From Section 3.1.2, 2D images and kinetics data are collected.

1. Subtract the second 2D image after washing from the third 2D image after the off-curve scanning to generate the net 2D image using the LabVIEW program. The net 2D image can be used to deduce the OIRD signal change on the antigen sample. Given that monoclonal antibodies have a high affinity for their specific antigen, the off-curves are minimal.

2. Extract the on- and off-curves from LabVIEW into OriginPro 9.0 (OriginLab, USA).

3. Fit the simulated curves with the observed on- and off-curves using the OriginPro program to calculate the k_{on} and k_{off} values, respectively (Fig. 3). *See* **Note 7** for additional details regarding fitting models.

4. Deduce the K_D value by taking the k_{off}/k_{on} ratio. The average K_D and relevant standards are calculated from the dilutions of monoclonal antibody used in the flow cell chambers.

3.2 Methylated DNA Motif–Protein Model

3.2.1 Printing

Methylated DNA motifs suspended in 50 % DMSO are printed on amine slides by a contact printing machine and exposed to 600 μJ UV for 3 min to immobilize and dried in a 37 °C incubator for 1 h.

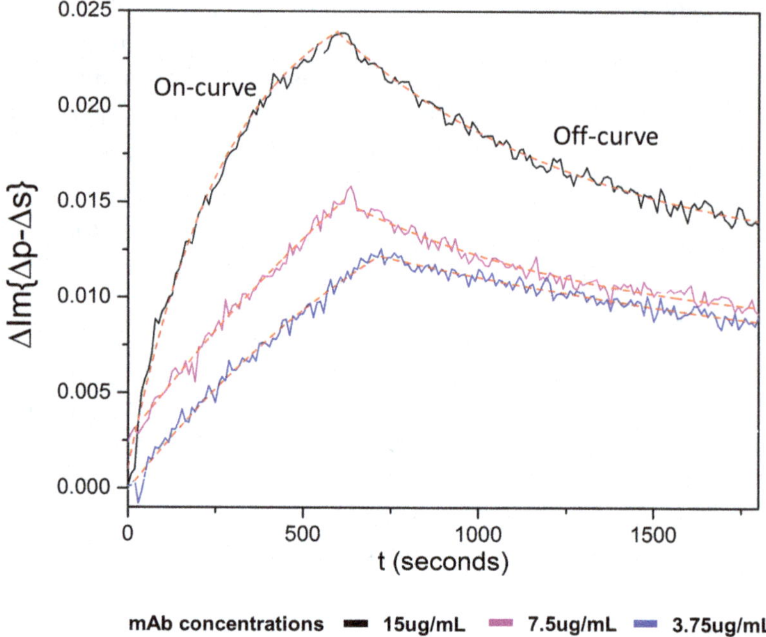

Fig. 3 The raw on- and off-curves (*color solid lines*) measured with the OIRD method. A human protein was first immobilized on the array and its monoclonal antibody was pumped into the reaction chamber at three different concentrations. The corresponding fitting curves are shown in *red dotted lines*

3.2.2 OIRD Detection and Data Analysis

The main procedures are identical to the antigen–monoclonal antibody model except the DNA motif slides are washed with EMSA buffer for the first wash at 1 mL/min for 10 min, and wash to generate the off-curves [19].

4 Notes

1. Common surface modifications for printing DNA are: poly-L-lysine, 3-glycidoxypropyltrimethoxysilane and aldehyde, 3-aminopropyltrimethoxysilane or carboxylic acid, etc. Here we choose amine surface for its easy manipulation and cost-effectiveness [17].

2. To maximize signal, the printing concentration should be saturated at the printing area. For proteins and DNA (~10–50 kDa), 0.1–0.5 mg/mL is sufficient. Sub-arrays are printed to be compatible with the flow-cell construction (Fig. 2).

3. The scanning program related with a stepping motor code in LABVIEW is easy to learn. The 2D image after printing will point out the start scanning coordinate for the real-time procedure.

4. The baseline and the next on-curve data are defined by the subtraction of average pixels (10–20) of the unprinted region adjacent the sample from average pixels (10–20) of the sample.

5. This scanning process of the printed spots is repeated every 10 s. The reflective light intensity proportionately corresponding to Im $\{\Delta_p - \Delta_s\}$ signals is directly collected to obtain the on-curves of the binding events.

6. 200 μL/min is the empirical result based on the flow-cell and the peristaltic pump. Experimentally, we determine that the flow rate should be a double the rate beyond which the association–dissociation curves are affected for the flow-cell used in the present experiment.

7. One 1:1 Langmuir model is applied in the fitting method. This model displays the simplest situation of an interaction between Ligand (L) and immobilized Receptor (R). The 1:1 Langmuir model was developed by Irving Langmuir in 1916. The fitting method is used and developed in SPR and other real-time detection biosensors [20, 21].

Acknowledgements

S.L. and H.Z. are supported in part by the NIH Common Fund grant U54RR020839.

References

1. Zhu H, Snyder M (2003) Protein chip technology. Curr Opin Chem Biol 7(1):55–63. doi:10.1016/S1367-5931(02)00005-4

2. Heller MJ (2002) DNA microarray technology: devices, systems, and applications. Annu Rev Biomed Eng 4(1):129–153. doi:10.1146/annurev.bioeng.4.020702.153438

3. Templin MF, Stoll D, Schrenk M, Traub PC, Vöhringer CF, Joos TO (2002) Protein microarray technology. Drug Discov Today 7(15):815–822. doi:10.1016/S1359-6446(00)01910-2

4. Schulman SG, Sharma A (1999) Introduction to fluorescence spectroscopy. Wiley, New York

5. Green R, Davies J, Davies M, Roberts C, Tendler S (1997) Surface plasmon resonance for real time in situ analysis of protein adsorption to polymer surfaces. Biomaterials 18(5):405–413

6. Abdiche Y, Malashock D, Pinkerton A, Pons J (2008) Determining kinetics and affinities of protein interactions using a parallel real-time label-free biosensor, the Octet. Anal Biochem 377(2):209–217. doi:10.1016/j.ab.2008.03.035

7. Hu S, Wan J, Su Y, Song Q, Zeng Y, Nguyen HN, Shin J, Cox E, Rho HS, Woodard C (2013) DNA methylation presents distinct binding sites for human transcription factors. Elife 2:e00726. doi:10.7554/eLife.00726

8. Landry JP, Fei Y, Zhu X (2012) Simultaneous measurement of 10,000 protein-ligand affinity constants using microarray-based kinetic constant assays. Assay Drug Dev Technol 10(3):250–259. doi:10.1089/adt.2011.0406

9. Liu S, Zhu J, He L, Dai J, Lu H, Wu L, Jin K, Yang G, Zhu H (2014) Label-free, real-time detection of the dynamic processes of protein degradation using oblique-incidence reflectivity difference method. Appl Phys Lett 104(16):163701. doi:10.1063/1.4873676

10. Lu H, Wen J, Wang X, Yuan K, Li W, Lu H, Zhou Y, Jin K, Ruan K, Yang G (2010) Detection of the specific binding on protein microarrays by oblique-incidence reflectivity

difference method. J Optic 12(9):095301. doi:10.1088/2040-8978/12/9/095301

11. Sun Y-S, Landry JP, Fei Y, Zhu X, Luo J, Wang X, Lam K (2008) Effect of Fluorescently Labeling Protein Probes on Kinetics of Protein-Ligand Reactions. Langmuir 24(23):13399–13405. doi:10.1021/la802097z

12. Xu W, Heng L, Juan W, Kun Y, Hui-Bin L, Kui-Juan J, Yue-Liang Z, Guo-Zhen Y (2010) Label-free and high-throughput detection of protein microarrays by oblique-incidence reflectivity difference method. Chin Phys Lett 27(10):107801

13. Chen F, Lu H, Chen Z, Zhao T, Yang G (2001) Optical real-time monitoring of the laser molecular-beam epitaxial growth of perovskite oxide thin films by an oblique-incidence reflectance-difference technique. J Opt Soc Am B 18(7):1031–1035. doi:10.1364/JOSAB.19.001218

14. Zhu X-D (2004) Oblique-incidence optical reflectivity difference from a rough film of crystalline material. Phys Rev B 69(11):115407. doi:10.1103/PhysRevB.69.115407

15. Chen F, Lu H, Zhao T, K-j J, Chen Z, Yang G-Z (2000) Real-time optical monitoring of the heteroepitaxy of oxides by an oblique-incidence reflectance difference technique. Phys Rev B 61(15):10404. doi:10.1103/PhysRevB.61.10404

16. Zhu X-D (2006) Comparison of two optical techniques for label-free detection of bio-molecular microarrays on solids. Optic Commun 259(2):751–753. doi:10.1016/j.optcom.2005.09.079

17. Bradley A, Cai WW (2000) Chemically modified nucleic acids and methods for coupling nucleic acids to solid support. Google Patents, Patent CA2326684C.

18. Gershon D (2002) Microarray technology: an array of opportunities. Nature 416(6883):885–891. doi:10.1038/416885a

19. Hu S-H, Xie Z, Blackshaw S, Qian J, Zhu H (2011) Characterization of protein–DNA interactions using protein microarrays. Cold Spring Harbor Protocols 2011 (5). doi:10.1101/pdb.prot5614

20. Langmuir I (1918) The adsorption of gases on plane surfaces of glass, mica and platinum. J Am Chem Soc 40(9):1361–1403

21. Myszka DG (2000) Kinetic, equilibrium, and thermodynamic analysis of macromolecular interactions with BIACORE. Methods Enzymol 323:325–340. doi:10.1016/S0076-6879(00)23372-7

Chapter 6

Label-Free Inhibition in Solution Assays for Fragment Screening

Stefan Geschwindner

Abstract

Fragment screening displays probably the most challenging aspect for the application of label-free technologies, as it requires reliable and specific detection of weakly binding molecules of low molecular weight to a large target protein. In the strive to increase the sensitivity of biosensor-based affinity screening technologies, novel approaches and assay configurations have been developed to not only increase assay sensitivity but also deliver information about the interaction site (that is, the specificity). By adapting the inhibition in solution assay from surface plasmon resonance, it is possible to conduct effective fragment screening campaigns using plate-based optical waveguide grating systems. This assay format allows for rapid ranking of fragment hits based on affinity that can serve as a starting point for a fragment-based drug discovery project or as an experimental assessment of the target ligandability. This chapter discusses practical aspects of assay development and screening and provides a step-by-step protocol that has been successfully used in fragment screening of PDE10A inhibitors.

Key words Fragment screening, Inhibition in solution, Optical waveguide grating, PDE10A, Surface plasmon resonance, Target definition compound

---

1 Introduction

The success of early drug discovery activities is very much influenced by the hit finding approach, the strategy that is taken to identify primary hits from corporate compound libraries that can serve as attractive starting points for lead identification and optimization activities. This has led to dynamic developments in assay technologies that either allow for screening of larger compound libraries (>1 million compounds) with increased sensitivity, specificity and throughput, or enable orthogonal screening confirmation using a readout and/or assay configuration that differs from the primary assay [1, 2]. Such orthogonal assays allow to effectively identify and dismiss false positives or to derive additional information

Ye Fang (ed.), *Label-Free Biosensor Methods in Drug Discovery*, Methods in Pharmacology and Toxicology, DOI 10.1007/978-1-4939-2617-6_6, © Springer Science+Business Media New York 2015

119

including binding stoichiometry, ligand-binding kinetics, and/or thermodynamics, all of which can be potentially considered as additional parameters in the lead selection process.

To meet the requirements for highly sensitive determination of ligand-binding characteristics, assay technologies frequently employ signal enhancers or labels and typically operate with radioactive (tritiated or iodinated ligands) or fluorescent probes. In contrast, label-free technologies, in particular optical biosensor systems, generally suffer from such possibilities of signal enhancement, although some recently introduced approaches involving label-enhanced surface plasmon resonance (SPR) hold promise but still require further investigation of their potential value [3]. Optical biosensor platforms such as SPR [4] or optical waveguide grating (OWG) [5–7] typically rely on small changes in the refractive index that are proportional to the mass increase caused by the binding of small molecules to a much larger macromolecular target. Instead of monitoring the consequences of a binding event through the use of signal amplifiers, those technologies directly monitor the binding of small molecules in a time-resolved fashion, which comes at the cost of working with low signal intensities, as the observed mass changes at the biosensor surface are typically small. Obviously, the biosensor signal is dependent not only on the molecular weight (MW) of the ligand but also on other factors including the amount of tethered and ligand-binding competent target proteins on the biosensor, the MW-ratio between the ligand and the macromolecule, and the dissociation binding constant K_D and the concentration of the ligand [8]. By looking at the MW-ratio as a function of ligand's K_D and concentration, it intuitively appears that the detection dynamic range becomes smaller with increasing MW of the macromolecule and decreasing MW of the ligand. This mass-sensitivity limit displays a particular challenge when working with fragments, the molecules that typically just constitute a fraction of a larger ligand and often display very low affinity down in the mM-regime [9]. As this mass sensitivity is of technical nature and characteristic to label-free optical biosensor systems and thus outside of the control of the user, the only available direct manipulation is around the assay configuration and setup in order to achieve the objective of sensitivity increase.

As fragment screening is nowadays well accepted as an important hit finding approach in support of modern drug discovery [10], it calls for novel biosensor approaches that enable the detection of minute changes in mass with acceptable assay reliability and sensitivity. One obvious strategy is to elevate the concentration of the ligand. However, the physical behavior of compounds and/or fragments often leads to situations, where the specific binding component only constitutes a minor fraction of the observed binding signal, making it difficult to analyze the specific binding component. Such physical behavior can even lead to the exclusion of such compound from further progression, if the unspecific binding

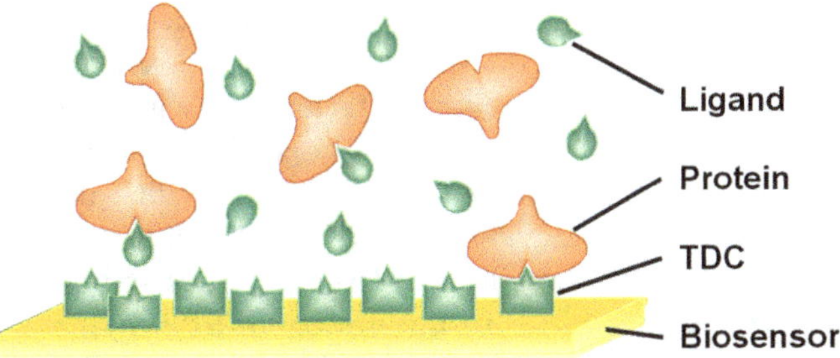

Fig. 1 Assay configuration for the inhibition in solution assay in flow-based systems. The biosensor-tethered target definition compound (TDC) enables to determine the exact concentration of free protein binding sites under conditions of mass-transport limitation. The reduction of free binding sites in the presence of a competing ligand leads to a proportional reduction in the binding signal that can be used to determine the specificity and affinity of the competing ligand

component exceeds the maximum binding signal expected for a 1:1 binding event, which would classify the compound as a super-stoichiometric binder. Thus, any increase in assay sensitivity would need to go hand in hand with improving the readout specificity and need to be reflected in the assay configuration.

The first-generation SPR instruments have had clear limitations in their mass sensitivity, making inhibition in solution assay (ISA) format an impactful strategy for the characterization of ligand binding [11]. In the ISA assay, instead of directly monitoring the binding of a small molecule, a tool compound is employed as a probe for the binding and is tethered to the biosensor surface. This tool compound, often designated as the target definition compound (TDC), provides the possibility to assess and measure the concentration of free protein binding sites when exposing the protein to the modified biosensor (Fig. 1) [12]. Performing assays in the presence of competing ligands will lead to a reduction of the available binding sites and consequently a decreased binding signal. The ISA also permits determination of dissociation constants K_D in flow-based SPR systems or IC_{50} values in plate-based OWG systems.

Key to establishing a suitable ISA is the identification of a TDC ligand that can be tethered to the biosensor without compromising binding mode and affinity. High affinities are usually advantageous, as this determines the lowest concentration of protein to be used in the assay in order to achieve a detectable binding signal. Good choices of ligands to be used as a TDC are substrate analogues or commercially available inhibitors that offer directed tethering via their primary amine attached to a short linker. Obviously, those moieties should be inert to interaction with the target, as any modification could lead to a significant drop in affinity. Alternatively, a primary amine function group can be introduced to an existing ligand by taking into account additional information about its binding mode or structure-activity relationships in order to minimize the interference with target binding. Recent examples on how this can be achieved on fluidics-based platforms include the evaluation of fragment hits against BACE-1 [13] as well as the analysis of peptide binding to Keap1 [14], both using tethered versions of large peptides acting as a TDC.

In fluidics-based SPR systems, the ISA setup enables a direct readout of the free protein concentration without disturbing the equilibrium between the ligand and the protein in solution. As there is effectively no direct competition between the TDC and the ligand in solution, concentration-response experiments will allow extraction of exact K_D-values for the ligand in solution. In plate-based systems, the affinity of the TDC will have an impact on the ability of small molecules to effectively displace the protein from the sensor, as there will be direct competition between the TDC on the biosensor and the ligand in solution. Although a reliable ranking of ligands based of their affinity is still possible, the values from such concentration-response experiments will rather represent an IC_{50} value, reflecting the dependence on assay conditions and particularly the TDC.

A typical assay procedure for fragment screening using plate-based OWG platforms and applying the ISA format is outlined in Fig. 2. After the covalent tethering of the TDC to the sensor surface, the target protein is added to each individual well at a concentration that causes a binding signal representing about 50 % of the total binding signal when using saturating concentrations of protein. After the equilibrium binding signal is reached, compounds are added to each individual well and will, upon competition with the TDC, lead to a reduced equilibrium binding signal that scales with the potency of the competing compound. The superiority of this assay configuration was previously confirmed by conducting a comparative study with a more traditional direct binding assay using human trypsin as a model system [9]. A tailored set of compounds was composed containing pools of confirmed trypsin inhibitors as well as non-actives and frequently hitting compounds based on previous high-throughput screening (HTS) results with trypsin. While the direct binding assay picked out a high number of false positive hits from the non-active and frequent hitter pool as well as simultaneously failed to identify a substantial number of compounds expected to be found as hits from the trypsin inhibitor set, the ISA showed a largely improved ability to identify true binders going along with a low rate for false positive binders. This indicates that the ISA provides a suitable format to identify fragments with good confidence.

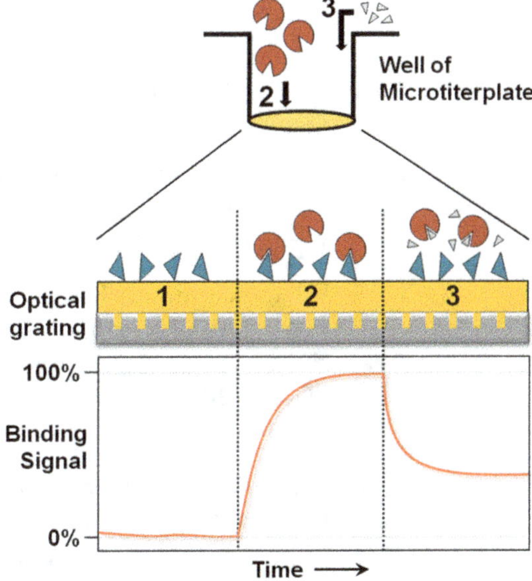

Fig. 2 Schematic representation of the ISA configuration and screening procedure on a plate-based OWG system. In (1), a TDC is covalently attached to the biosensor and washed with buffer until a stable signal is obtained, defining the 0 % binding baseline. After addition of the protein in (2), the specific interaction with the TDC is leading to an increase in the signal with the new equilibrium binding signal defining 100 %. The addition of a competing compound in (3) will lead to a partial displacement of the protein from the sensor resulting in a reduction of the binding signal that is proportional to the affinity of the competing compound

Phosphodiesterase 10A (PDE10A) is an important therapeutic target for schizophrenia and cognitive disorders, as inhibitors of its enzymatic activity provide a novel therapeutic mechanism and thus a clinical profile possibly different from these validated antipsychotic drugs [15, 16]. We have previously developed on OWG ISA for PDE10A, which offers an increased dynamic range compared to a direct binding assay, allowing for the detection of fragment affinities in the mM-regime without compromising the throughput of the plate-based platform [17]. This method was used to screen a tailored fragment library against human PDE10A.

This chapter describes a step-by-step protocol on how the OWG ISA is applied to effectively screen the fragment library to find small-molecule starting points that can act as inhibitors of PDE10A enzyme activity. The primary results are also discussed in the context of other fragment screening technologies to highlight the potential of the OWG ISA for high-throughput fragment screening applications.

2   Materials

1. 384-well GA4-biosensor plates (SRU Biosystems, Woburn, MA, USA).

2. *N*-Hydroxysulfosuccinimide (S-NHS) (Sigma-Aldrich, St. Louis, MO, USA).

3. 1-Ethyl-3-[3-dimethylaminopropyl]carbodiimide (EDC) (Sigma).

4. Ethanolamine (>98 %), Sodium acetate, HEPES (4-(2-hydroxyethyl)-1-piperazineethanesulfonic acid), dimethyl-sulfoxide (DMSO; >99.7 %), polyethylene glycol sorbitan monolaurate (Tween 20) (Sigma).

5. BIND Reader 384/1536 Turbo system (SRU Biosystems).

6. GraphPad Prism 5 Software (Graph Pad Software Inc., La Jolla, CA, USA).

7. PDE10A compound library. This library was selected from our generic fragment screening library according to ligand-, structure-, and diversity-based selection criteria and contained in total 3,000 fragments. Of those, 1,700 have been selected based on similarity to a group of about 7,000 known PDE inhibitors, 300 were selected based on available structural information of drug-like molecules that have been crystallized with PDE10A, and the residual 1,000 were selected according to diversity considerations.

8. PDE10A protein (produced in-house). PDE10A was produced according to [17]. In brief, the PDE10A construct (amino acid residues 449–789) was co-expressed with protein chaperones in BL21-Gold (DE3) *E. coli* cells at low temperature to enable proper folding of active PDE10A. This HIS-tagged protein was purified to homogeneity by a combination of Ni-NTA and ion-exchange chromatography and the tag was released by treatment with TEV protease prior to a final purification step using Ni-NTA.

9. The TDC (*N*-[2-(2-aminoethoxy)ethyl]-2-(2′-ethoxybiphenyl-4-yl)-6-fluoro-3-methylquinoline-4-carboxamide) containing a linker enabling the covalent attachment via a free primary amine was derived from a known PDE10A inhibitor according to [17]. The optimal positioning of the linker was rationalized by using X-ray crystallography information revealing the binding mode of the parental compound and thus offered opportunity for modifications that do not compromise the binding mode significantly. Figure 3 shows the required chemical modification to this PDE10A inhibitor to convert it into a suitable TDC for the screening assay. The synthetic route is detailed in [17].

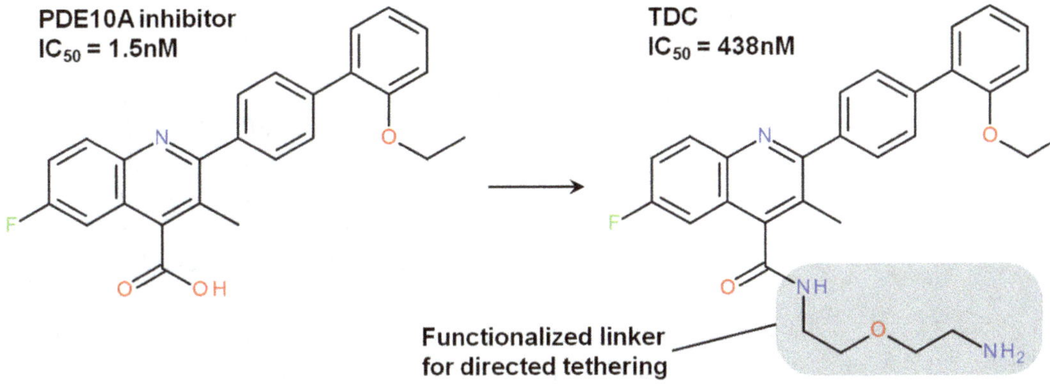

Fig. 3 Conversion of a PDE10A inhibitor into a TDC to enable development of an OWG ISA for PDE10A. The primary amine that is introduced via a well-positioned linker enables the directed tethering of the molecule for a range of biosensor platforms. The inhibition data are determined by monitoring the effect on the enzymatic assay as described in [17]

3 Methods

3.1 Tethering of the TDC

In preparation for the fragment screening, the following steps describe the process how to tether the TDC to the GA4-biosensor surface.

1. Wash the GA4 384-well plate three times with deionized water (approximately 50 µl per well) and use the BIND Reader to obtain a baseline signal. The acquisition is done in Turbo mode with two acquisitions per minute over the entire 384-well plate and remains the same throughout this procedure.

2. Prepare the TDC in 10 mM sodium acetate, pH 5.6 to a final concentration of 100 µM. Each 384-well plate requires about 7 ml of TDC solution for the generation of the modified biosensor surface.

3. Prepare a mixture of EDC and S-NHS by mixing 1.9 ml of a 10 mM S-NHS-solution with 200 µl of a 650 mg/ml solution of EDC and add 17.9 ml of deionized water. This will enable to activate 3 GA4 384-well plates. It may be scaled according to the number of plates needed for screening.

4. Add 20 µl of the EDC/NHS mixture immediately into each well of the GA4 384-well plate and incubate for 15 min.

5. Remove all solution to apparent dryness by flick and tap. Attention: do not wash the wells, since wash could deactivate the surface.

6. For the covalent coupling of the TDC, add 20 µl of the TDC solution prepared in step 2 to the individual wells of the plate. As negative control for the level of unspecific protein binding, leave some wells unmodified by adding 20 µl of 10 mM sodium acetate, pH 5.6 depleted of the TDC.

7. Monitor the time course of immobilization by continuous data acquisition.

8. Stop after 30 min incubation time, wash the plate three times with HBS-P buffer (10 mM HEPES, 150 mM NaCl, 0.005 % (v/v) Tween 20, pH 7.4; approximately 50 µl per well) to remove unbound TDC and take another measurement to determine the final immobilization level. Typical levels of the change in the peak wavelength value (PWV) are 1,000–1,500 picometers (pm).

9. To block remaining activated groups, remove the HBS-P buffer and add 20 µl of 0.4 M ethanolamine per well for 30 min.

10. To prepare the plates for the subsequent fragment screening, wash the plate three times with HBS-P buffer as in step 7 and add finally 22.5 µl HBS-P supplemented with 1 % (v/v) DMSO for the final signal stabilization (30 min).

3.2 Fragment Screening

Fragment screening is performed by starting from a 384-well mother plate containing 1 µl of a 100 mM solution of the respective fragment in 100 % DMSO. In the first step, the fragments are diluted in buffer to a working concentration of 1 mM. In a subsequent step, PDE10A protein is added to the TDC-modified GA4-plate to reach an equilibrium binding signal. After the addition of the 1 mM fragment solution to reach a final concentration of 100 µM, eventually a new equilibrium binding signal is obtained that is dependent on the inhibitory potential of the respective fragment. The data acquisition is done in Turbo mode with two acquisitions per minute over the entire 384-well plate and remains the same throughout this screening procedure.

1. Add 99 µl of HBS-P buffer to 1 µl of each 100 mM fragment solution in 100 % DMSO provided in a 384-well plate to reach a working concentration of 1 mM in HBS-P buffer with 1 % (v/v) DMSO.

2. Prepare a solution of PDE10A in HBS-P plus 1 % (v/v) DMSO at a concentration of 12 µM. Each 384-well plate requires about 2 ml of PDE10A solution for the screening.

3. Add 4.5 µl of the PDE10A solution to the equilibrated, TDC-modified GA4-plate and wait until a new equilibrium binding signal is obtained reflecting the specific interaction of PDE10A with the TDC. Typically, a new equilibrium signal is obtained after 25–30 min with a ΔPWV in the range of 500–600 picometers (pm).

4. Add 3 µl of the fragment solution prepared in step 1 to reach a final screening concentration of 100 µM in the well. Monitor the change in the equilibrium binding signal until a new stable signal is obtained, which typically takes 5–10 min.

5. Calculate the displacement of PDE10A from the TDC-modified sensor upon addition of the fragment, and plot as percent of residual PDE10A binding signal in relation to the maximum equilibrium binding signal (=100 %) obtained after addition of the PDE10A protein (Fig. 2).

3.3 Fragment Validation and IC_{50} Determination

The validation of the original fragment hits is performed by conducting a four concentration-response experiment. Increasing concentrations of selected primary fragment hits are added stepwise to a PDE10A-equilibrated, TDC-modified GA4-plate. The respective equilibrium binding signals from each step are used to calculate the IC_{50} value that can be used for affinity ranking and comparison with enzyme inhibition data.

1. Tether the TDC to a GA4-biosensor surface according to the previously described procedure (Section 3.1).

2. Add 26.4 μl HBS-P supplemented with 1 % (v/v) DMSO and incubate for 30 min to reach for the final signal stabilization.

3. Add 99 μl of HBS-P buffer to 1 μl of each 100 mM fragment solution in 100 % DMSO provided in a 384-well plate to reach a working concentration of 1 mM in HBS-P buffer with 1 % (v/v) DMSO.

4. Prepare a solution of PDE10A in HBS-P plus 1 % (v/v) DMSO at a concentration of 18 μM.

5. Add 3.6 μl of the PDE10A solution to the equilibrated, TDC-modified GA4-plate and wait until a new equilibrium binding signal is obtained.

6. Add 1.5 μl of the fragment solution prepared in step 3 and monitor the change in the binding signal until a new, stable equilibrium binding signal is obtained.

7. Repeat step 6 three times, each time recording the change in the equilibrium binding signal (signal should decrease stepwise).

8. Plot the increasing fragment concentrations (47.6, 90.9, 130.4, and 166.6 μM) against the respective equilibrium binding signals and use a standard software package (e.g., GraphPad Prism) for data analysis in order to provide a numerical solution for the IC_{50} value.

---

4   Results

The screening of the 3,000 fragment library at 100 μM concentration resulted in 395 initial fragment hits (=13.2 % hit rate) by setting the hit cut-off criterion to those compounds that reduced the residual binding of PDE10A to the biosensor surface to a level of

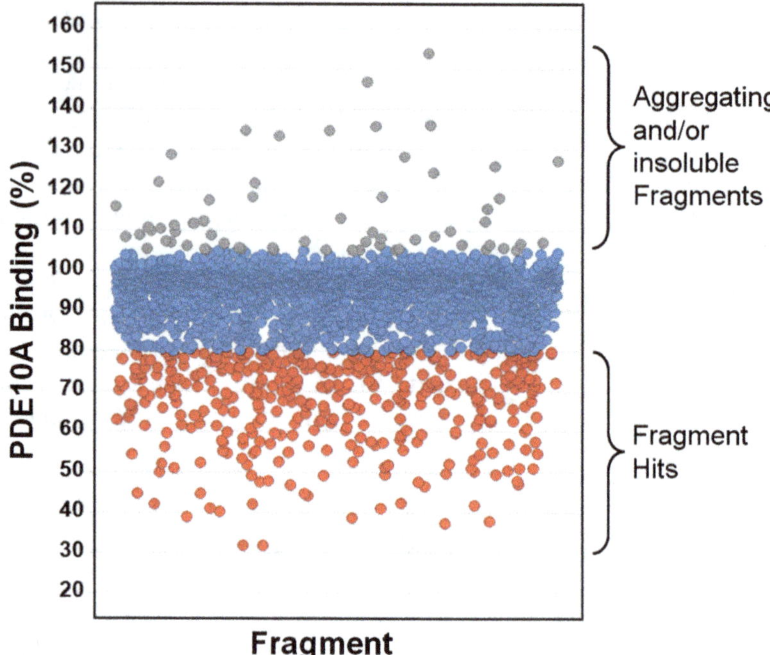

Fig. 4 Graphical results of the primary fragment screening in the OWG assay. PDE10A binding percentage is defined by the OWG signal prior to addition of PDE10A (defined as 0 % binding) in relation to the equilibrated OWG signal after addition of PDE10A (defined as 100 % binding). The graph shows the remaining binding percentage of PDE10A after addition of the fragments. Fragments that reduce the PDE10A binding to the biosensor after addition of the compound to 80 % or less were selected as primary hits (*red color*), resulting in the initial identification of 395 fragments. The OWG assay could also identify fragments that have issues relating to aggregation and/or insolubility under the experimental conditions (*grey color*)

80 % or less (lower values indicate more extensive binding by the fragment to PDE10A) (Fig. 4). We also observed 40 fragments (1.3 %) that showed an *increase* of the PDE10A residual binding signal. Such behavior typically indicates fragment aggregation or solubility issues; such information usually helps to eliminate unsuitable fragments from further consideration. As described earlier, the 3,000 fragments have been selected according to ligand-, structure-, and diversity-based selection criteria. The hit rates in those different pools have been 11.4 %, 21.1 %, and 11.3 %, respectively.

From the 395 initial fragment hits, 368 have been selected for a determination of their IC_{50} values to allow for an affinity ranking. All of the selected hits were found to be able to displace PDE10A from the biosensor in a concentration-dependent manner, indicating a very high confirmation rate. The calculated IC_{50} values were in the range of 40 μM to 2 mM, indicating an excellent sensitivity of the developed and applied screening method for the detection of weak binders. To further validate the fragment hits, we employed an orthogonal enzyme assay, which is generally an important step in fragment-based lead generation. Enzymatic assays can be particularly challenging for fragment screening, as they are frequently compromised by the need to use relatively high ligand concentrations in order to detect their typically weak activity. Nevertheless, we were able to implement an enzymatic assay that tolerated a relatively high ligand concentration and applied it to test a representative subset of the fragment hits [17].

The correlation between the IC_{50} values from the enzymatic assay and the OWG ISA is shown in Fig. 5. Results showed that the correlation is not ideal but sufficient to add confidence in the hit validity. One reason for the poor correlation could be the differences between the full-length PDE10A used in the enzymatic assay and the truncated PDE10A used in the OWG assay. Nonetheless, some of the identified and validated fragment hits displayed very attractive and novel starting points for further hit expansion and chemistry design which was greatly facilitated by structural binding information from X-ray crystallography (data not shown).

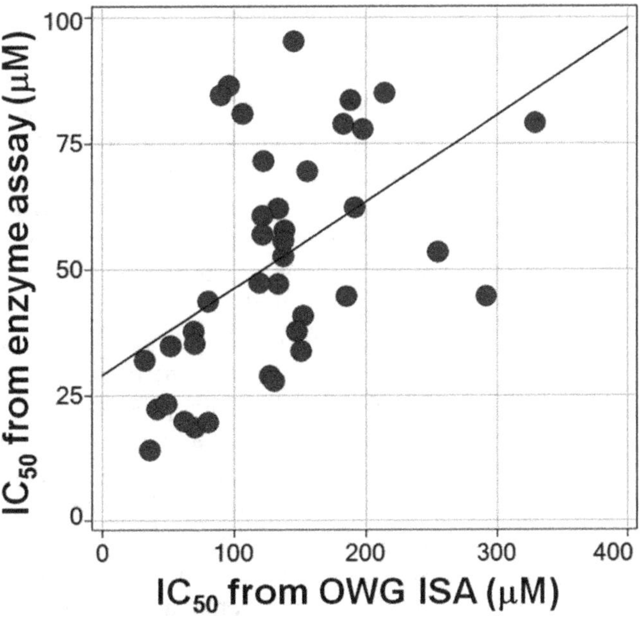

Fig. 5 Correlation between results for the plate-based OWG ISA screening assay and the enzymatic inhibition assay for a representative subset of fragment hits. The linear regression line is shown

5 Discussion

In order to address challenges related to sensitivity and throughput in current fragment screening applications, a novel fragment screening methodology employing a plate-based optical biosensor system was developed. The principles of this inhibition in solution assay (ISA) configuration rely on the ability of a free ligand in solution to displace a large target-protein molecule from a modified biosensor surface through specific and direct competition. The observed mass changes are, dependent on the molecular weight of the ligand and the target protein, about 100 times larger as compared to a direct binding assay format that measures the direct binding of a small molecule, qualifying the ISA as an excellent screening tool, particularly for small molecules. The assay principles have been applied to screen a tailored fragment library of 3,000 members against PDE10A, which resulted in the identification of 395 fragment hits (13.2 % hit rate). The relatively high hit rate can be partially attributed to the increased dynamic range and sensitivity of this assay format as compared to direct binding assays, and partially due to the enrichment from the library design in combination with the high ligandability of PDE10A as a target. Interestingly, the vast majority of the primary fragment hits are validated in dose–response experiments and all members from a selected subset are confirmed as being able to reduce the enzymatic activity of PDE10A in a concentration-dependent manner, building further confidence in the screening approach.

In contrast to fluidics-based SPR systems, the parallelization enabled through the plate-based format of the OWG platform greatly facilitates an effective screening of large fragment libraries without compromising on the ability to detect even weakly binding fragments with good confidence. The key for the ISA to enable screening lies in the identification and design of a suitable compound (TDC) that can be tethered to the biosensor surface in a way that still allows high-affinity target protein binding. By combining information about the chemical structure of available inhibitors with binding information on the molecular level as provided by X-ray crystallography, we have been able to devise a way for synthesizing a suitable TDC that could be used during the screening of a PDE10A fragment library. In this context it is important to note that the required protein concentration for achieving a good binding signal will reciprocally scale with the potency of the TDC; that is, more protein will be required if the affinity of the TDC gets weaker to achieve the same signal. Thus, it is important to strive for high-affinity TDCs, as this will have direct consequences on the required reagent amounts and might exclude some targets from screening of larger fragment libraries due to limitations in protein quantities. In the case of PDE10A, a total amount of

0.8 mg protein was used per 384-well plate, meaning the entire fragment screen consumed about 7 mg of protein. Noticeably, the fluidics-based systems typically consume much less protein (probably 100-fold in the given example) due to their sequential, iterative interrogation of the same biosensor surface with varying ligand solutions, which can be seen as re-using the same protein after washing away unbound ligand. On the flipside, this apparently leads to an increase in screening time, as only one or at best eight different analytes (that is, compounds) can be experimentally assessed simultaneously using currently available high-throughput SPR systems. Some compounds might display some unwanted binding effects, often referred to as promiscuous or aggregation-based binding, that can compromise the ligand-binding competency of the tethered target protein for subsequent binding experiments. We have seen that some of the fragments (1.3 %) showed indeed an increased binding signal that would speak to that point. Those could be problematic in fluidics-based system further reducing the throughput due to loss in surface activity.

References

1. Holdgate GA, Anderson M, Edfeldt F, Geschwindner S (2010) Affinity-based, biophysical methods to detect and analyze ligand binding to recombinant proteins: matching high information content with high throughput. J Struct Biol 172(1):142–157. doi:10.1016/j.jsb.2010.06.024

2. Holdgate G, Geschwindner S, Breeze A, Davies G, Colclough N, Temesi D, Ward L (2013) Biophysical methods in drug discovery from small molecule to pharmaceutical. Methods Mol Biol 1008:327–355. doi:10.1007/978-1-62703-398-5_12

3. Granqvist N, Hanning A, Eng L, Tuppurainen J, Viitala T (2013) Label-enhanced surface plasmon resonance: a new concept for improved performance in optical biosensor analysis. Sensors 13(11):15348–15363. doi:10.3390/s131115348

4. Jonsson U, Fagerstam L, Ivarsson B, Johnsson B, Karlsson R, Lundh K, Lofas S, Persson B, Roos H, Ronnberg I (1991) Real-time biospecific interaction analysis using surface plasmon resonance and a sensor chip technology. Biotechniques 11(5):620–627

5. Cunningham BT, Li P, Schulz S, Lin B, Baird C, Gerstenmaier J, Genick C, Wang F, Fine E, Laing L (2004) Label-free assays on the BIND system. J Biomol Screen 9(6):481–490. doi:10.1177/1087057104267604

6. Fang Y, Ferrie AM, Fontaine NH, Mauro J, Balakrishnan J (2006) Resonant waveguide grating biosensor for living cell sensing. Biophys J 91(5):1925–1940. doi:10.1529/biophysj.105.077818

7. Fang Y, Li G, Ferrie AM (2007) Non-invasive optical biosensor for assaying endogenous G protein-coupled receptors in adherent cells. J Pharmacol Toxicol Methods 55(3):314–322. doi:10.1016/j.vascn.2006.11.001

8. Dalvit C (2009) NMR methods in fragment screening: theory and a comparison with other biophysical techniques. Drug Discov Today 14(21–22):1051–1057. doi:10.1016/j.drudis.2009.07.013

9. Geschwindner S, Carlsson JF, Knecht W (2012) Application of optical biosensors in small-molecule screening activities. Sensors 12(4):4311–4323. doi:10.3390/s120404311

10. Silvestre HL, Blundell TL, Abell C, Ciulli A (2013) Integrated biophysical approach to fragment screening and validation for fragment-based lead discovery. Proc Natl Acad Sci U S A 110(32):12984–12989. doi:10.1073/pnas.1304045110

11. Karlsson R, Kullman-Magnusson M, Hamalainen MD, Remaeus A, Andersson K, Borg P, Gyzander E, Deinum J (2000) Biosensor analysis of drug-target interactions: direct and competitive binding assays for

investigation of interactions between thrombin and thrombin inhibitors. Anal Biochem 278(1):1–13. doi:10.1006/abio.1999.4406

12. Karlsson R, Roos H, Fägerstam L, Persson B (1994) Kinetic and concentration analysis using BIA technology. Methods 6(2):99–110. doi:10.1006/meth.1994.1013

13. Geschwindner S, Olsson LL, Albert JS, Deinum J, Edwards PD, de Beer T, Folmer RH (2007) Discovery of a novel warhead against beta-secretase through fragment-based lead generation. J Med Chem 50(24):5903–5911. doi:10.1021/jm070825k

14. Chen Y, Inoyama D, Kong AN, Beamer LJ, Hu L (2011) Kinetic analyses of Keap1-Nrf2 interaction and determination of the minimal Nrf2 peptide sequence required for Keap1 binding using surface plasmon resonance. Chem Biol Drug Des 78(6):1014–1021. doi:10.1111/j.1747-0285.2011.01240.x

15. Chappie T, Humphrey J, Menniti F, Schmidt C (2009) PDE10A inhibitors: an assessment of the current CNS drug discovery landscape. Curr Opin Drug Discov Devel 12(4): 458–467

16. Siuciak JA (2008) The role of phosphodiesterases in schizophrenia : therapeutic implications. CNS Drugs 22(12):983–993. doi:10.2165/0023210-200822120-00002

17. Geschwindner S, Dekker N, Horsefield R, Tigerstrom A, Johansson P, Scott CW, Albert JS (2013) Development of a plate-based optical biosensor fragment screening methodology to identify phosphodiesterase 10A inhibitors. J Med Chem 56(8):3228–3234. doi:10.1021/jm301665y

Chapter 7

Silicon Photonic Micro-Ring Resonators for Drug Screening and Kinetic Analysis

Muzammil Iqbal, Rufus W. Burlingame, Randy Romero, Annabel Wang, Tyler Grove, and Martin A. Gleeson

Abstract

Genalyte has developed a turnkey silicon photonic chip sensing platform (Maverick™) for rapid detection of multiple biological analytes from a drop of sample. We present here the system applied to multiplex detection of antibodies in serum, the detection of receptor–ligand interactions, and the kinetic characterization of binding. The core of the technology is a silicon microchip, on the surface of which we pattern 128 microscopic ring resonators covered by a single microfluidic channel. The rings are individually functionalized to bind antigens for detecting serum analytes directly, antibodies for detecting immune response, or other biomarkers of interest in a sample that is pumped through the channel over the rings. The frequency of each ring's optical resonance is exquisitely sensitive to the mass of bound analyte. A laser in the Maverick instrument interrogates the 128 rings almost simultaneously to quantify the presence of analytes. Currently, each assay is performed in quadruplicate, with 2 flow channels per chip, providing 15 multiplexed assays plus 1 control in each channel. Twelve chips are packaged into a consumable cartridge that can measure 24 samples. A 96-well plate with foil cover holds the reagents for all the tests, including 24 wells with a buffer solution, into which the operator loads the samples. The user needs only to collect a few drops of sample, transfer them to the sample well, insert the measurement cartridge and the well plate into the unit, and press start. The instrument performs all fluid operations internally, connecting dedicated probes from the measurement cartridge to the appropriate wells in the plate and pumping the sample and reagents through the microfluidic channels on the sensor chips as required by the assay protocol.

Key words Drug screening, Kinetics, Protein interactions, Photonic ring resonance

---

1 Introduction

Historically, drug discovery has been concerned about finding small molecules that interact with the active site of biologically important targets [1]. Currently, because of the revolutionary advances in genetics and molecular biology over the last two decades, much of drug discovery is now focused on macromolecular interactions [2]. Some of these protein drugs are human monoclonal antibodies and soluble receptors against clinically important

Ye Fang (ed.), *Label-Free Biosensor Methods in Drug Discovery*, Methods in Pharmacology and Toxicology,
DOI 10.1007/978-1-4939-2617-6_7, © Springer Science+Business Media New York 2015

cytokines that are used to treat chronic diseases such as rheumatoid arthritis [3] and Crohn's disease [4], among others.

Besides characterizing known targets, novel protein-protein interactions have been identified by homology to known proteins [2], structure-based drug design [5], and large-scale protein arrays optimized to detect novel binding partners [6, 7]. This chapter focuses on the use of a novel label-free, real-time detection system to discover protein-protein interactions and characterize their binding properties.

Silicon photonic ring resonators have been investigated for applications in bio-sensing for the past decade and are particularly attractive because of their exquisite sensitivity. Genalyte is the first company to develop and produce a commercially available sensing platform based on silicon photonic ring resonators. Leveraging silicon manufacturing technology, many ring resonator sensors can be lithographically printed on a silicon-on-insulator (SOI) substrate producing a disposable chip. This complements high sensitivity of the sensor with high throughput and multiplexing capability, which is desirable for most research and clinical diagnostic applications. By employing economies of scale, cost per sensor chip is reduced to a point where large-scale commercial use becomes feasible. The sensing platform technique is described in detail in Section 2.

Sensors based on silicon photonic ring resonators function by detecting the changes in interaction between light circulating inside the sensor and matter deposited on the sensor surface. Ring resonators have the ability to trap light of a particular wavelength (resonance) when the light source is tuned to a cavity mode. Binding of biological material results in a localized change in refractive index on the sensor surface, which affects the circulating optical field extending beyond the sensor boundary. This has the effect of shifting the resonance to longer wavelengths in case of matter deposition and shorter wavelengths in case of matter depletion. The shift is directly proportional to the amount of material bound. Specificity is achieved by attaching a capture probe to the surface of the ring. The probe binds with its matching ligand as it flows over the sensor in liquid phase, and continuous monitoring of shift in resonance wavelength leads to real-time detection without the need for a tag, label, or reporter molecule. The sensing platform is agnostic of the composition and nature of probe molecule so long as it has good specificity and affinity for its target. Capture of protein, antibody, antigen, glycoprotein, glycans, and nucleic acid targets, both DNA for SNP analysis, and miRNA and tmRNA have been demonstrated [8–12]. Since each sensor is interrogated individually and there is no source of signal from tags or labels, multiple sensors can be assembled in the same channel with each dedicated to report on a specific analyte with no cross talk.

Real-time analysis of binding interactions allows for a rapid iterative development of surface assay conditions, and has been used to develop zwitterionic polymer modifications to reduce nonspecific binding in undiluted human serum [13], the monitoring and characterization of surface-initiated polymerization, polymer growth [14], and definition of efficient bio-conjugation conditions [15].

A detailed characterization of the sensor properties was revealed through empirical determination. The $(1/e)$ decay length of the optical field beyond the sensor boundary was calculated to be 63 nm [16]. Therefore, ring resonator-based sensors favor surface biological interactions which are on the order of tens of nanometers. This contrasts with surface plasmon resonance (SPR)-based technologies where the evanescent field extends several hundreds of nanometers and so is perturbed by signal from the extended surrounding environment. In terms of absolute mass, the limit of detection has been measured at 1.5 pg/mm^2, which for a ring with a surface area of 66 μm^2 translates to 125 attograms, equivalent to the mass of about 500 IgG antibodies binding to the surface [16].

Kinetic analysis of binding interactions is reported here (*see* Section 3) and has been demonstrated for protein [17] and nucleic acid interactions [9, 18].

In complex undefined samples such as biological fluids, abundant low affinity-binding components create a nonspecific signal, which limits the ability to perform multiplex analysis. This challenge has been resolved with secondary detection schemes that increase the specificity of signal and amplify the specific response [19, 20]. For low-abundance analytes, a variety of additional amplification strategies using robust and well-characterized reagents have been employed. These include biotinylated secondary antibodies used in conjunction with streptavidin micro-beads [21], and most recently the use of a localized enzymatic reaction to create a precipitate with a horseradish peroxidase/streptavidin fusion protein [22]. This approach has increased the sensitivity of detection in complex biological samples down to single-digit picograms per milliliter levels. An interesting developing application is the analysis of lipid bilayer nanodiscs which can be used to perform analysis of membrane-embedded proteins. The nanodisc-supported lipid bilayer has a natural affinity for the oxide-passivated surface of silicon. Membrane proteins assembled in the nanodisc lipid bilayer are stable and capable of binding proteins in a receptor-specific manner. Concentration-dependent binding of soluble protein with its target receptor and the ability to monitor binding rates in a multiplex format combined with the small amount of reagents required represent significant advancements in drug screening capability. This should be of particular interest in comparison of closely related membrane signaling families, and analysis of drugs for manipulation of a target pathway [23].

2 Mode of Operation

Ring resonators belong to a class of resonant cavity sensors that is highly sensitive to changes in refractive index. Fabry-Perot oscillators [24–26], microspheres [27, 28], micro-discs [29], and photonic crystal cavities [30] are some other examples of integrated resonant interferometers that are suited for high-performance sensing applications. Ring resonators rely upon the interaction of the evanescent tail of an optical mode confined inside a guiding medium, with liquid-phase sample in close proximity [31–33]. In bio-sensing applications, a change in refractive index is caused by binding of analyte molecules in sample to the area above the ring resonator through specific capture by previously deposited probe molecules on the ring surface. In essence, the complex formed through this binding event displaces the lower refractive index carrier media (typically water; $n = 1.33$), thereby changing the refractive index of cladding medium around the ring. This causes a displacement of cavity resonance wavelength, which is directly proportional to the total mass of bound molecules per unit surface area. During an assay, continuous monitoring of the sensor return spectrum leads to measurement of wavelength shift, which qualitatively and quantitatively represents reaction dynamics.

Silicon photonics technology offers the desirable attributes of low manufacturing cost, low sensor-to-sensor variation, ease of light coupling, and co-integration of interrogation optoelectronics. Advances in photolithography have enabled wafer-scale printing of highly uniform submicron optical features on silicon, which is suitable for high-volume manufacturing. Ring resonators built on this platform exhibit excellent optical properties, such as high cavity $Q > 40,000$ and extinction ratio (ER) better than –10 dB when implemented in the relatively simple configuration of a single feed and ring waveguide [16]. Ring diameter can be chosen to produce a free spectral range (FSR) that is attainable by most commercially available continuously tuned laser systems.

Efficient and robust light coupling into and out of the sensor chip is crucial to produce a reliable sensing platform. This is achieved by utilizing photonics grating couplers, which exhibit small footprint, low insertion loss, and low back-scatter. Additionally, grating couplers easily lend themselves to free-space light coupling with systems built from off-the-shelf optics.

Due to small sensor footprint ($\sim$200 μm^2), an array of sensors can be formed on a single chip. Before the assay, each sensor can be functionalized with a unique probe. During an assay, each sensor can be interrogated individually, leading to multiplexed analysis. Construction of multiple flow channels can selectively expose portions of a chip to mutually exclusive samples, allowing multiple samples to be run in a single test. Furthermore, small sensor dimensions lead to smaller flow channels requiring small sample volumes to flow over the chip, which is typically less than 100 μl. At protein concentrations greater than 1 μg/ml, primary binding between analyte and a specific probe produces adequate signal to measure both reaction kinetics and the total mass binding to the probe directly. In experiments where concentrations are less than 100 ng/ml, a secondary amplification step can be seamlessly integrated into the assay protocol. It should be noted that no operator intervention or additional off-line steps are needed for a typical protocol consisting of introduction of buffer, primary binding, secondary amplification, and washing.

Uniformity inherent in manufacturing of sensor arrays yields low variability between sensors. Combining low sample volume, ability to multiplex, fast time to result, and high sensitivity makes ring resonator-based biosensors a viable technology for research and diagnostic applications.

2.1 Theory of Ring Resonators

Similar to most resonant cavity sensors [34], ring resonators are capable of sensing small refractive index changes in their surroundings. Optical energy is transferred into the ring waveguide via evanescent coupling between the ring and a linear feed waveguide. Figure 1a shows a ring resonator formed with linear and ring waveguides, which are geometrically identical and are placed in close proximity, where the tangential spacing is a few hundred nanometers. In such a configuration, light energy from the linear waveguide will "leak" into the ring and excite a circulating guided wave mode, which recedes in energy by the same amount after one round trip in the ring. Three factors that affect coupling strength include ring-to-linear waveguide spacing, dielectric constant of the intervening medium, and refractive index contrast for each waveguide.

Ring resonators are typically interrogated by light from a continuously tunable laser. When light is tuned to a resonant wavelength, coupling into the ring is maximized and all light is

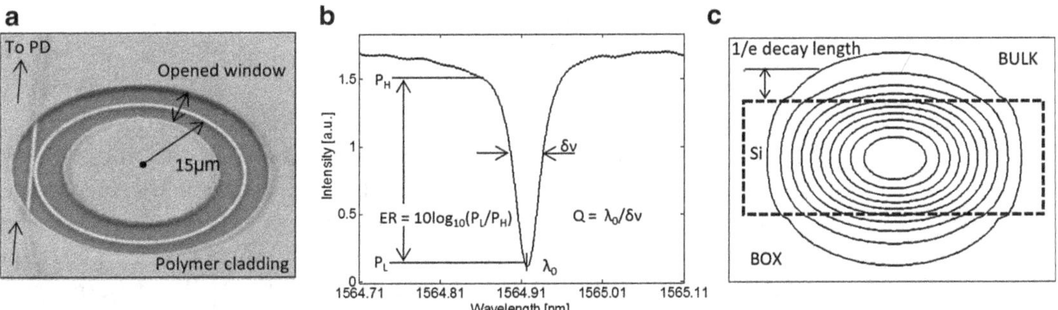

Fig. 1 (**a**) SEM micrograph of Genalyte's ring resonator biosensor, (**b**) spectrum of a ring resonator obtained from a tunable laser sweep, and (**c**) FDTD mode profile of a single-mode silicon waveguide

extinguished at the output of the linear waveguide. This condition is called critical coupling [35], where all light is trapped inside the ring for the duration that the light source dwells on a resonant wavelength. During this time the coupling loss between the feed and the ring waveguide equals the round trip propagation loss inside the ring. The transmitted power at the output of the linear waveguide yields a transfer function depicting inverted peaks in the cavity spectrum at the resonant wavelengths (Fig. 1b). For a continuously tuned source, continuity of the transmission spectrum results in a Lorentzian line shape for cavity resonance peaks. This is crucial when accurate measurement of the location of resonance peaks is required, and precludes the use of discretely stepped lasers. In an ideal configuration where the coupling between two waveguides is loss-less, light is completely extinguished at resonant wavelength at the output of the feed waveguide when critical coupling occurs. The extinction ratio (ER) is a quantity that is typically used to quantify the extent of critical coupling in non-ideal (actual) situations. Extinction ratios of better than −10 dB are adequate for producing highly accurate measurements of peak locations and their shifts during an assay.

It should be noted that cavity mode of the ring is a periodic function that repeats at integer multiples of a resonant wavelength. Wavelength spacing between adjacent peaks is referred to as the free spectral range and is dependent on ring diameter and the "effective index" of the ring waveguide. For high-refractive-index contrast systems, such as silicon-air or silicon-water, optical mode in the ring waveguide closely resembles the profile of a mode confined in the linear waveguide. This allows for utilization of a 2-D finite-difference time-domain (FDTD) mode solver to achieve optimal design parameters. Genalyte's ring resonators are designed for the center wavelength of 1,550 nm with waveguide dimensions of 200 nm × 500 nm. The notion of effective index is understood by studying the profile of the optical mode produced by FDTD mode solver (Fig. 1c). For Genalyte's production devices, effective index of 2.34 is measured, with confinement factors of 0.7624, 0.1193, 0.1088, and 0.0094 for silicon, buried oxide (BOX), bulk, and sensing regions, respectively [16].

For biological binding assays, continuous increase of mass on the ring surface will result in a continuous shift of the resonant wavelength, which is a direct measurement of change in effective index, which is proportional to the total mass of bound molecules.

To achieve critical coupling, the gap between the feed waveguide and the ring must be set based on the chip manufacturing process being utilized. In practice, gaps ranging between 180 and 240 nm have resulted in an extinction ratio (ER) of better than −10 dB. This type of process control is well within the bounds of a modern lithographic process, which typically has tolerance well below 10 nm. A typical sensor transmission spectrum is shown in Fig. 1b, where cavity $Q = 43,000$, ER < −15 dB, and FSR = 5.98 nm.

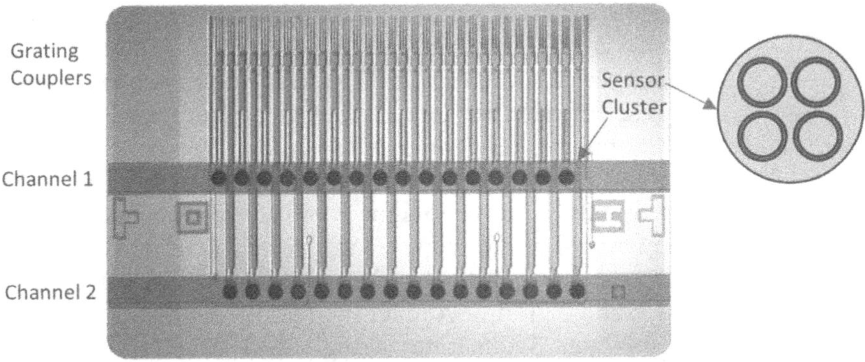

Fig. 2 Schematic of a sensor array featuring 32 sensor clusters split between two flow channels

2.2 Chip Architecture

In its current configuration, Genalyte's sensor chip comprises 136 ring resonator biosensors. During manufacturing, the entire chip is spin coated with a thin film of a perfluoropolymer cladding. Using photolithography and etching, annular windows are opened over 32 clusters, each consisting of 4 rings, such that the ring surface is exposed to sample flowing through the fluidic channels. These unclad sensors are arranged in quadruplicates forming a total of 32 clusters split between two flow channels (Fig. 2). The remaining rings are used to correct assay results for thermally induced drift.

A device called a grating coupler is used to facilitate light entering and leaving the chip. All input and output grating couplers are placed at the chip edges, which are left optically accessible to the free-space optical scanner. More specifically, grating couplers are formed by etching optical grates into multimode expansion sections at the end of silicon waveguides. Input and output grating couplers, multimode expansion sections, multimode waveguide sections, single-mode feed waveguide, and a single-mode ring waveguide are stitched together to form one sensor loop. Light from the tunable laser enters into one set of grating couplers that direct it into waveguides in the chip. The light passes by the ring resonators where very particular wavelengths are captured, and continues on to the outgoing waveguide which is connected to an output grating coupler that emits back into free space where it is collected by the observing optical scanner.

2.3 Scanning Instrumentation

To interrogate sensors during an assay, a free-space optical scanner is used. The scanner provides laser light to the chip and facilitates efficient coupling between free-space and guided-wave optical modes through the grating couplers. As such, Genalyte's grating couplers are designed to accept an optical power distribution exactly equal to that of a C-band, polarization maintaining single-mode optical fiber. A coupling incidence angle of approximately 12° is used and maximum insertion loss per coupling is better than −6 dB.

In order to maximize coupling efficiency, the mode overlap integral requires the beam emerging from the optical scanner to meet strict specifications. These include spot diameter, encircled energy distribution, wave-front error, numerical aperture, and the chief ray angle of the incident beam. Optics inside the scanner is carefully designed to meet these requirements. Grating couplers are highly sensitive to light polarization, so linearly polarized light is provided to the chip, where extinction of unwanted polarization is better than –18 dB. Additionally, our system routinely achieves an average grating coupler insertion loss of –5.5 dB.

Figure 3 illustrates a high-level depiction of the free-space optics scanner, which employs two tip-tilt beam steering mirrors to direct the free-space beam spot from one sensor to the next. The scanner has the ability to hold a position accuracy of ±2 μm when dwelling on an input grating coupler, which meets the mode overlap

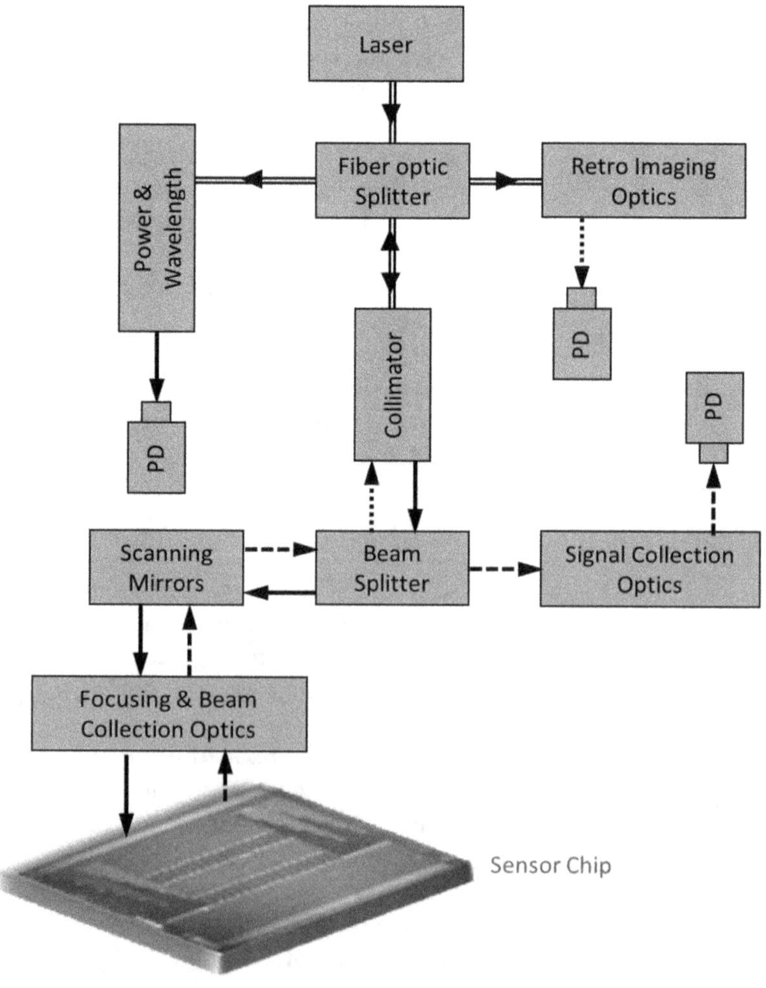

Fig. 3 Architecture of optics scanner depicting key components and functions

requirements. It should be noted that noise in positioning accuracy of the beam spot over a grating coupler directly translates into intensity noise on the output spectrum, when insertion loss grows geometrically as a function of spatial misalignment.

Light returned from the chip is captured by the scanner and co-propagates with the incoming beam, until it is split and routed to a photodetector through the beam conditioning optics (Fig. 3). To elicit a response from a sensor under test, the scanner dwells on the input grating coupler of a sensor loop for the duration of a tunable laser wavelength scan. The laser completes the scan in a pre-specified interval and triggers data acquisition electronics to capture and process the observed spectra. In the meantime, the scanner moves to the next available sensor to perform another scan.

When a chip is first placed in the instrument, tip-tilt mirrors are used to perform a raster scan, creating an image of its surface by looking at reflections from the beam spot. Every coincidence between the beam and a grating coupler results in light insertion into the sensor loop, which is subsequently detected by the observing photodetector. Automated software then identifies the location of "bright spots" in the raster image in terms of their position on the chip. This form of active alignment is considerably faster than other methods, and allows for discovery of sensors with relaxed constraints on chip placement with respect to the scanner.

Genalyte's Maverick Detection System integrates the functions described above into a simple and easy-to-use workflow. The chips are arrayed into a consumable cartridge that holds 12 chips. Each chip has two channels. Using a custom-designed main controller board, the instrument control functions for an assay are exercised according to a pre-defined assay protocol. The user has the ability to use different protocols for each of the 12 chips available in an array. Analyte or samples are introduced over each chip via aspiration tubes connected to syringe pumps through the flow channels. A three-axis robot aligns the desired wells of a 96-well plate with the aspiration tubes during the assay. As an assay is being run on a chip, the spectra from each sensor are acquired as wavelength shift over time and processed by electronics on the main controller board. The data are transmitted to an accompanying computer that hosts a software application used for instrument control, data visualization, and data storage.

The optical architecture of the Maverick™ Detection System is designed to support up to eight instruments, which are cascaded in a chain. The instrument that houses the tunable laser and other expensive optical components is called a "Master Module," whereas the remaining seven instruments share these components through an umbilical interconnection system, and are referred to as "Expansion Modules." In order to achieve this, a fiber-optic distribution network is used that splits tunable laser light and supplies it to the individual instrument.

3 Methods

3.1 Functionalization of Chips

Genalyte uses a robotic analyte spotter from Scienion [36] to precisely position every analyte onto the silicon chip. The current chip contains 32 separate clusters with 4 rings per cluster to measure binding reactions, plus 8 rings for temperature and leak controls. The chip is divided into 2 channels with 16 clusters per channel. Each cluster can be coated with a unique analyte. The Sciflexarrayer (spotter) is capable of dispensing drops of defined volume, 200–600 pL per drop, and the total volume spotted on a cluster may be increased by dispensing several drops. The spotter utilizes multiple cameras to ensure quality control of the drops dispensed and the quality control of the spotted targets [37]. Genalyte chips contain two specific fiducial marks that the camera recognizes to ensure precise and reproducible placement of every analyte on each chip.

Genalyte's Photonic Ring Sensors come with a protective layer of photoresist to protect the chips from possible environmental damage before use. This photoresist layer must be removed with organic solvent before use. Chips may also be treated with acid or aminosilane depending on the surface chemistries ultimately used for the chips. This process is performed by placing chips in a chip rack and submerging the chips in acid or organic solvent, treating them with aminosilane if desired, washing them, and finally drying with nitrogen gas.

Once the surface of the chips is activated, several chemistries can be used for coupling analytes to the chip surface. Most simply, the analyte can be spotted directly onto the silicon surface, or directly onto the surface that has been pretreated with aminosilane [38]. Covalent coupling of analytes to the aminosilane can be accomplished with cross-linkers such as BS3, GMBS, and EDC (available from Thermo/Pierce) or other cross-linkers, depending on the desired specificity and properties.

The protein analytes being spotted onto chips must be diluted to a designated concentration range using a stabilizer. The designated concentration range should be optimized for saturating the photonic rings with either antibodies or other proteins. A stabilizer must be used to ensure stability of the spotted analyte since there is no further treatment to the chips, once spotted. Glycerol is generally, but not always, required and is only used to increase the amount of time the spotted analyte is allowed to bind to the rings in solution. When DNA is spotted onto the chips no stabilizer is needed. After the spotting process, the chips are assembled into a consumable microfluidic array cassette containing 12 chips that can be run on the Maverick™ platform.

3.2 Multiplex Measurement of Antibodies

One use of the Maverick™ instrument is multiplex measurement of antibodies. The first autoimmune application is detecting autoantibodies against six extractable nuclear antigens (ENAs), SS-A, SS-B, Sm, RNP, Scl-70, and Jo-1. All components of the assay apart from the test samples are provided in a kit format with qualified and calibrated reagents. Barcode tracking and software management of all robotic steps ensure standardized flow times and correct reagent selection. The system is designed to require minimal operator attention and apart for sample addition to the loading tray, the other steps are automated.

1. The six nuclear antigens, SS-A, SS-B, Sm, RNP, Scl-70, and Jo-1, are provided as prespotted over the rings in each channel of the chip using a Scienion spotter (*see* Section 3.1). Thus, two samples can be tested simultaneously on each chip (*see* **Note 1**).

2. The user adds 2 µl of patient sample to each of the sample wells (columns 1, 4, and 7) in the 96-well plate that comes preloaded with 95 µl of sample buffer in the well, and mixes it 10 times. The chip array and the sample plate are loaded into the instrument.

3. The instrument aspirates the diluted patient sample and flows it over the chip for 3 min. Primary binding of molecules to the spots can be detected at this stage (Fig. 4).

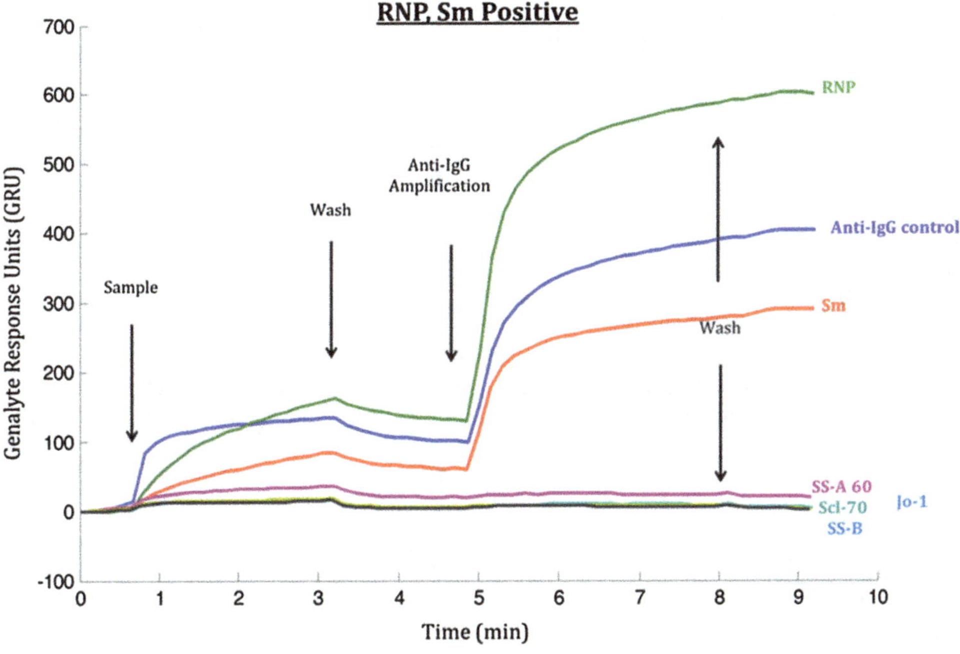

Fig. 4 Sensogram profile for an RNP- and Sm-positive sample run over an ENA 6 chip. Response in GRUs is continuously monitored for each sensor. Each sensor is functionalized with its indicated antigen or with an anti-IgG-positive control. Sample is introduced and after 2.5 min is followed by a wash with buffer. Anti-IgG then flows for 3 min and then a final wash in buffer with end point read. This particular sample is positive for anti-RNP and anti-Sm and negative for the other markers

4. The instrument moves the 96-well plate containing the reagents and aspirates wash buffer from column 2, which is automatically flowed over the chip for 1.5 min at a flow rate of 30 μl/min.

5. The instrument moves the 96-well plate to column 3 and anti-human IgG is flowed over the chip in a step that gives both amplification and specificity, since only IgG bound to the antigens over the sensors is amplified by the anti-IgG reagent (Fig. 4). The test only takes 10 min for two samples (*see* **Note 2**).

The assays have over two orders of magnitude analytical measuring range, which means that the concentration of the autoantibodies can be quantified (Fig. 5). Linear regression of values in ELISA compared to PRI show R^2 values around 0.90 (Fig. 6). Agreement between ELISA and PRI of positive and negative results for the six assays ranges from 95 to 100 %. Precision studies yielded percent CVs less than 3 % for highly positive samples and less than 8 % for moderately positive samples.

A similar application is the detection of autoantibodies to tumor-associated antigens [39]. In this case antigens that are associated with tumors are spotted on the chip. Diluted sera are flowed

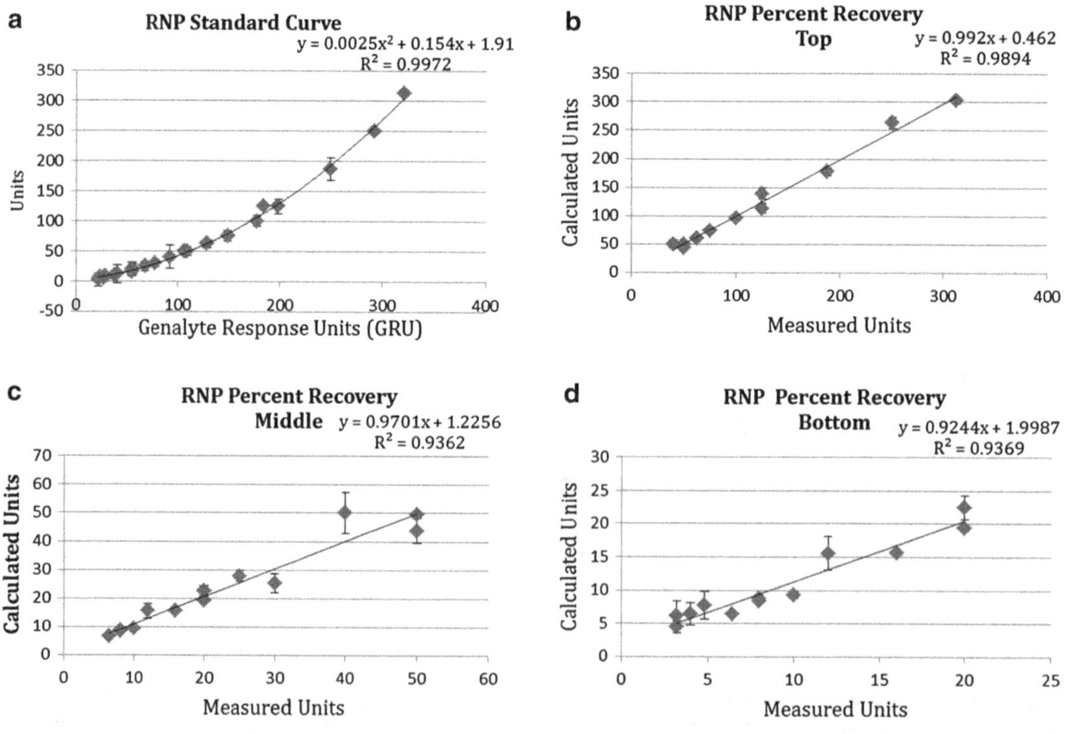

Fig. 5 (**a**) Standard curve for RNP assay. The standard curve for anti-RNP assay is provided (**a**) for calculated units versus measured GRUs (units). (**b–d**) Show the linearity of the percent recovery shown by plotting calculated versus measured values for ranges at the upper, middle, and lower range of the curve

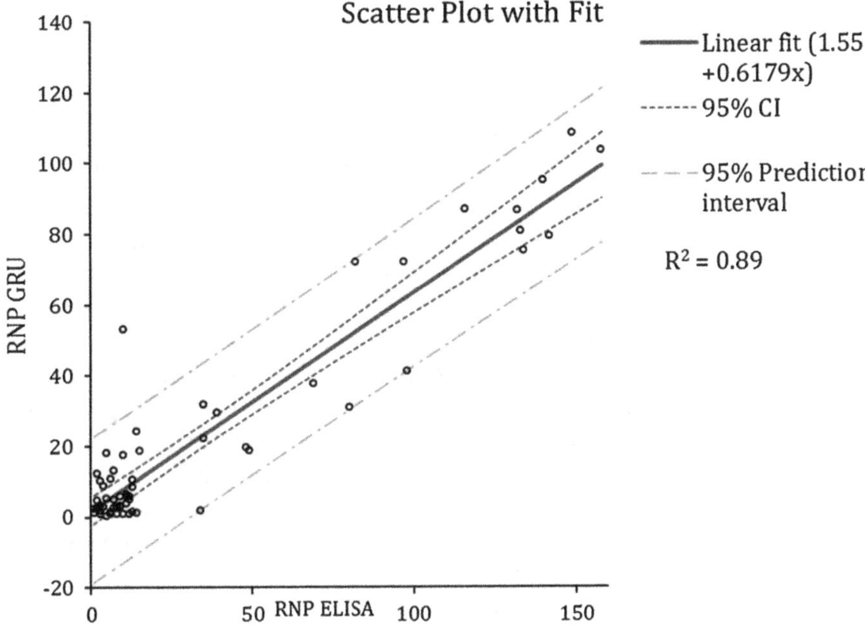

Fig. 6 Linear regression of ELISA units versus GRU with 95 % confidence intervals. Linear regression comparison with ELISA. Samples tested for anti-RNP by PRI and ELISA are compared on a scatterplot. A linear fit with 95 % confidence intervals calculated by the program Analyse—it is drawn through the plot

over the chip and amplified for specific IgG binding to the antigens as described above. The goal of this approach is to develop a multiplex assay that can reliably differentiate people with cancer from non-cancer patients with high sensitivity and specificity.

A further application is a chip that has six capture reagents to six different tags. Currently, the tags are biotin, fluorescein, digoxigenin, polyethylene glycol, Fc portion of IgG, and poly-histidine. In this assay one or more proteins, each with a unique tag, are flowed over the chip and captured by the appropriate reagent. Then the experimental reagents are flowed over the chip to measure binding to any of the captured proteins. This technique allows the users to create their own custom chip without the need to spot novel reagents onto the chip directly.

3.3 Detecting Anti-drug Antibodies

Maverick™ system permits the simultaneous detection of the isotype and IgG subclass of anti-drug antibodies (ADA) in patients who have received treatment with some of the new biologic drugs such as Humira® and Remicade®. These drugs are human monoclonal antibodies against tumor necrosis factor alpha (TNFα), and are used to treat people who have rheumatoid arthritis, and Crohn's disease. Some of the patients become refractory to the effects of the drug, and many of them have developed antibodies against the drug. It is often difficult to measure these ADA since they are bound up by the free drug [3, 4], which acts as a specific liquid-phase inhibitor of antibody by its target.

1. Prespotted chips are provided in an array with anti-Fc-specific antibodies to IgG1, IgG2, IgG3, IgG4, IgA, IgM, and IgE spotted over microring sensors in each chip flow channel.

2. Prepare the patient sample using an affinity capture and elution (ACE) procedure. This procedure is universal to detect any ADA as long as a biotinylated form of the drug is available. Specifically, 50 µl of human serum is spiked with 20 µg/ml of biotinylated drug, followed by glycine buffer pH 2.3 to dissociate any ADA/drug complexes that might be present. The sample is then neutralized with Tris buffer pH 8 to allow the unlabeled drug and the biotinylated drug to compete for binding onto ADA. All biotinylated drug, with or without bound anti-drug antibodies, is removed from the sera by incubating with streptavidin-coated paramagnetic beads for 15 min, and washing three times with PBS-Tween. After the third wash the ADA molecules are eluted from the beads with glycine buffer pH 2.3, the beads are removed, and the eluted antibodies are neutralized with Tris pH 8. The remaining portions of the assay are performed automatically once the eluted antibody sample is loaded into the reagent tray. The instrument follows the set flow instructions.

3. The eluted antibodies are aspirated by the instrument and flowed over the human anti-isotype chips for 7 min, allowing any antibodies present to be captured by their Fc region by the appropriate antibodies on the chip.

4. The instrument moves the 96-well plate and aspirates the wash solution, which contains a low concentration of human IgG. This solution is flowed over the chip for 2 min to wash away any loosely bound antibodies and to block free antibody-binding sites on the chip.

5. The specificity and amplification of the captured antibodies are measured by first flowing biotinylated drug over them that is aspirated from wells in the third column of the 96-well plate, followed by streptavidin-coated nanobeads from wells in the fourth column. The signal is automatically read by the onboard software.

6. The specific signal is the value obtained by subtracting the baseline from before streptavidin-coated nanobead amplification from the baseline after streptavidin-coated nanobead amplification to obtain the specific signal.

In model systems with monoclonal antibodies (AbDSerotec) to either Humira® or Remicade® (AbD Serotec), used as an ADA mimic, sensitivity for ADA in the presence of 20 µg/ml of free drug is 60 ng/ml. At 250 ng/ml of ADA, the free drug tolerance is greater than 40 μg/ml. This technique yields high sensitivity to detect ADA, even in the presence of free drug, enabling appropriate modification of treatment for individuals who are not responding to the drug because they have ADA.

3.4 Protein Library Screening

Maverick system permits the screening of a protein library for detecting low levels of protein-protein binding. In this format, although the concentration of the binding reagent is too low to be seen by direct primary binding, it can still be measured by signal amplification with reagents such as unconjugated antibodies, phycoerythrin conjugated to an antibody or streptavidin, or nanobeads coupled to an antibody, protein A/G, or streptavidin. An example of a model system for screening a protein library for detecting low levels of protein-protein binding is the interaction between CD200-Fc and CD200R-Fc [40, 41].

1. Spot recombinant human CD200R-Fc on the chip.

2. Prepare solution of recombinant human CD200-Fc (R&D Systems). Both CD200 and CD200R are cloned with the human IgG Fc region. The Fc region is both a recognition tag as well as a structural feature that causes the molecules to self-assemble into dimers.

3. Flow CD200-Fc at concentrations from 20 μg/ml down to 40 ng/ml over a chip spotted with CD200R-Fc.

4. Detect the primary binding. The primary binding more than 20 times background was readily observed at 1 μg/ml, but not seen at 100 ng/ml (Table 1).

Table 1
CD200R-Fc titration

CD200R-Fc Conc. (μg/ml)	CD200-Fc capture
40	167
20	155
10	136
5	127
2.5	99
1.25	75
0.63	47
0.31	31
0.16	18
0.08	15
0.04	5
0	2

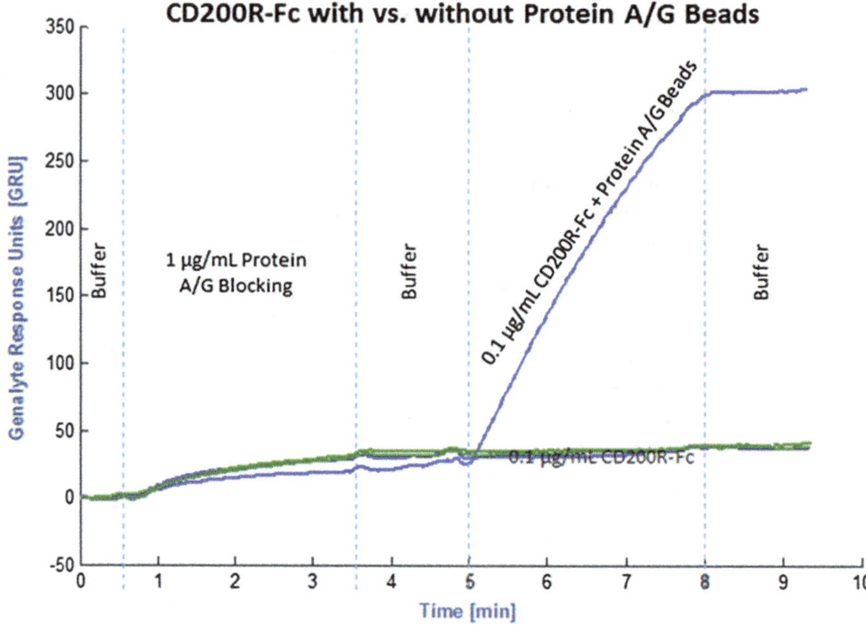

Fig. 7 CD200-Fc and CD200R-Fc were spotted onto chips. CD200R-Fc was flowed over at 100 ng/ml with and without protein A/G beads. To ensure protein-protein interaction, protein A/G was first used to block the Fc region of the capture protein

Table 2
CD200R-Fc with and without protein A/G beads

CD200R-Fc incubated with and without protein A/G beads	CD200-Fc capture	CD200R-Fc capture
100 ng/ml with protein A/G beads	279	6
100 ng/ml	5	14

However, when binding was amplified by nanobeads coated with protein A/G, binding of CD200R-Fc to CD200-Fc more than 50 times background was detected at 100 ng/ml (Fig. 7 and Table 2). A cartoon showing the molecular interactions described above is depicted in Fig. 8.

With an amplification step, the sample of interest can be tested at approximately 100 ng/ml. Each channel requires 70 µl of sample. Thus, to screen for potential interactions of a protein with 384 other proteins, only 168 ng of reagent is needed to flow over the chips in the array (0.07 ml × 24 channels × 100 ng/ml). Scaling up to testing a library of 1,000 proteins for interactions with each of the other 1,000 proteins would only require about 3 µg of each

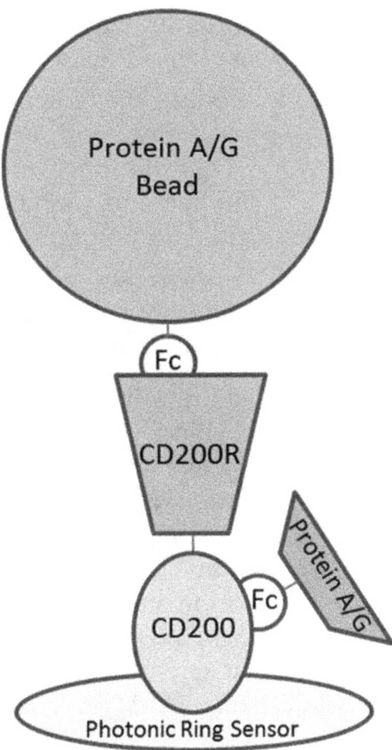

Fig. 8 Cartoon of a labeled receptor binding to its ligand on the solid phase, with amplification by a protein A/G beads

protein. This includes 2.5 µg to spot the chips for 3,000 arrays (1,000 proteins/384 proteins per array = 2.6 arrays, round up to 3 arrays per sample × 1,000 samples = 3,000 arrays), and 504 ng of sample to run over the 3 arrays (168 ng/array × 3 arrays = 504 ng). The Maverick system makes efficient use of valuable reagents.

3.5 Determining Binding Kinetics of Protein-Protein Interactions

Once potential protein-protein interactions have been discovered with the initial screening step, the kinetics and affinity constants of the interaction can also be determined using the Maverick detection technology. In an assay using purified proteins, the primary binding that is measured directly must be caused by the known analytes in the system and with appropriate controls can be attributed to specific protein-protein interactions. The same model system used above to screen for potential binding events at low concentration, CD200R-Fc and CD200-Fc, has also been used to demonstrate the ability to directly measure kinetic properties, such as association rate constant (k_a), dissociation rate constant (k_d), and the equilibrium rate constants (K_D).

1. Spot CD200-Fc onto the chips at saturating concentrations.

2. Flow CD200R-Fc over the chip for 3 min at concentrations ranging from 40 to 0.04 µg/ml. This corresponds to 266–0.266 nM using a molecular weight of 150 kDa for CD200R-FC.

3. Wash the chip for 6 min with the same buffer used in the binding step.

4. Monitor the biosensor response throughout the assays, so the association and dissociation process of CD200R-Fc and CD200-Fc interaction can be monitored in real time. The binding and washing steps are referred to as the adsorption and desorption process, respectively.

5. Fit the sensogram with a robust non-linear least square fitting algorithm to obtain association rate constant (k_a), dissociation rate constant (k_d), and equilibrium rate constants (K_D).

Figure 9 shows assay sensograms where signal growth represents protein binding to sensor surface and signal decay characterizes protein depletion during the wash step. In addition, the adsorption and desorption curves are individually fitted to an analytical model described in [18], with aid of a robust non-linear least square fitting algorithm. Coefficients of the fitted model are interpreted as the association and dissociation rate constants, which lead to the measurement of the equilibrium rate constant. Using this technique kinetic rate constants were found to be $K_a = 2.6 \times 10^{-3}$ M^{-1} s^{-1}, $K_d = 1.5 \times 10^5$ M^{-1} s^{-1}, and $K_D = 1.66 \times 10^{-8}$ M^{-1} s^{-1}.

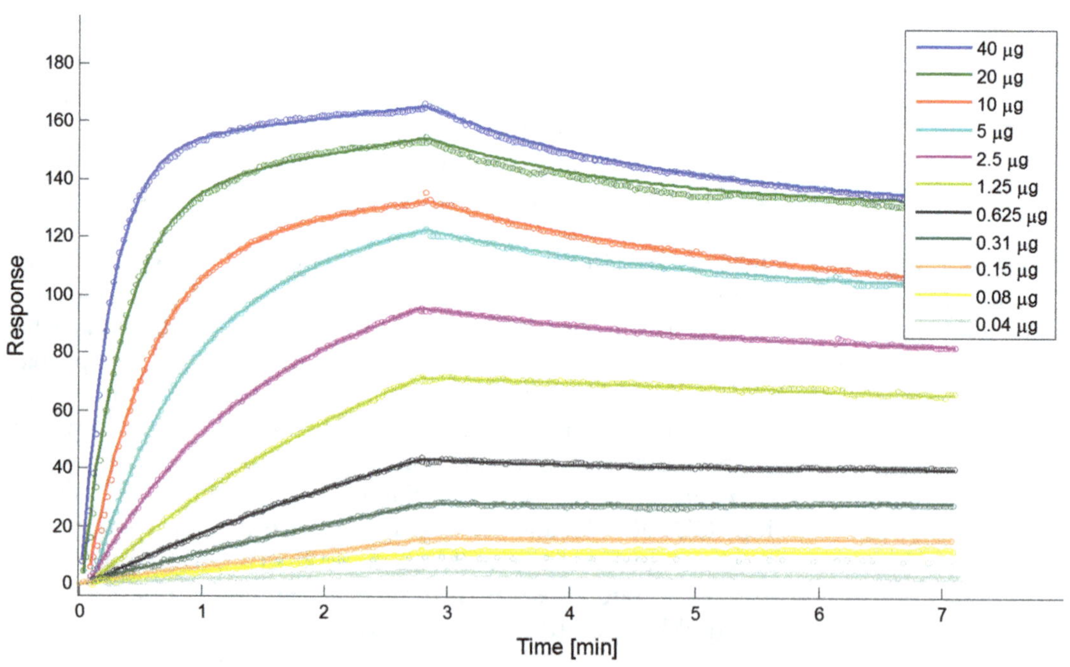

Fig. 9 Sensogram data for serial dilutions of CD200R-Fc analyte binding to CD200-Fc capture probe (line marker "o"). Raw data fitted to a well-known kinetic model for adsorption and desorption curves separately (*solid lines*). Concentration spread is *color coded* and depicted in *legend inset*

4 Notes

1. The specifics of the Maverick™ detection system allow for very small amount of reagents to be used for screening. The amount of probe on each cluster of the chip is about 1 nl of solution at 250 µg/ml of protein. The Scienion spotter works with 10 µl of sample in the nozzle, or 2.5 µg of protein, which is enough to spot 5,000 chips with 2 clusters per chip. The current version of the chip can be spotted with 16 different solid-phase proteins (or other macromolecules) per channel, and there are 2 channels per chip. There are 12 chips per array. On one end of the spectrum, 24 different samples can be tested on 16 different solid-phase reagents per array. On the other end, 1 sample can be tested on 384 different solid-phase reagents per array.

2. Any protein-protein interaction of sufficiently high affinity can be measured by the Maverick™. When the protein is sufficiently large and in a relatively high concentration, such as autoantibodies found in patients with autoimmune disease, the binding interaction can be measured directly. In this assay the amplification with anti-human IgG is more important for determining the specificity of the primary binding from a complex matrix like serum than it is for amplifying the binding signal. For example, IgM, IgA, or some other serum protein could bind to an ENA bound to the chip, causing a primary signal. However, only bound IgG will yield amplification by the anti-IgG step.

References

1. McFedries A, Schwaid A, Saghatelian A (2013) Methods for the elucidation of protein-small molecule interactions. Chem Biol 20(5):667–673. doi:10.1016/j.chembiol.2013.04.008

2. Makley LN, Gestwicki JE (2013) Expanding the number of "druggable" targets: non-enzymes and protein-protein interactions. Chem Biol Drug Des 81(1):22–32. doi:10.1111/cbdd.12066

3. Hetland ML, Christensen J, Tarp U, Dreyer L, Hansen A, Hansen T, Kollerup G, Linde L, Lindegaard HM, Poulsen UE, Schlemmer A, Jensen DV, Jensen S, Hostenkamp G, Østergaard M, on Behalf of All Departments of Rheumatology in Denmark (2010) Direct comparison of treatment responses, remission rates, and drug adherence in patients with rheumatoid arthritis treated with adalimumab, etanercept, or infliximab: results from eight years of surveillance of clinical practice in the nationwide Danish DANBIO registry. Arthritis Rheum 62(1):22–32. doi:10.1002/art.27227

4. Colombel JF, Sandborn WJ, Reinisch W, Mantzaris GJ, Kornbluth A, Rachmilewitz D, Lichtiger S, D'Haens G, Diamond RH, Broussard DL, Tang KL, van der Woude CJ, Rutgeerts P, for the SONIC Study Group (2010) Infliximab, azathioprine, or combination therapy for Crohn's disease. N Engl J Med 362(15):1383–1395. doi: 10.1056/NEJMoa0904492

5. Lounnas V, Ritschel T, Kelder J, McGuire R, Bywater RP, Foloppe N (2013) Current progress in structure-based rational drug design marks a new mindset in drug discovery. Comput Struct Biotechnol J 5:e201302011. doi:10.5936/csbj.201302011

6. Gonzalez LC (2012) Protein microarrays, biosensors, and cell-based methods for secretome-wide extracellular protein–protein interaction mapping. Methods 57:448–458. doi:10.1016/j.ymeth.2012.06.004

7. Ramani SR, Toma I, Lewin-Koh N, Wranik B, DePalatis L, Zhang J, Eaton D, Gonzalez LC

(2012) A secreted protein microarray platform for extracellular protein interaction discovery. Anal Biochem 420(2):127–138. doi:10.1016/j.ab.2011.09.017

8. Iqbal M, Gleeson MA, Spaugh B, Tybor F, Gunn WG, Hochberg M, Baehr-Jones T, Bailey RC, Gunn LC (2010) Label-free biosensor arrays based on silicon ring resonators and high-speed optical scanning instrumentation. IEEE J Sel Top Quantum Electron 16:654–661. doi:10.1109/JSTQE.2009.2032510

9. Qavi AJ, Mysz TM, Bailey RC (2011) Isothermal discrimination of single-nucleotide polymorphisms via kinetic desorption and label-free detection of DNA using silicon photonic microring resonator arrays. Anal Chem 83(17):6827–6833. doi:10.1021/ac201659p

10. Qavi AJ, Bailey RC (2010) Multiplexed detection and label-free quantitation of microRNAs using arrays of silicon photonic microring resonators. Angew Chem Int Ed Engl 49(27):4608–4611. doi:10.1002/anie.201001712

11. Washburn AL, Luchansky MS, Bowman AL, Bailey RC (2010) Quantitative, label-free detection of five protein biomarkers using arrays of silicon photonic microring resonators. Anal Chem 82(1):69–72. doi:10.1021/ac902451b

12. Scheler O, Kindt JT, Qavi AJ, Kaplinski L, Glynn B, Barry T, Kurg A, Bailey RC (2012) Label-free, multiplexed detection of bacterial tmRNA using silicon photonic microring resonators. Biosens Bioelectron 36(1):56–61. doi:10.1016/j.bios.2012.03.037

13. Kirk JT, Brault ND, Baehr-Jones T, Hochberg M, Jiang S, Ratner DM (2013) Zwitterionic polymer-modified silicon microring resonators for label-free biosensing in undiluted human plasma. Biosens Bioelectron 42:100–105. doi:10.1016/j.bios.2012.10.079

14. Limpoco FT, Bailey RC (2011) Real-time monitoring of surface-initiated atom transfer radical polymerization using silicon photonic microring resonators: implications for combinatorial screening of polymer brush Growth Conditions. J Am Chem Soc 133(38):14864–14867. doi:10.1021/ja205358g

15. Byeon JY, Limpoco FT, Bailey RC (2010) Efficient bioconjugation of protein capture agents to biosensor surfaces using aniline-catalyzed hydrazone ligation. Langmuir 26(19):15430–15435. doi:10.1021/la1021824

16. Luchansky MS, Washburn AL, Martin TA, Iqbal M, Gunn LC, Bailey RC (2010) Characterization of the evanescent field profile and bound mass sensitivity of a label-free silicon photonic microring resonator biosensing

platform. Biosens Bioelectron 26(4):1283–1291. doi:10.1016/j.bios.2010.07.010

17. Marty MT, Sloan CD, Bailey RC, Sligar SG (2012) Nonlinear analyte concentration gradients for one-step kinetic analysis employing optical microring resonators. Anal Chem 84(13):5556–5564. doi:10.1021/ac300478f

18. Byeon JY, Bailey RC (2011) Multiplexed evaluation of capture agent binding kinetics using arrays of silicon photonic microring resonators. Analyst 136(17):3430–3433. doi:10.1039/c0an00853b

19. Qavi AJ, Kindt JT, Gleeson MA, Bailey RC (2011) Anti-DNA:RNA antibodies and silicon photonic microring resonators: increased sensitivity for multiplexed microRNA detection. Anal Chem 83(15):5949–5956. doi:10.1021/ac201340s

20. Luchansky MS, Bailey RC (2011) Rapid, multiparameter profiling of cellular secretion using silicon photonic microring resonator arrays. J Am Chem Soc 133(50):20500–20506. doi:10.1021/ja2087618

21. Luchansky MS, Washburn AL, McClellan MS, Bailey RC (2011) Sensitive on-chip detection of a protein biomarker in human serum and plasma over an extended dynamic range using silicon photonic microring resonators and submicron beads. Lab Chip 11:2042–2044. doi:10.1039/c1lc20231f

22. Kindt JT, Luchansky MS, Qavi AJ, Bailey RC (2013) Subpicogram per milliliter detection of interleukins using silicon photonic microring resonators and an enzymatic signal enhancement strategy. Lab Chip 11(12):2042–2044. doi:10.1039/c1lc20231f

23. Kuhnline Sloan CD, Marty MT, Sligar SG, Bailey RC (2013) Interfacing lipid bilayer nanodiscs and silicon photonic sensor arrays for multiplexed protein-lipid and protein-membrane protein interaction screening. Anal Chem 85(5):2970–2976. doi:10.1021/ac3037359

24. Mitchell G (1989) A review of Fabry-Perot interferometer sensors. Proc Phys 44: 450–457

25. Murphy K, Gunther M, Vengsarkar A, Claus R (1991) Quadrature phase-shifted, extrinsic Fabry-Perot optical fiber sensor. Opt Lett 16(4):273–275. doi:10.1364/OL.16.000273

26. Brandenburg A, Edelhauser R, Hutter F (1991) Gas sensor based on an integrated optical interferometer. SPIE Chem Med Sensing 150:148–159. doi:10.1117/12.47133

27. Arnold S, Khoshima M, Teraoka I, Holler S, Vollmer F (2003) Shift of whispering gallery modes in microspheres by protein adsorption. Opt Lett 28(4):272–274. doi:10.1364/OL.28.000272

28. Hanumegowda N, Stica C, Patel B, White I, Fan X (2005) Refractometric sensors based on microsphere resonators. Appl Phys Lett 87:201107. doi:10.1063/1.2132076

29. Boyd R, Heebner J (2001) Sensitive disk resonator photonic biosensor. Appl Opt 40(31):5742–5747. doi:10.1364/AO.40.005742

30. Chow E, Grot A, Mirkarimi L, Sigalas M, Girolami G (2004) Ultracompact biochemical sensor built with two-dimensional photonic crystal microcavity. Opt Lett 29(10):1093–1095. doi:10.1364/OL.29.001093

31. Ksendzov A, Lin Y (2005) Integrated optics ring-resonator sensor for protein detection. Opt Lett 30(24):3344–3346. doi:10.1364/OL.30.003344

32. De Vos K, Bartolozi I, Schacht E, Bienstman P, Baets R (2007) Silicon-on-insulator microring resonator for sensitive and label-free biosensing. Opt Express 15(12):7610–7615. doi:10.1364/OE.15.007610

33. Kwon M, Steir W (2008) Microring-resonator-based sensor measuring both the concentration and temperature of a solution. Opt Express 16(13):9372–9377. doi:10.1364/OE.16.009372

34. Armani A, Kulkarni R, Fraser S, Flagan R, Vahala K (2007) Label-free, single-molecule detection with optical microcavities. Science 317(5839):783–787. doi:10.1126/science.1145002

35. Yariv A (2000) Universal relations for coupling of optical power between microresonators and dielectric waveguides. Electron Lett 36:321–322. doi:10.1049/el:20000340

36. Eickhoff H, Malik A (2013) Planar protein arrays in microtiter plates: development of a new format towards accurate, automation-friendly and affordable (A(3)) diagnostics. Adv Biochem Eng Biotechnol 133:149–165. doi:10.1007/10_2012_148

37. Kirk JT, Fridley GE, Chamberlain JW, Christensen ED, Hochberg M, Ratner DM (2011) Multiplexed inkjet functionalization of silicon photonic biosensors. Lab Chip 11(7):1372–1377. doi:10.1039/c0lc00313a

38. Zhu M, Lerum MZ, Chen W (2012) How to prepare reproducible, homogeneous, and hydrolytically stable aminosilane-derived layers on silica. Langmuir 28(1):416–423. doi:10.1021/la203638g

39. Zhang J-Y, Casiano CA, Peng X-X, Koziol JA, Chan EKL, Tan EM (2003) Enhancement of antibody detection in cancer using panel of recombinant tumor-associated antigens. Cancer Epidemiol Biomarkers Prev 12(2):136–143

40. Hatherley D, Cherwinski HM, Moshref M, Barclay AN (2005) Recombinant CD200 Protein does not bind activating proteins closely related to CD200 Receptor. J Immunol 175:2469–2474. doi:10.4049/jimmunol.175.4.2469

41. Voulgaraki D, Mitnacht-Kraus R, Letarte M, Foster-Cuevas M, Brown MH, Barclay AN (2005) Multivalent recombinant proteins for probing functions of leucocyte surface proteins such as the CD200 receptor immunology. Immunology 115(3):337–346. doi:10.1111/j.1365-2567.2005.02161.x

Chapter 8

Optical Waveguide Light-Mode Spectroscopy for Ion Channel Profiling

Inna Székács

Abstract

Ion channel-based biosensors using label-free optical waveguide light-mode spectroscopy (OWLS) technique provide a sensitive measurement method of trans-channel ion transport, and allow further development in utilization of ion channels as models for pharmacological purposes (drug design targeting ion channels or diagnostic applications in clinical trials). This chapter describes a sensor setup for supported cell-derived membrane fragments deposited onto a hydrophilic polytetrafluoroethylene membrane with further separation from the OWLS sensor surface by a thin polyethylene terephthalate membrane. This approach provides spatial separation between the lipid layer and the sensor surface, and also allows space for possible extramembranous domains of the inbuilt membrane channel proteins. Influx of Cl^- ions through $GABA_A$ channels in the presence or absence of GABA and channel blocking agent bicuculline is measured by changes of the optical characteristics in the evanescent field at near proximity of the OWLS sensor surface.

Key words Ion channel, Optical biosensor, Optical waveguide light-mode spectroscopy, Supported lipid membrane

1 Introduction

The development of sensitive, real-time, and high-throughput approaches for screening of candidate substances affecting ion channels is becoming increasingly important in current rational drug design processes. Numerous drugs can act on membrane-embedded or membrane-associated proteins including membrane receptors, metabolite transporters, and ion channels. Optical biosensors are a highly effective tool in the characterization of such drug-protein interactions [1]. Incorporation of ion channels into the lipid bilayer on the sensor surface provides the platform for development of biosensors based on mimicking signals of ion channels in living cells. Ion channel-based biosensors are created either by self-assembly of pore-forming peptides of smaller molecular size such as gramicidin [2–4], melittin [5, 6], alamethicin [7, 8],

Ye Fang (ed.), *Label-Free Biosensor Methods in Drug Discovery*, Methods in Pharmacology and Toxicology, DOI 10.1007/978-1-4939-2617-6_8, © Springer Science+Business Media New York 2015

and others [9, 10] or by incorporation of large transmembrane ion channel proteins [11, 12] onto the sensor surface. The biological activity of ion channels requires an appropriate lipid environment to preserve spatial conformation and proper conditions to allow assembling of the subunits of the multi-unit functional molecular complexes.

Artificial biomembrane constructions (liposome arrays, planar lipid bilayer, and supported lipid bilayer) have been developed and applied in multitude of techniques and experimental designs [13, 14]. The use of liposomes attached directly to the sensor surface in the biosensor approach presents some difficulties in the experiments (bulk composition effects), e.g., liposome motion, fusion or detachment, and ionic changes inside or outside of vesicles potentially generating significant changes in the refractive index and thus causing serious limitations to the rapid measurement of transport processes. An alternative approach to the use of liposomes for ion channel-ligand interaction studies is the application of planar lipid membranes. The artificial lipid layer platform enables variations of experimental conditions, but also challenges with several difficulties in sensor technology, including errors in the continuity of the lipid layers, as well as their mechanical instability and short lifetime. Lipid layer structures can be created by using the Langmuir-Blodgett method or by fusing liposomes on hydrophilic or hydrophobic solid surfaces [15]. The success of the preparation of supported lipid bilayers depends on several factors, such as surface charge, lipid composition, size of the liposomes, and other experimental conditions including pH and ionic strength [15, 16]. The significant drawback of the design based on solid supported lipid bilayers is that it cannot provide the appropriate space between the sensor surface and the lipid layer to accommodate extramembrane parts of transmembrane proteins. To overcome these shortcomings, several methodologies have been developed to place lipid layers at a distance from the sensor surface [17–19]. Due to their chemical stability, as well as variable porosity and hydrophobicity, Teflon polymers (polytetrafluoroethylene, PTFE) and copolymers (e.g., ethylene tetrafluoroethylene, ETFE) are well applicable as holders in supported lipid layer-based sensors. In situ-prepared Teflon films with multiple microfabricated pores were applied for the stable formation of planar lipid bilayers [7]. Alternatively, a porous Teflon surface was created on commercially available ETFE films using tungsten wire heated tips for pore formation [20]. Moreover, hydrophilic and hydrophobic Teflon filters with different pore sizes were also utilized as membrane holders to support the formation of artificial lipid bilayers with built-in functional ion channels [12, 21].

Ion flux through ion channels embedded in the lipid layer can be monitored by measuring electrochemical (as conductivity) or optical (as refractive index) parameters. The commonly used electrophysiological technique for studying ion channel activity and measuring the kinetics of ion channels is the patch clamp method pioneered by Neher and Sakman [22]. Optical detection-based techniques, such as surface plasmon resonance [23] or optical waveguide light-mode spectroscopy (OWLS) [24] sensors, detect physical changes of light in a narrow evanescent field over the sensor surface. Thus, these optical biosensors provide real-time information on molecular interactions without labeling of the interacting molecules [1].

Various techniques were utilized for lipid layer deposition [25, 26] and for monitoring functions of inbuilt ion channels [12, 27] in OWLS-based assay systems. This chapter describes an OWLS measurement system for detecting the channel functions of the GABA$_A$ ($\alpha5$, $\beta2$, $\gamma2$) receptor in the presence or absence of γ-aminobutyric acid (GABA) and the competitive GABA-blocker bicuculline [12]. In the sensor design, the lipid bilayer is kept at a distance from the detection proximity of the sensor surface by inserting membrane sheets, so the lipid bilayer is outside of the sensing volume. The upper (PTFE) membrane towards the external medium supports the formation of lipid layers containing the ion channels to be investigated, and provides an environment for the extramembrane part of protein. The lipid layer, supported by the PTFE membrane, ideally provides full insulation by eliminating the bulk permeation of electrolytes. In real applications this insulation may be imperfect that may contribute to background signal intensity. The bottom (polyethylene terephthalate, PET) membrane facing towards the sensor excludes lipid vesicles from the detection field of the sensor, but allows passive migration of ions through the lipid layers favorably via the opening of ion channels to the sensor surface.

2   Materials

Reagents are available from Sigma-Aldrich (Hungary), unless stated otherwise. All buffer solutions are made in deionized distilled water (18.2 MΩ cm at 25 °C) and filtered through 0.22 μm Millex®GP filter (Millipore, Hungary) prior to use. Buffer solutions are stored at 4 °C and used within 1 month upon preparation.

2.1   Buffers

1. Artificial cerebrospinal fluid (ACSF): 145 mM NaCl, 3 mM KCl, 1 mM MgCl$_2$, 2 mM CaCl$_2$, 10 mM D-glucose, 10 mM HEPES, pH 7.4.

2. Cl$^-$-free ACSF: 140 mM Na-acetate, 5 mM KH$_2$PO$_4$, 0.8 mM MgSO$_4$, 1.8 mM Ca-acetate, 10 mM D-glucose, 10 mM HEPES, pH 7.4 (*see* **Note 1**).

2.2 Reagents

2.2.1 Reagents for Liposome Preparation

1. Egg yolk lecithin (composition: 70 % phosphatidylcholine, 10 % phosphatidylethanolamine, and 20 % other lipids including neutral lipids; Avanti Polar Lipids, Alabaster, AL, USA).

2. Texas Red® DHPE (1,2-dihexadecanoyl-sn-glycero-3-phosphoethanolamine, triethylammonium salt; Invitrogen, Carlsbad, CA, USA).

2.2.2 Reagents for Cell Membrane Assay

1. Protease inhibitor cocktail tablets (Complete Mini, Roche, Hungary).

2. γ-Aminobutyric acid (GABA).

3. Bicuculline (*see* **Note 2**).

2.3 Membrane Sheets

1. PET membrane (RoTrac®; thickness 23 μm, with regular pores of 50 nm diameter; Oxyphen AG, Switzerland).

2. PTFE membrane (LCR; thickness 140 μm, virtual pore diameter 450 nm; Millipore, Hungary).

2.4 Cell Line

1. Cell lines expressing $GABA_A$ ($\alpha5$, $\beta2$, $\gamma2$) receptors (*see* **Note 3**).

2.5 Equipment

1. OWLS 110 instrument with OW 2400 grating coupler sensors and BioSense 2.6 software (MicroVacuum Ltd, Budapest, Hungary).

---

3 Methods

3.1 Liposome Preparation

For cell membrane modeling it is very important to use liposomes consisting of single phospholipid bilayer—unilamellar vesicles. In this approach unilamellar liposomes are used for fusing with cell-derived membranes containing ion channels. The protocol below describes a simple and rapid method for liposome preparation from egg yolk lecithin according to Moscho et al. [28].

1. Dissolve egg yolk lecithin in chloroform-methanol (9:1) mixture at a concentration of 2 mg/ml.

2. Dissolve Texas Red DHPE in chloroform-methanol (9:1) mixture at a concentration of 1 mg/ml.

3. Add 1.1 μl of the abovementioned Texas Red DHPE solution to 2 ml of the egg yolk lecithin solution (*see* **Note 4**).

4. Add 2 ml of the lipid mixture to a 100 ml round-bottomed flask.

5. Layer 7 ml of the corresponding buffer above the organic solution (the density of the organic solution is higher than that of the buffer) and remove the organic solvent from the rotating flask immersed into a 30 °C water bath under reduced pressure (final vacuum < 20 mmHg) (*see* **Note 5**).

6. Dispense the remaining turbid suspension (~6 ml) into 1.5 ml Eppendorf tubes, and centrifuge at 2,085 $\times g$ for 10 min.

7. Collect the pellets and suspend them in 600 µl buffered saline (*see* **Note 5**).

8. Check the quality of the liposome preparation by phase-contrast or confocal fluorescence microscope. Avoid the high proportion of multilamellar liposomes. Liposomes prepared with this method contain mainly large (LUV) and giant (GUV) unilamellar vesicles.

3.2 Preparation of Cell Membrane Extracts

Instead of using ion channel proteins in purified form for insertion into liposomes or artificial lipid layers, cell-derived membrane fractions enriched genetically in a given transmembrane channel can be used. That helps multi-unit transmembrane channel to keep its native structure and activity. In the mammalian brain $GABA_A$ receptors are the major mediators of inhibitory neurotransmission. The GABA-gated ion channel upon activation selectively conducts Cl^- through its pore. The $GABA_A$ receptor contains the binding site for GABA that also binds several drugs such as bicuculline. Moreover, the channel activity may be allosterically modulated by a number of drugs. The following protocol describes preparation of cellular membrane fractions from HEK293 cells expressing transmembrane $GABA_A$ ($\alpha5$, $\beta2$, $\gamma2$) receptors.

1. Wash the adherent cells 3× with PBS.

2. Detach cells from the culture surface with 1 mM EDTA-PBS (pH 7.4).

3. Centrifuge 15 ml of the cell suspension (at least 6.7×10^6 cells/ml density) at $200 \times g$ for 10 min at 4 °C (*see* **Note 6**).

4. Resuspend the pellets in tenfold volume (approximately 200 µl) of ice-cold buffered saline containing protease inhibitors (applied according to the manufacturer's instruction).

5. Rupture cells by three freezing-thawing cycles using a dry ice for 2 min and 37 °C water bath for 5 min (*see* **Note 7**).

6. Centrifuge the suspension at $1,100 \times g$ for 10 min at 4 °C to remove larger cell debris and nuclei.

7. Centrifuge supernatant at $21,000 \times g$ for 20 min at 4 °C to sediment mitochondria (*see* **Note 8**).

8. Use the supernatant containing fragments of mixed cellular membranes in the OWLS assays (*see* **Note 9**).

3.3 Application of Cell-Derived Membrane Fraction onto the PTFE/PET Membranes

1. Mix 50 µl aliquot of the cell membrane fraction (obtained in Section 3.2) with equal volume of liposomes (obtained in Section 3.1) and incubate at room temperature for 2 h.

2. Cut out the PTFE and the PET membranes to appropriate size (12 mm × 8 mm) to fit the OWLS chip and put into the Cl^--free ACSF buffer.

3. Place a piece of PET membrane onto a sensor surface with carefully preventing ingress of air bubbles (*see* **Note 10**).

4. Layer a piece of the PTFE membrane above the PET membrane with carefully preventing ingress of air bubbles (*see* **Note 10**).

5. Place the OWLS chip with membranes into the sensor holder.

6. Inject 100 µl of mixed liposome-cell membrane suspension into the OWLS cuvette using Hamilton syringe, and incubate it for 2 h at room temperature (*see* **Note 11**).

7. After sedimentation, wash the cuvette with Cl^--free ACSF until stable NTM and NTE values.

3.4 Application of Compounds Affecting Ion Channel Activity

1. Prepare a solution of 100 µM GABA in ACSF buffer (Cl^--containing).

2. Prepare a solution of 100 µM bicuculline in ACSF buffer (Cl^--containing) (*see* **Note 2**).

3. Prepare a solution of 100 µM GABA and 100 µM bicuculline in ACSF buffer (Cl^--containing) (*see* **Note 2**).

4. Inject the above three test solutions consecutively into the flow stream of Cl^--free ACSF. Start each injection after the return of the original NTM and NTE baseline (Fig. 1).

3.5 OWLS Assay [29]

The OW 2400 sensor chip, used in the OWLS110 biosensor system, consists of a 12 mm×8 mm substrate glass slide covered with a thin SiO_2-TiO_2 waveguide film (refractive index: nf = 1.77 ± 0.03) with a 12 mm×2 mm optical grating (2,400 lines/mm). The optical grating incouples the light of a He-Ne laser at a given resonance angle into the waveguide layer [30, 31]. Total internal reflection of light creates an evanescent field in a small (typically 150–200 nm) sensing volume above the sensor surface, decreasing exponentially with the distance from the waveguide. Incoupling is a resonance phenomenon that occurs at two well-defined angles of incidence of the laser beam: one for transverse electric (TE) and the other for transverse magnetic (TM) mode. This angle depends on optical features of the sensor surface (optical grating on the surface and refractive index of the sensor layer) and on the refractive index of the medium covering the surface of the waveguide. By varying the angle of incidence of the laser light, the spectrum (both electric and magnetic modes) can be obtained, from which the effective refractive indices and, in turn, analyte concentrations in the medium are calculated [32]. To accelerate detection velocity, chose one side (positive or negative) of the obtained spectrum with two bigger peaks (NTM and NTE) and select a range of $\pm0.2°$ around the incoupling angles; thus 10 data points/min can be reached.

The glass sensor chip is placed on the sensor holder (type SH-0812-08) and is tightened to its sealing O-ring. The sensor

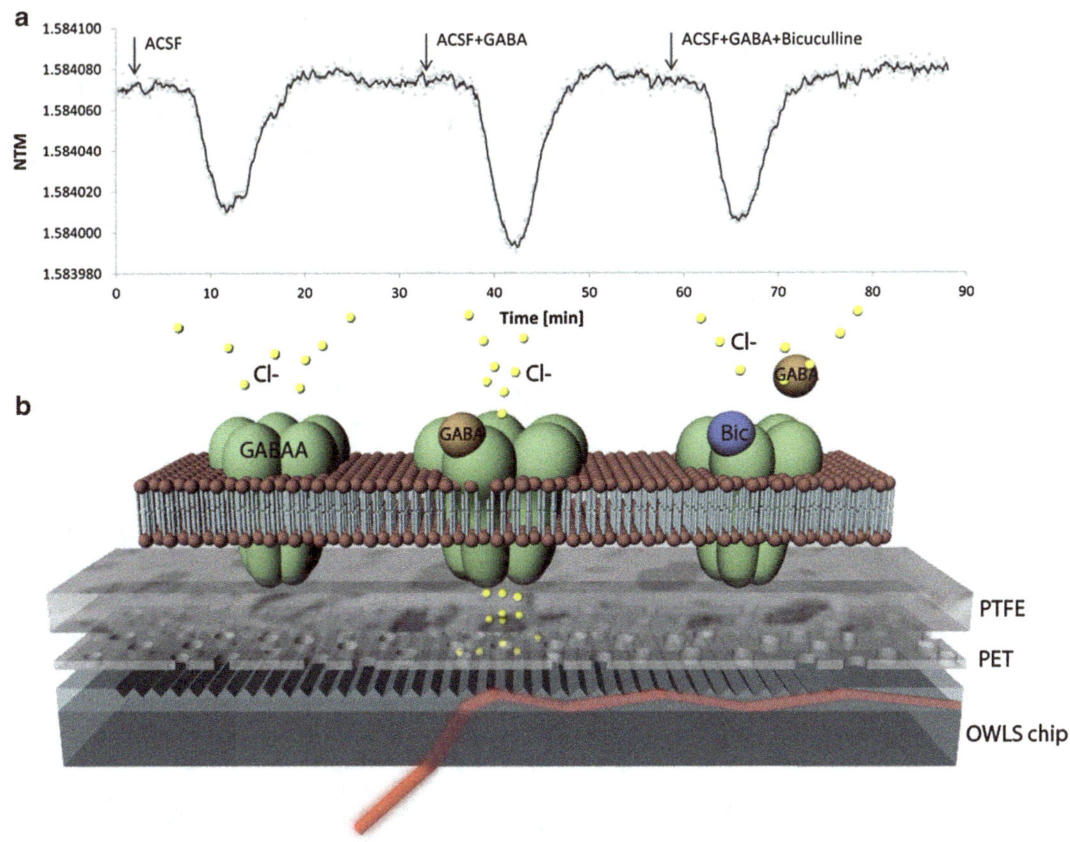

Fig. 1 Demonstration of Cl⁻ channel functions of cell-derived GABA_A receptors in the membrane-supported OWLS sensor setup. (**a**) Representative OWLS NTM recording in Cl⁻-free ACSF running buffer with injection of Cl⁻-containing ACSF without GABA (ACSF) (*left*), with GABA (ACSF + GABA) (*middle*), and with GABA and channel blocker bicuculline (ACSF + GABA + bicuculline) (*right*). (**b**) Illustration of the OWLS sensor setup for supported cell-derived membrane fragments containing GABA_A channel. A thick PTFE membrane is placed on the top of a thin PET membrane for complete separation of lipid material from the sensor surface. Closed GABA_A channel in ACSF running buffer in the absence of GABA (*left*), open GABA_A channel (allowing Cl⁻ influx) in the presence of GABA (*middle*), closed GABA_A channel in the presence of GABA antagonist bicuculline competing GABA off the receptor site (*left*)

holder forms a flow cell above the glass sensor with a volume of 12 μl. The glass sensor chip and the sensor holder form an integrated unit, which is placed in the OWLS instrument during measurement. All assays are carried out in a flow-injection system at continuous buffer flow at a rate of 23 μl/min, and 22 °C, with continuous recording of both NTE and NTM signals in the OWLS system in all individual experiments. Background signal corresponding to the refractive index of the Cl⁻-free ACSF buffer (baseline) is recorded in the absence of GABA_A channel agonists or antagonists. Signal development upon injection of 100 μl aliquots of a given test solution into the running buffer stream through the injector valve is recorded in time, and signal intensity is followed in each injection experiment until the baseline is stabilized again (Fig. 1). From the measured mode spectra deposited mass, refractive indices, effective refractive indices, and thickness of deposited material on the sensor surface can be determined using BioSense application.

4   Notes

1. *Warning*: To avoid contamination of the Cl⁻-free ACSF buffer with Cl⁻ ions, do not use HCl if acidification is required. Use $NaHCO_3$ instead.

2. Prepare 100 mM stock solution of bicuculline in dimethyl sulfoxide (DMSO), and dissolve this stock solution 1:1,000 in ACSF buffer to obtain the working concentration of bicuculline of 100 μM. Thus, the maximal concentration of DMSO in the final working solution is 0.1 %, known as not affecting the measurement. Working solutions should be prepared and used on the same day due to the extreme instability of bicuculline at physiological pH. Store stock solutions as aliquots in tightly sealed vials at –20 °C up to 1 month.

3. A $GABA_A$-expressing cell line reported previously in this sensor format [12] was human embryonic kidney (HEK293) cell line, expressing α5, β2, and γ2 subunits of human $GABA_A$ receptors (established by researchers of EGIS Pharmaceutical Inc., Hungary). Human $GABA_A$ (α5, β2, γ2) receptor cell line can be also purchased from ChanTest (Cleveland, Ohio; Catalog #: CT6119).

4. Texas Red-labeled liposomes are used to check the lipid coverage of the holder membrane by fluorescence microscope. Store Texas Red desiccated at –20 °C, and protect Texas Red and Texas Red-labeled liposomes from light.

5. Prepare liposomes in the same buffer as the running buffer to avoid refractive index changes due to possible differences in ionic strength.

6. The cell pellets can be frozen at this point if necessary or be directly used for membrane preparation.

7. Alternatively, the cells may be homogenized.

8. Purity of the preparation may be further improved by additional centrifugation of the supernatant at $100,000 \times g$ for 1 h and subsequent resuspension of the pellet in buffer.

9. If samples are not being analyzed immediately, store at –20 °C until assaying.

10. Air bubbles in the system can dramatically change optical sensing. To avoid the ingress of air bubbles between the sensor surface and the PET membrane, as well as between the two (PET and PTFE) membranes, put one drop of Cl⁻-free ACSF buffer onto the sensor surface, and carefully layer the PET membrane on it; and again put another drop of the buffer onto the PET membrane, and carefully layer the PTFE membrane on it. To avoid desiccation of the membranes, assemble the cuvette immediately upon placing the membrane sheets.

11. The supported lipid bilayer prepared by this method, of course, does not eliminate the possibility of the presence of intact liposomes on the membrane support, despite the washing procedure that is supposed to remove all excess liposomes. This, however, does not represent a problem in the measurement process, as even unruptured liposomes improve the insulation of supported layer.

Acknowledgments

The author expresses her sincere appreciation to her coworkers in the study that resulted in the original publication related to this protocol report. Particular thanks are due to Emilia Madarász (Institute of Experimental Medicine, Hungarian Academy of Sciences, Budapest, Hungary), István Szendrő and Katalin Erdélyi (Microvacuum Ltd., Budapest, Hungary), Pál Gróf and Nóra Kaszás (Semmelweis University, Budapest, Hungary), as well as Ferenc A. Anthony, Balázs Mihalik, and Ágnes Pataki (EGIS Pharmaceutical Co., Budapest, Hungary) for their contribution, technical support, and helpful discussions in the OWLS technique, liposome preparation, and HEK293 cell line, expressing GABAA ($\alpha5$, $\beta2$, $\gamma2$) receptors, respectively. The material support by Oxyphen GmbH (Zürich, Switzerland) by providing samples of RoTrack membranes is also acknowledged.

References

1. Fang Y (2007) Label-free optical biosensors in drug discovery. Trends Bio/Pharm Ind 3:34–38

2. Cornell BA, Braach-Maksvytis VLB, King LG, Osman PDJ, Raguse B, Wieczorek L, Pace RJ (1997) A biosensor that uses ion-channel switches. Nature 387:580–583. doi:10.1038/42432

3. Misra N, Martinez JA, Huang SCJ, Wang Y, Stroeve P, Grigoropoulos CP, Noy A (2009) Bioelectronic silicon nanowire devices using functional membrane proteins. Proc Natl Acad Sci U S A 106:13780–13784. doi:10.1073/pnas.0904850106

4. Wright LS, Harding MM (2000) Detection of DNA via an ion channel switch biosensor. Anal Biochem 282:70–79. doi:10.1006/abio.2000.4568

5. He L, Robertson JWF, Li J, Kärcher I, Schiller SM, Knoll W, Naumann R (2005) Tethered

bilayer lipid membranes based on monolayers of thiolipids mixed with a complementary dilution molecule. 1. Incorporation of channel peptides. Langmuir 21:11666–11672. doi:10.1021/la051771p

6. Brändén M, Dahlin S, Höök F (2008) Label-free measurements of molecular transport across liposome membranes using evanescent-wave sensing. ChemPhysChem 9:2480–2485. doi:10.1002/cphc.200800614

7. Mayer M, Kriebel JK, Tosteson MT, Whitesides GM (2003) Microfabricated Teflon membranes for low-noise recordings of ion channels in planar lipid bilayers. Biophys J 85:2684–2695. doi:10.1016/S0006-3495(03)74691-8

8. Yin P, Burns CJ, Osman PDJ, Cornell BA (2003) A tethered bilayer sensor containing alamethicin channels and its detection of amiloride based inhibitors. Biosens Bioelectron 18:389–397. doi:10.1016/S0956-5663(02)00160-4

9. Bayley H (1999) Designed membrane channels and pores. Curr Opin Biotechnol 10:94–103. doi:10.1016/S0958-1669(99)80017-2

10. Majd S, Yusko EC, Billeh YN, Macrae MX, Yang J, Mayer M (2010) Applications of biological pores in nanomedicine, sensing, and nanoelectronics. Curr Opin Biotechnol 21:439–476. doi:10.1016/j.copbio.2010.05.002

11. Ramsden J, Hucho F, Vogel H (1992) Membrane protein receptors in supported lipid bilayers as biosensors. In: Scheller F, Schmid RD (eds) Biosensors: fundamentals, technologies and applications, vol 17, Gbf Monographs. VCH Publishers, New York, pp 435–441

12. Székács I, Kaszás N, Gróf P, Erdélyi K, Szendrő I, Mihalik B, Pataki A, Antoni FA, Madarász E (2013) Optical waveguide lightmode spectroscopic techniques for investigating membrane-bound ion channel activities. PLoS One 8:12013. doi:10.1371/journal.pone.0081398

13. Bally M, Bailey K, Sugihara K, Grieshaber D, Vörös J, Städler B (2010) Liposome and bilayer arrays towards biosensing applications. Small 6:2481–2497. doi:10.1002/smll.201000644

14. Heimburg T (2010) Lipid ion channels. Biophys Chem 150:2–22. doi:10.1016/j.bpc.2010.02.018

15. Castellana ET, Cremer PS (2006) Solid supported lipid bilayers: from biophysical studies to sensor design. Surf Sci Rep 61:429–444

16. Richter RP, Bérat R, Brisson AR (2006) Formation of solid-supported lipid bilayers: an integrated view. Langmuir 22:3497–3505. doi:10.1021/la052687c

17. Heyse S, Vogel H, Sänger M, Sigrist H (1995) Covalent attachment of functionalized lipid bilayers to planar waveguides for measuring protein binding to biomimetic membranes. Protein Sci 4:2532–2544. doi:10.1002/pro.5560041210

18. Kugler R, Knoll W (2002) Polyelectrolyte-supported lipid membranes. Bioelectrochemistry 56:175–178. doi:10.1016/S1567-5394(02)00031-2

19. Jadhav SR, Sui D, Garavito RM, Worden RM (2008) Fabrication of highly insulating tethered bilayer lipid membrane using yeast cell membrane fractions for measuring ion channel activity. J Colloid Interf Sci 322:465–472. doi:10.1016/j.jcis.2008.02.064

20. Kitta M, Tanaka H, Kawai T (2009) Rapid fabrication of Teflon micropores for artificial lipid bilayer formation. Biosens Bioelectron 25:931–934. doi:10.1016/j.bios.2009.08.021

21. Phung T, Zhang Y, Dunlop J, Dalziel J (2011) Bilayer lipid membranes supported on Teflon filters: a functional environment for ion channels. Biosens Bioelectron 26:3127–3135. doi:10.1016/j.bios.2010.12.013

22. Neher E, Sakmann B (1992) The patch clamp technique. Sci Am 266:44–51

23. Homola J (2006) Surface plasmon resonance based sensors. Springer, Berlin

24. Vörös J, Ramsden JJ, Csúcs G, Szendro I, De Paul SM, Textor M, Spencer ND (2002) Optical grating coupler biosensors. Biomaterials 23:3699–3710

25. Merz C, Knoll W, Textor M, Reimhult E (2008) Formation of supported bacterial lipid membrane mimics. Biointerphases 3:FA41–FA50. doi:10.1116/1.2896119

26. Horváth R, Fricsovszky G, Papp E (2003) Application of the optical waveguide lightmode spectroscopy to monitor lipid bilayer phase transition. Biosens Bioelectron 18:415–428. doi:10.1016/S0956-5663(02)00154-9

27. Sugihara K, Delai M, Szendro I, Guillaume-Gentil O, Vörös J, Zambelli T (2012) Simultaneous OWLS and EIS monitoring of supported lipid bilayers with the pore forming peptide melittin. Sensor Actuat B Chem 161:600–606. doi:10.1016/j.snb.2011.11.007

28. Moscho A, Orwar O, Chiu DT, Modi BP, Zare RN (1996) Rapid preparation of giant unilamellar vesicles. Proc Natl Acad Sci U S A 93:11443–11447

29. MicroVacuum. http://owls-sensors.com. Accessed Sep 2014

30. Tiefenthaler K, Lukosz W (1989) Sensitivity of grating couplers as integrated-optical chemical sensors. J Opt Soc Am B 6:209–220

31. Ramsden J (1993) Review of new experimental techniques for investigating random sequential adsorption. J Stat Phys 73: 853–877

32. Székács A, Adányi N, Székács I, Majer-Baranyi K, Szendro I (2009) Optical waveguide light-mode spectroscopy immunosensors for environmentalmonitoring.ApplOpt48:B151–B158. doi:10.1364/AO.48.00B151

Part III

Cell Phenotypic Profiling and Screening

Label-Free Profiling of Endogenous Receptor Responses in Primary Isolated Cardiac Cells

Douglas G. Tilley, Ashley A. Repas, and Rhonda L. Carter

Abstract

Label-free detection systems have been available and utilized for several years in the pharmacological exploration of receptor responses to ligand stimulation. While a vast majority of studies have investigated signaling responses in cell lines stably expressing a receptor of interest, relatively fewer studies have used label-free technology to examine endogenous receptor responses in primary cells with more physiologic relevance. The exploration of cardiac receptor biology is fraught with challenges, primarily stemming from the difficulty in maintaining isolated adult cardiac myocytes under cell culture conditions in sufficient quantity and for extended periods that may be required for various assays. However, isolated rat neonatal cardiac myocytes and fibroblasts offer an alternate approach that allows in vitro investigation of primary cardiac cells for several days to weeks. For use with label-free technologies, primary cardiac cells provide a unique opportunity to explore the impact of various ligands on endogenous cardiac receptor responses, which in the case of myocytes may also be directly applicable to regulation of contractile function. In this chapter we provide a detailed methodology for the isolation of primary cardiac myocytes and fibroblasts and discuss their use in label-free assays, using the Epic BT resonant waveguide grating biosensor system as an example, with a particular consideration toward cardiac cell density and phenotypic modulation of cells in culture.

Key words Cardiac fibroblast, Cardiac myocyte, Cell phenotype, Endogenous receptors, Primary cell isolation, Resonant waveguide grating biosensor

---

1   Introduction

Label-free platforms, increasingly common in basic science research, allow an agnostic approach to determine the overall biological response to ligand stimulation, which can be compared across ligands and dissected with various pharmacologic or genetic tools. Cardiovascular pharmacology studies have long relied upon specific signaling readouts to define their importance in the regulation of cardiac function, which may not be representative or indicative of the overall contribution of various pathways to the response. Thus, label-free systems provide an invaluable resource with which to explore cellular responses to ligand stimulation in primary isolated cardiac cells.

Ye Fang (ed.), *Label-Free Biosensor Methods in Drug Discovery*, Methods in Pharmacology and Toxicology, DOI 10.1007/978-1-4939-2617-6_9, © Springer Science+Business Media New York 2015

Rat neonatal cardiac fibroblasts (RNCF) and myocytes (RNCM) are widely used in cardiovascular research to understand the impact of various ligands and receptor systems at the cellular level, though with the recognition that the results attained do not necessarily represent those of a fully differentiated adult cardiac cell. However, as primary cardiac cells, they are relatively simple to attain and maintain in cell culture for several days. In the case of RNCF, the cells may be passaged several times and maintained in cell culture for weeks, with the caveat that they undergo modulation toward a myofibroblast phenotype [1]. Of note, this property can be exploited to study changes in primary cardiac fibroblast responses to various ligands throughout different stages of phenotypic switch. RNCM can be maintained in culture for a few days, and if isolated and seeded properly will begin to beat spontaneously, a property that can also be used to assess signaling responses to various pharmacologic agents via label-free systems.

This chapter describes in detail the methodology used to isolate and culture primary RNCF and RNCM for use in label-free assays, with specific examples provided using β-adrenergic receptor (βAR) and epidermal growth factor receptor (EGFR) responses to ligands as measured via dynamic mass redistribution (DMR) with the Epic BT resonant waveguide grating (RWG) biosensor system. Special considerations for cell density and passaging are highlighted.

2 Materials

2.1 Buffers and Cell Culture Media

1. *ADS Buffer*: ADS buffer is prepared in advance (Table 1) and stored at 4 °C until required. Following preparation of ADS buffer, adjust pH to 7.35 using 10 N NaOH, sterile filter, and store at 4 °C.

Table 1
Components required for 1 L ADS buffer

Component	Quantity	Final concentration
NaCl	6.78 g	116 mM
HEPES	4.76 g	20 mM
Na_2HPO_4	0.1136 g	0.8 mM
Glucose	1.01 g	5.6 mM
KCl	0.4026 g	5.4 mM
$MgSO_4 \cdot 7H_2O$	0.1792 g	0.8 mM
H_2O	To 1 L	–

Table 2
Components required for 70 mL ADS enzyme solution

Component	Quantity	Final concentration
Pancreatin (Sigma Cat# P3292)	42 mg	0.6 mg/mL
Collagenase II (Worthington Cat# LS004176)	17,500 U (*see* **Note 1**)	250 U/mL
CaCl$_2$ (50 mM stock)	35 µL	25 µM
ADS buffer	To 70 mL	–

Table 3
Components required for 500 mL F-10 complete media

Component	10 % HS/5 % FBS (mL)	5 % FBS (mL)	0 % FBS (mL)
Horse serum (HS)	50	0	0
Fetal bovine serum (FBS)	25	25	0
Antibiotic-antimycotic (100×)	5	5	5
F-10 Medium (Corning Cellgro)	420	470	495

2. *ADS Enzyme Solution*: Enzymes should be added to required amount of ADS buffer fresh on the day of the cell isolation procedure (Table 2). 70 mL can be made in one Erlenmeyer flask for use in the digestion of hearts from two litters of neonatal rat pups. Place ADS enzyme solution in rotator at 4 °C for 1 h or until all crystals have dissolved, then sterile filter, and keep in tissue culture hood for use in primary cell isolation and preparation.

3. *F-10 Complete Media*: Required for RNCM and is prepared in advance and stored at 4 °C. Different % serum concentrations required for post-isolation RNCM culture steps in the procedure are indicated in Table 3.

4. *Minimal Essential Medium (MEM) Complete Media*: Required for RNCF and is prepared in advance and stored at 4 °C. Different % serum concentrations required for post-isolation RNCF culture steps in the procedure are indicated in Table 4.

2.2 DMR Assay Buffer, Microplates, and Instruments

1. Hanks' Balanced Salt Solution (HBSS): 1× with calcium and magnesium, but no phenol red.
2. HEPES buffer: 1 M HEPES, pH 7.1.

Table 4
Components required for 500 mL MEM complete media

Component	10 % FBS (mL)	5 % FBS (mL)	0 % FBS (mL)
Fetal bovine serum (FBS)	50	25	0
Antibiotic-antimycotic (100×)	5	5	5
MEM (Corning Cellgro)	445	470	495

3. Assay-buffered vehicle solution: 1× HBSS, 10 mM HEPES, pH 7.1.

4. Corning® Epic® 384 well fibronectin-coated cell assay microplate (Corning Incorporated, Corning, NY, USA).

5. Corning 384-well polypropylene compound storage plate.

6. Matrix 16-channel electronic pipettor (Thermo Fisher Scientific, Hudson, NH).

7. Epic® BT system (Corning).

3 Methods

3.1 Preparation for Primary Cardiac Cell Isolation

For the isolation of primary cardiac myocytes and fibroblasts from rat neonates, proper sterile technique is essential to ensure that the cells do not become contaminated from the materials used, or carcasses generated, during the procedure, which could negatively impact cell recovery, cell growth, and study outcomes.

1. Place F-10 complete media and 50 mL FBS in water bath at 37 °C.

2. Fill 1 L and 500 mL beakers with 500 mL and 300 mL of 70 % ethanol, respectively.

3. Sterilize cell culture hood by wiping down with 70 % ethanol.

4. Place absorbent pad and biohazard carcass bag in culture hood.

5. Wipe down solution bottles (ADS buffer, ADS enzyme solution, F-10 complete media, MEM complete media) and materials (scissors, razor, forceps, flasks, 50 mL conicals, culture plates) with 70 % ethanol and place in culture hood.

3.2 Isolation of Rat Neonatal Hearts

The purpose of this section is to excise, clean, and mince rat neonate hearts in preparation for enzymatic digestion. It is essential to perform these steps with clean, sterile tools and materials in a sterile culture hood and prevent contamination of the freshly isolated hearts by contact with neonates/carcasses that have not been dipped in EtOH.

1. Add 7 mL ADS buffer and 7 mL ADS enzyme solution to bottom portion of a 10 cm plate.

2. Add 10 mL ADS buffer to the top portion of a 10 cm plate (not on ice).

3. Dip each pup into medium-sized beaker containing 300 mL of 70 % EtOH.

4. Decapitate pups with large scissors, heads into biohazard bags.

5. Dip each body into the large-sized beaker containing 500 mL of 70 % EtOH.

6. Make an incision from neckline down toward abdomen with small scissors over a 15 cm plate; holding arms back will allow the heart to emerge from excision site.

7. Place excised hearts in 10 cm plate with 10 mL ADS buffer.

8. Remove any extra tissue/atria/blood clots from the hearts and transfer to the 10 cm plate containing ADS buffer/enzyme solution.

9. Using a razor and forceps, cut each heart into small pieces (at least six).

10. Transfer the minced hearts in the ADS buffer/enzyme solution to a 125 mL Erlenmeyer flask with stopper; make sure that stopper is tight fitted (*see* **Note 2**).

3.3 Digestion of Rat Neonatal Hearts

Digestion of the heart tissue will ultimately provide isolated cardiac myocytes and fibroblasts for culture; however only healthy cells will survive and attach to the culture plates once isolated. To ensure healthy yields of cells one must be mindful to perform the steps gently and consider the importance of cell viability versus absolute number of cells attained from the digest.

1. Shake flask at 55 rpm in 37 °C shaking water bath for 10 min.

2. Add 15 mL F-10 complete media and 4 mL FBS to each of 4× 50 mL conicals and place in a 37 °C humidified incubator with 5 % CO_2 with caps loosely tightened.

3. Remove flask from shaking water bath and carefully aspirate and discard supernatant.

4. Add 10 mL ADS enzyme solution and pipette up and down 6–7 times with a 25 mL pipette (*see* **Note 3**).

5. Shake flask at 55 rpm in 37 °C shaking water bath for 15 min.

6. Transfer supernatant to one of the 50 mL conicals and put in the incubator with a loose-fitting cap.

7. Repeat steps 3–5 three more times (*see* **Note 4**).

3.4 Isolation of RNCM and RNCF

The purpose of this step is to concentrate and isolate the cardiac cells attained via enzymatic digestion from the remaining heart tissue, and commence separation of the myocytes and fibroblasts.

To attain the best yield of isolated cells possible, care must be taken to perform the cell filtration slowly.

1. Centrifuge the 4× 50 mL conicals at 1,000 rpm for 5 min.

2. Aspirate and discard supernatants from each conical.

3. Gently resuspend each pellet in 4 mL FBS with a 10 mL pipette and combine into one tube.

4. Centrifuge cells at 1,000 rpm for 5 min.

5. Place a 70 µm cell strainer onto a clean 50 mL conical and prime with 1 mL F-10 complete media.

6. Aspirate supernatant when cells are done spinning.

7. Resuspend pellet in 5 mL F-10 complete media for one litter, and 8 mL for two litters.

8. SLOWLY (dropwise) strain cells into primed conical (*see* **Note 5**).

9. Wash the pellet conical in ~2 mL F-10 complete media for 1 L (or 4 mL for 2 L) and put through cell strainer slowly.

10. Wash the strainer with ~2 mL F-10 complete media for 1 L (or 4 mL for two litters).

11. Add contents of conical to Nunc NUNCLON DELTA 10 cm plates (1 plate per litter) and incubate for 1 h 45 min (*see* **Note 6**).

12. Put MEM complete media for RNCF in 37 °C water bath to warm up during this incubation step.

3.5 Separation of RNCM and RNCF

At this stage, the cardiac myocytes are separated from the fibroblasts. Keep in mind that the purity of each cell population can vary depending on the length of time given for the incubation step.

1. Slowly pipette the media from the Nunc plate up and down five times to gently, but thoroughly, wash the plate and transfer to a new 50 mL conical.

2. Repeat wash step with an additional 4 mL F-10 complete media to ensure removal of all RNCM and add to the same 50 mL conical (*see* **Note 7**).

3. Add 8 mL MEM complete media to Nunc plate now enriched with RNCF and place in a 37 °C humidified incubator with 5 % CO_2.

3.6 Seeding of RNCM in DMR Assay Plates

In this step, freshly isolated primary RNCM are seeded into the DMR assay plate, where they will be maintained in culture for up to 3 days. The primary considerations to ultimately attain successful DMR responses with the RNCM preparation are to seed the cells at an appropriate density and perform the necessary media replacement steps.

1. Obtain a cell count from the RNCM/F-10 complete media suspension to calculate volume of suspension required to seed 2×10^4 cells in 40 μL per well of a 384-well DMR assay plate (*see* **Notes 8** and **9**).

2. Seed RNCM at 2×10^4 cells per 40 μL in each well of a Corning® Epic® 384 Well Fibronectin-Coated Cell Assay Microplate (*see* **Note 10**).

3. Once RNCM are seeded, store microplate in a 37 °C humidified incubator with 5 % CO_2.

4. After 24 h, remove media from wells and replace with 40 μL per well of F-10 complete media (5 % FBS) (*see* **Note 11**).

5. 24 h prior to label-free assay, remove 5 % FBS-containing media from wells, replace with 40 μL per well of serum-free F-10 media (*see* **Notes 11** and **12**), and return microplate to 37 °C humidified incubator with 5 % CO_2 overnight.

3.7 Seeding of RNCF in DMR Assay Plates

Unlike RNCM, RNCF can be maintained in culture for weeks and passaged several times. Depending on the study goals, it may be desirable to test the DMR responses in RNCF at various passages. However, the steps below specifically outline the procedure for seeding primary RNCF to perform the DMR assay within the same time frame as RNCM. As with RNCM, cell density and media replacement are important considerations.

1. 24 h following RNCF isolation, replace the MEM complete media (10 % FBS) with 5 % FBS-containing MEM (*see* **Note 13**).

2. 24 h prior to label-free assay, remove media, rinse with serum-free MEM, add 5 mL trypsin-EDTA, and place in a 37 °C humidified incubator with 5 % CO_2 for 5–10 min, after which the cells will detach.

3. Transfer cell suspension to a 15 mL conical and centrifuge for 3 min at 1,000 rpm. Aspirate the supernatant and resuspend the pellet in 10 mL of 5 % FBS-containing MEM.

4. After attaining a cell count, seed RNCF using a microplate dispenser to attain 2×10^4 cells/per well in 40 μL into Corning® Epic® 384 Well Fibronectin-Coated Cell Assay Microplates (*see* **Note 9**) and return to 37 °C humidified incubator with 5 % CO_2.

5. After 4–6 h, replace the 5 % FBS-containing MEM with serum-free MEM and return to humidified incubator overnight (*see* **Note 12**).

3.8 Preparation of DMR Plates for Assay

By this stage in the process, the primary cardiac cells have been seeded in the assay plates, possibly pretreated with G protein uncouplers for a prolonged period, and are ready for testing. The main consideration here is to allow the microplate to equilibrate following buffer replacement to allow baseline DMR levels to normalize prior to addition of test agents.

1. On the day of assay, remove media from microplate wells and rinse three times with pre-warmed (37 °C) HBSS containing 20 mM HEPES (40 µL/well).

2. Following the final addition of HBSS/HEPES buffer, allow microplate to equilibrate for 1 h in the EPIC® Benchtop (BT) system (Corning®) at 37 °C.

3.9 Drug Additions and EPIC® BT Settings

This is the final step in the use of primary cardiac cells for the measurement of DMR responses to stimulation of endogenous receptors. The main consideration at this stage is that all required buffer/vehicle/agonist/antagonist controls are included in the study design to allow proper data analysis following completion of the assay.

1. Set scan speed and begin run; a scan speed of 3 s/scan with 4 scans/data point results in each data point being attained every 12 s.

2. Attain baseline DMR readings for 5 min.

3. Pause the run.

4. Remove the microplate, and add the first set of compounds, 10 µL/well, using a liquid handler (5× concentrations of antagonists or buffer/vehicle controls).

5. Return the microplate to the EPIC BT system.

6. Resume the run for another 30 min.

7. Pause the run again.

8. Remove the microplate, and add the second set of compounds, 10 µL/well, using the liquid handler (6× concentrations of agonists or buffer/vehicle controls).

9. Return the microplate to EPIC BT system and resume run, capturing data points for another 60 min, or until responses attained are sufficient for analysis, after which the run can be stopped.

10. Normalize DMR responses (change in pm shift) to compounds with corresponding buffer or antagonist additions for further analysis (*see* **Note 14**).

4 Notes

1. The U/mg of collagenase attained from suppliers varies from lot to lot; therefore the mg amount of collagenase required for ADS enzyme solution needs to be calculated specifically for each lot purchased.

2. When transferring the minced hearts in the ADS buffer/
   enzyme solution to an Erlenmeyer flask, *do not* pipette up and
   down to mix as this will destroy cardiomyocytes. A prolonged
   gentle digestion of the minced hearts as outlined in the protocol will provide a much higher yield of healthy cardiomyocytes
   than trying to break apart the heart pieces via pipetting.

3. In this step, the minced heart samples have undergone digestion with the ADS buffer/enzyme solution, which is removed
   and replaced with fresh ADS enzyme solution for further
   digestion. When resuspending the tissue/cell material at the
   bottom of the flask, a gentle pipetting up and down is beneficial to begin to mix the contents for better enzyme digestion.
   Pipetting up and down should only be done 6–7 times, again
   to prevent too much trauma to the cardiomyocytes. As this
   step is repeated, the solution should become more cloudy than
   chunky as the tissue becomes more thoroughly digested.

4. The replacement of ADS enzyme solution and repeated incubation at 37 °C in a shaking water bath for 15 min should be
   performed at least three times, but not more than five times. If
   repeated less, the tissue will not be digested as thoroughly,
   leading to a lower yield of cells. However, after each repeat of
   the digestion, the supernatant containing the digested cells is
   collected in a 50 mL conical and incubated at 37 °C until completion of the digestion steps. Therefore, the more the digestion steps are repeated, the longer the cells sit prior to plating,
   increasing the chance of cell death and lowering the overall
   yield of healthy cells at the completion of the isolation procedure. Thus, five repeats of the digestion steps should be the
   maximal number performed. Only four 50 mL conicals are
   prepared for collecting the supernatant after each digestion
   step; therefore if a fifth digestion is performed, the final supernatant collected should be split evenly among the four conicals
   prior to centrifugation.

5. It is important to add the resuspended cell/tissue solution
   SLOWLY into the strainer. Dropwise addition of the solution
   will allow prevent conglomeration of the remaining tissue
   chunks that would prevent the cells from passing efficiently
   through the strainer.

6. This step is essential for separating the RNCM and RNCF
   populations. The RNCF will preferentially adhere to the
   Nunc NUNCLON DELTA 10 cm plates, whereas the
   RNCM will not adhere and can be removed via pipetting off
   the solution after the incubation time. The time of incubation is important to consider as too long an incubation
   (>2 h) will allow RNCM to begin to adhere to the plate,
   thus reducing the yield. Conversely, too short an incubation

time (<1.5 h) will not allow efficient clearance of RNCF from the solution; if the cell solution collected at the end of the incubation contains both cell populations, the RNCF can quickly overgrow the RNCM.

7. DO NOT SPIN DOWN the 50 mL conical containing the harvested RNCM as this can destroy them, thereby reducing the yield of viable cells.

8. A typical digestion of the hearts from one to two litters of neonatal rats will yield approximately $2.5–4.0 \times 10^6$ RNCM/ mL. Therefore, the concentration of cells should end up higher than that required for seeding and can be adjusted via dilution. For even cell coverage of the microplate wells, it is recommended to seed the cells using a microplate dispenser rather than a repeater pipette.

9. For both RNCM and RNCF it is recommended to seed at a minimal density of at least 2×10^4 cells/well of a 384-well microplate. Cell density has been previously shown to play a significant role in determining the detected responses to ligand stimulation using label-free detection methods [2], and we have also demonstrated a cell density-dependent increase in DMR detection to βAR agonists, wherein the magnitude of DMR signal increased and variability decreased as RNCF density reached 2×10^4 cells/well at the time of seeding [3]. RNCF will proliferate in cell culture, so seeding at higher densities could lead to overcrowding and alterations in cell response to ligand. Seeding density is also an important consideration for attaining healthy RNCM preparations. Since primary cardiomyocytes do not proliferate in culture, seeding RNCM at a density of at least 2×10^4 cells/well will promote their survival and recovery of spontaneous beating. Both cell density and spontaneous beating of the RNCM can be observed in the wells through a light microscope. Further, RNCM spontaneous beating can be measured by label-free systems, as shown in Fig. 1a, and even altered by pharmacologically targeting components of the β-adrenergic receptor (βAR) signaling pathway. Spontaneous beating could be prevented by treatment of RNCM with the Gs protein uncoupler cholera toxin for 18 h (B) or via acute addition of the βAR antagonist propranolol (C), while acute treatment with the phosphodiesterase 4D inhibitor rolipram to prevent cAMP degradation (D) enhanced the beating.

10. When seeding primary cardiac cells for assessment with Corning's® Epic® BT the Corning® Epic® 384 Well Fibronectin-Coated Cell Assay Microplates are recommended for use as the fibronectin will aid in cell adherence. For RNCF this is

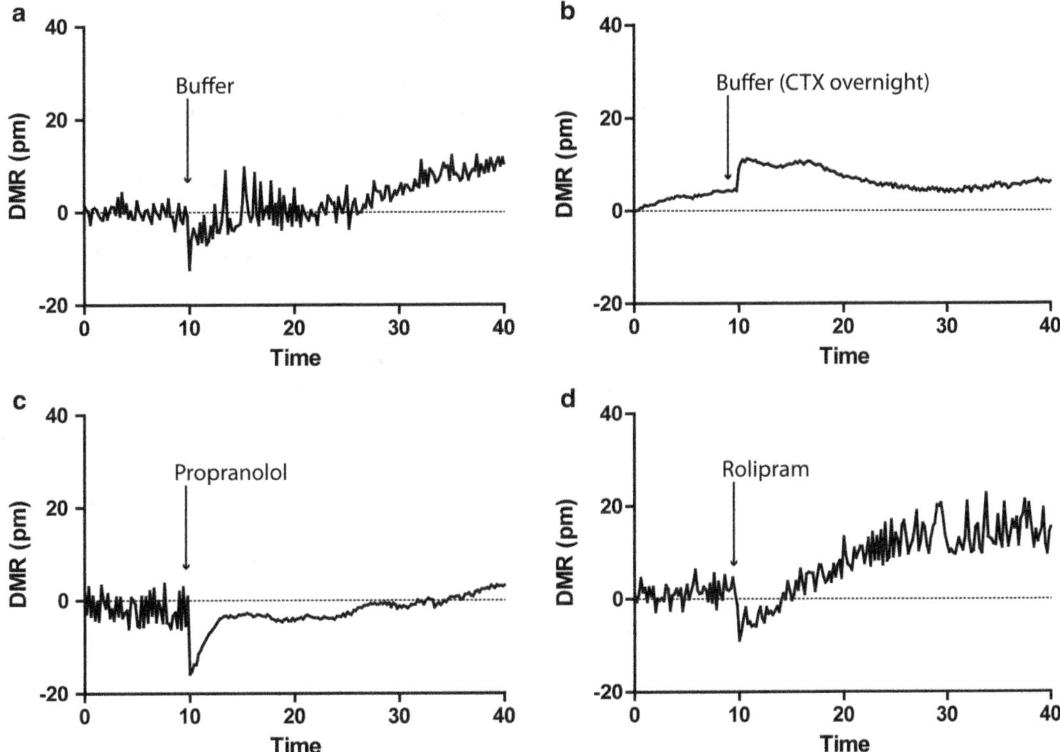

Fig. 1 Dynamic mass redistribution (DMR) tracings of RNCM spontaneous beating. RNCM were seeded at 2×10^4 cells/well in Corning® Epic® 384 Well Fibronectin-Coated Cell Assay Microplates. Baseline reads were obtained for 10 min prior to addition of buffer (0.1 % DMSO) or inhibitors. (**a**) Spontaneous beating of RNCM is observable in RNCM both before and after buffer addition. (**b**) RNCM treated with cholera toxin (CTX, 100 ng/mL for 18 h) did not have detectable spontaneous beating. (**c**) RNCM have spontaneous beating at baseline that is ablated upon addition of the βAR antagonist propranolol (1 μM). (**d**) Spontaneous beating of RNCM is enhanced following treatment with the phosphodiesterase 4D inhibitor rolipram (1 μM)

the substrate of choice. Fibronectin is not typically used for seeding primary cardiomyocytes, where collagen or laminin are more common substrates; however the RNCM do adhere well to the bottom of the fibronectin-coated microplates and will still attain the spontaneous beating typical of a successful cell isolation and seeding at an appropriate density.

11. Removal of the F-10 complete media (10 %HS/5 % FBS) and replacement with F-10 complete media (5 % FBS) 24 h after primary isolation are essential to reduce to the proliferative capacity of any RNCF that did not adhere to the Nunc plates during cell separation, thereby preventing their expansion and maintaining a culture of primarily RNCM. As discussed in **Note 9**, a successful healthy RNCM preparation should begin

to beat spontaneously. Areas where spontaneous beating is not present could represent contaminating RNCF. If this becomes a problem, the incubation time of the cells on the Nunc plates can be adjusted as discussed in **Note 6**. Further, serum can be reduced to 0.2 %, or withdrawn completely, for the last 18–24 h prior to label-free assay to ensure RNCF growth arrest.

12. If toxins (i.e., cholera toxin or pertussis toxin) are to be used to assess the impact of uncoupling G proteins on ligand responses in cardiac cells, they should be premixed with the serum-free media prior to addition to the wells to attain a final concentration of 100 ng/mL. An 18-h incubation should be sufficient to confirm G protein inhibition [3, 4] (Fig. 1b).

13. Primary RNCF can be maintained in culture for days to weeks; however, their phenotype becomes altered toward a myofibroblast phenotype over time [1]. As their phenotype becomes altered in vitro, receptor expression patterns and resulting responses to ligands may change. For instance, β2AR expression in RNCF decreased rapidly in culture, losing approximately 50 % of its expression by 6 days post-isolation, which correlated with a significant reduction in DMR response detected in response to βAR agonist stimulation [3]. Similarly, EGFR expression (Fig. 2a) and responsiveness (Fig. 2b, c) also decrease by about half in RNCF cultured for 6 days compared to 3 days post-isolation. Thus, careful characterization of how phenotypic modulation of primary RNCF may alter a pathway of interest should be taken into consideration for label-free assays and a consistent post-isolation time point selected to ensure consistent results. Conversely, the ability of primary RNCF to undergo phenotypic modulation in culture may provide an opportunity to explore how this process impacts endogenous signaling pathways over time.

14. Aside from phenotypic modulation that can alter endogenous responses to ligands, primary cardiac cells also are associated with biological variability due to their isolation from different batches of neonatal rat pups. Since primary cell preparations can also vary in terms of number and quality of cells attained, which can impact their responses to ligands [3], results obtained from an individual cell preparation should be considered a single experiment, regardless of how many replicates per compound are tested. Thus, an n of 3 would be attained from 3 distinct cell preparations. Consistent primary isolation will not only increase the yield of healthy cardiac cells but will also help decrease the variability of their biological responses to ligand stimulation.

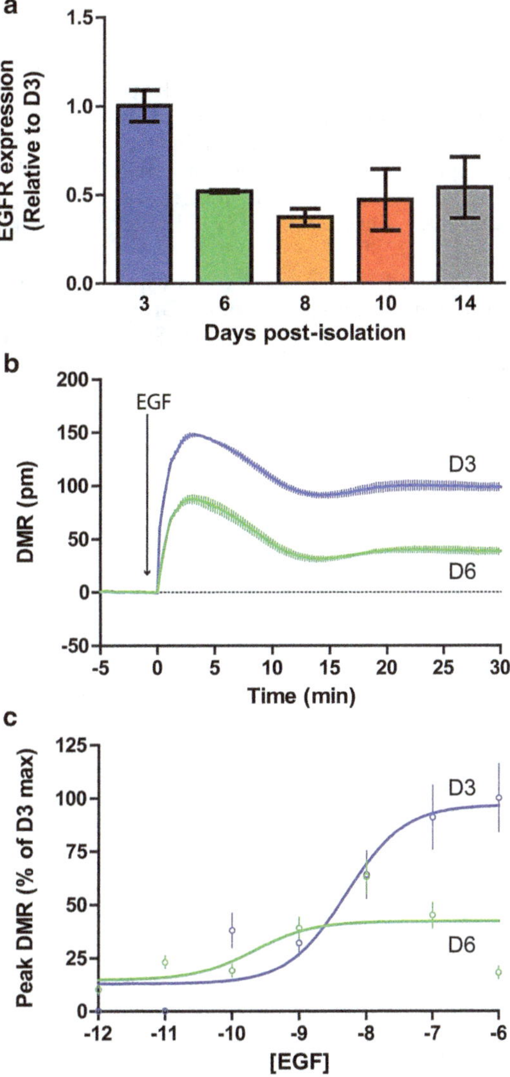

Fig. 2 Loss of responsiveness to epidermal growth factor in primary RNCF over days of in vitro cell culture. (**a**) Real-time PCR data show a rapid and sustained loss (~50 %) of detectable epidermal growth factor receptor (EGFR) gene expression following 3 days of primary RNCF culture. Real-time PCR was performed using assay primers for EGFR (Fwd: CCAAGCCCACTTGAGGATATT; Rev: TGGGATCCAGAGACCCTTATAC) and glyceraldehyde 3-phosphate dehydrogenase (GAPDH; Fwd: GCAAGCATACTGAGAGCAAGAG; Rev: GGATGGAATTGTGAGGGAGATG) at an annealing temperature of 60.0 °C. Data from samples were analyzed in triplicate. All RT-PCR data were analyzed using Applied Biosystems Comparative CT Method ($\Delta\Delta$CT) and EGFR gene expression analysis was normalized to GAPDH. Data are presented as relative quantity (RQ) values with RQmin and RQmax as error bars. (**b**) Dynamic mass redistribution (DMR, pm shift) responses in RNCF at 3 days and 6 days post-isolation were recorded following stimulation with EGF (100 nM), where D6 RNCF displayed a reduced response. Tracings are mean ± SEM ($n=3$). (**c**) Summarized concentration–DMR response curves for EGF in D3 versus D6 RNCF. Data are expressed as % of peak EGF (D3) response; mean ± SEM, $n=3$ per concentration point

References

1. Santiago JJ, Dangerfield AL, Rattan SG, Bathe KL, Cunnington RH, Raizman JE, Bedosky KM, Freed DH, Kardami E, Dixon IM (2010) Cardiac fibroblast to myofibroblast differentiation in vivo and in vitro: expression of focal adhesion components in neonatal and adult rat ventricular myofibroblasts. Dev Dyn 239(6):1573–1584. doi:10.1002/dvdy.22280

2. Fang Y (2006) Label-free cell-based assays with optical biosensors in drug discovery. Assay Drug Dev Technol 4(5):583–595. doi:10.1089/adt.2006.4.583

3. Carter RL, Grisanti LA, Yu JE, Repas AA, Woodall M, Ibetti J, Koch WJ, Jacobson MA, Tilley DG (2014) Dynamic mass redistribution analysis of endogenous beta-adrenergic receptor signaling in neonatal rat cardiac fibroblasts. Pharmacol Res Perspect 2(1):24. doi:10.1002/prp2.24

4. Schroder R, Janssen N, Schmidt J, Kebig A, Merten N, Hennen S, Muller A, Blattermann S, Mohr-Andra M, Zahn S, Wenzel J, Smith NJ, Gomeza J, Drewke C, Milligan G, Mohr K, Kostenis E (2010) Deconvolution of complex G protein-coupled receptor signaling in live cells using dynamic mass redistribution measurements. Nat Biotechnol 28(9):943–949. doi:10.1038/nbt.1671

Chapter 10

Surface Plasmon Resonance to Study Cell Signaling and GPCR Functional Selectivity in Live Cells

Philippe Bourassa, Thomas Söllradl, Jean-Sébastien Maltais, Paul G. Charette, Louis Gendron, and Michel Grandbois

Abstract

Surface plasmon resonance spectroscopy (SPR), a technique widely used for the study of biomolecular interactions, was recently demonstrated as a valuable label-free method to monitor live cell responses in real time. In contrast to molecular and biochemical assays, which rely on the detection of a unique marker such as cAMP, protein phosphorylation, or intracellular calcium, SPR is capable to detect and follow cell responses integrating the modulation of all signaling pathways. In recent studies, our group and others showed that SPR is a sensitive tool to study a broad range of cellular events on different timescales, ranging from rapid receptor-mediated responses (seconds to minutes) to long-lasting processes such as programmed cell death which typically occur over several hours. SPR allows the study of cellular responses evoked by different types of ligands through the analysis of parameters extracted from the SPR sensorgrams. For example, we previously showed that SPR allows the study of cellular responses evoked by the activation of G protein-coupled receptors (GPCRs) such as mu opioid receptor, protease-activated receptor-1, and angiotensin receptor type 1. Using pharmacological inhibitors it is possible to delineate the contribution of specific signaling pathways to the overall SPR response. Given the growing interest surrounding GPCR functional selectivity, this chapter describes how SPR spectroscopy can be used to study signaling cascades in living cells and, by way of consequence, functional selectivity.

Key words Cell signaling, G protein-coupled receptor, Functional selectivity, Living cells, Surface plasmon resonance, SPR sensorgram analysis

1 Introduction

Over the past decades, surface plasmon resonance spectroscopy (SPR) has emerged as a sensitive tool to study biomolecular interactions such as the binding affinity of a given ligand for its receptor [1, 2] or the detection of antibody–antigen interactions [3]. More recently, SPR was found to be a sensitive and reliable approach to study signaling pathways and their phenotypic outputs in living cells [4–9]. This is of particular interest with the emergence of functional selectivity, also known as biased signaling, a novel

Ye Fang (ed.), *Label-Free Biosensor Methods in Drug Discovery*, Methods in Pharmacology and Toxicology, DOI 10.1007/978-1-4939-2617-6_10, © Springer Science+Business Media New York 2015

183

concept of G protein-coupled receptor (GPCR) signaling [10] which assumes the existence of GPCR ligands able to activate distinct signaling pathways. With their ability to probe global and integrated cellular responses (i.e., multiple signaling cascades at once), label-free biosensing techniques such as SPR spectroscopy are well indicated in GPCR functional selectivity studies. In this perspective, multiple commercial optical based detection systems are available for label-free readout of cellular activity such as the BIND (SRU Biosystems) [11] and EPIC (Corning) [12]. Commercial SPR systems such as the Biacore (Biacore Life Sciences) and Horiba (HORIBA Scientific) are also available and could be easily adapted for the purpose of cell signal monitoring.

SPR is a phenomenon occurring at the interface between a metal (i.e., gold) and a dielectric material such as air, water, or any biological materials. SPR consists of the resonant excitation of surface plasmons by an optical radiation at the metallic surface, which results in a well-defined evanescent field protruding the dielectric medium. The evanescent field has a maximal intensity at the metal surface and decays exponentially away from the surface, yielding a probe range of ca. 200 nm above the interface when using visible wavelengths (Fig. 1a). If the refractive index properties of the interface change (e.g., when biomolecules or cells are present at the sensor surface), the plasmon resonance conditions change, which is the basis of SPR measurement. Thus, SPR has the ability to measure, in real time and label-free, biomolecular interactions or any other event leading to interfacial refractive index changes. Taking advantage of the label-free nature of SPR, it is possible to detect a wide array of cellular events, which is often an asset over selective biochemical assays. Indeed, virtually all cellular processes involving dynamic mass redistribution (i.e., membrane and/or protein movements) within the range of the evanescent field will generate a change in the interfacial refractive index. In a typical SPR experiment performed on living cells, the signal integrates the sum of the contribution on the refractive index, either increase or decrease, of cellular processes occurring within the sensing region. Previous experimental data have shown that cell responses involving cell contraction, loss of cell-cell contacts, or decrease in cell adhesion generate a reduction in the refractive index, resulting in lower resonance angle and measured reflectance. In contrast, we observed that the refractive index is increased when cell processes include events such as cell spreading, proliferation, higher cell-cell contacts, and stronger adhesion to the surface, leading to a higher resonance angle and measured reflectance (Fig. 1b). Therefore, integrated cell response measurement such as the one obtained by SPR allows to address the global signaling properties of a given ligand, in real time.

Monitoring SPR signals in real time has allowed to study complex cellular processes such as responses to active toxins [7] and

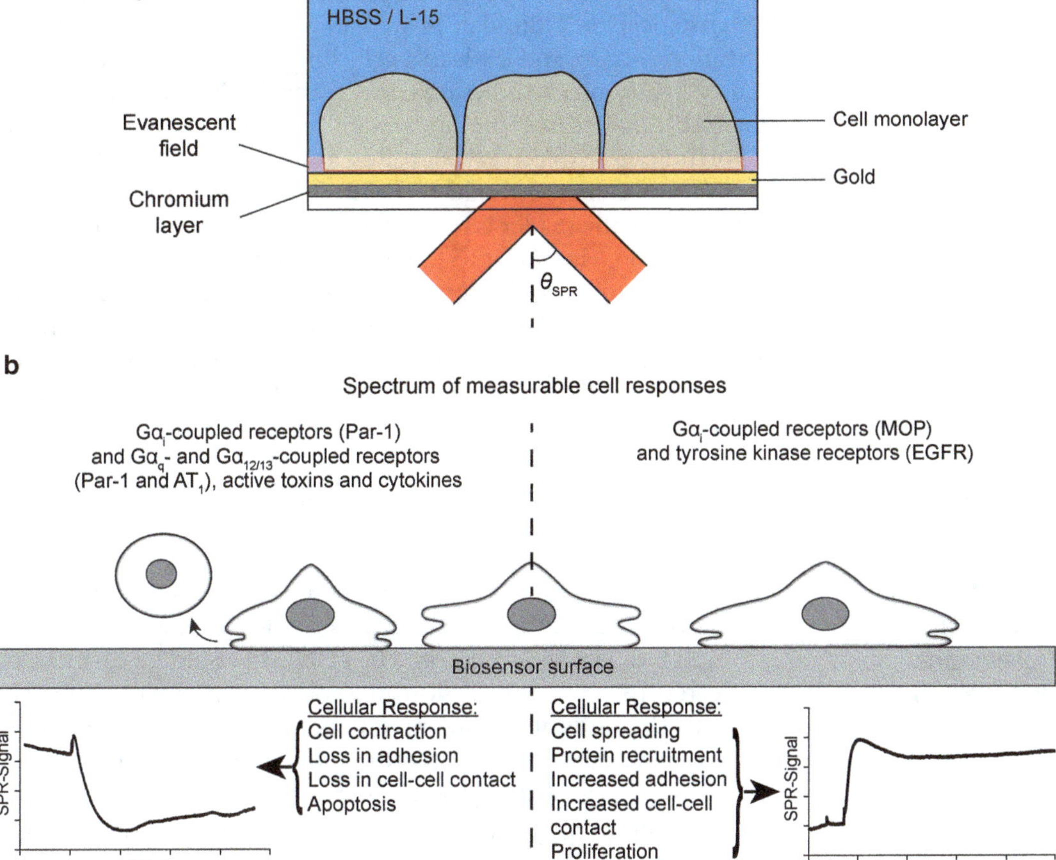

Fig. 1 Cell-based SPR sensing. (**a**) Schematic representation of the cell monolayer cultured on an SPR sensor surface. (**b**) Depending on the receptor activated, various SPR responses can be obtained. *Left*: Receptors leading to apoptosis or contraction of the cell body (i.e., death receptors DR4 and DR5, protease-activated receptor-1 (Par-1), and angiotensin receptor type 1 (AT1) produce a decrease in reflectance. *Right*: Activation of receptors such as mu opioid receptor (MOP) and epidermal growth factor receptor (EGFR) produce an increase in reflectance due to cell spreading and proliferation. This figure was reproduced from Ref. [6] with permission from Springer Science + Business Media

cytokine-induced programmed cell death [8] for time periods ranging from minutes to several hours. We also previously demonstrated that SPR can detect a wide diversity of cellular signals mediated by GPCRs such as the angiotensin receptor type 1 (AT1) [6], the protease-activated receptor-1 (Par-1) [7], and the mu opioid receptor (MOP) [9] (Fig. 1b). A significant advantage of SPR is that it can probe yet unknown signaling. For example, we found that antagonists assumed to be neutral for the mu opioid receptor behave either as partial or inverse agonists in native conditions [9]. Interestingly, such signaling was undetectable with the latest generation of BRET-based biosensors [9]. SPR also revealed that a specific

G protein can lead to opposite responses, depending on the receptor. For instance, the stimulation of Par-1 by thrombin triggers the activation the $G\alpha_i$ and leads to a cell contraction whereas the activation of MOP, also a $G\alpha_i$-coupled receptor, leads to a cell spreading (Fig. 1b). Label-free methods such as SPR therefore offer the opportunity to explore cell signaling at its functional level.

We use a custom-build SPR instrument, described in [7, 8]. Additionally, the reader is referred to a previous volume of Springer Protocols and Methods [13] for a detailed description of an instrument similar to ours. For the purpose of this chapter, we emphasize all the required steps for the realization of SPR experiments on living cells, which can be divided in three general steps: the preparation of the sensor chip, cell culture, and acquisition and analysis of the signal.

2 Materials

2.1 Cell Culture and System Requirements for Cell-Based SPR Sensing

1. A primary cell line endogenously expressing a receptor of interest or adherent cell line, such as HEK293, stably expressing high levels of the receptor: The cell line should be easily transfected using a transfection method that minimally interferes with the integrity of the membrane and a plasmid containing the gene coding the receptor under the control of a strong promoter (*see* **Notes 1** and **2**).

2. Cell culture media such as Dulbecco's Modified Eagle Medium (DMEM, Life technologies, Burlington, Canada), supplemented with 10 % of heat-inactivated fetal bovine serum and 50 mg/l gentamicin (*see* **Note 3**).

3. Solutions of extracellular matrix (ECM) to promote cell adhesion and growth on the SPR gold substrate such as a fibronectin (5 µg/ml) and gelatin (200 µg/ml) solutions, which are prepared by adding prepared by adding 80 g of gelatin (BD, Franklin Lakes, NJ) to 400 ml of distilled water. This solution is then autoclaved and 2 mg of sterile fibronectin (Sigma-Aldrich, St. Louis, MO) is added. Single-use aliquots are prepared and stored at –20 °C until use. Other coatings such as poly-L- or poly-D-lysine and laminin are commercially available and can be used (*see* **Note 4**).

4. A temperature-stabilized SPR system to ensure stable 37 °C throughout the experiment (*see* **Note 5**).

2.2 SPR Experiments

1. Buffered media designed for atmospheric equilibration such as HEPES-buffered salt solution (HBSS; 20 mM HEPES, 120 mM NaCl, 5.3 mM KCl, 1.8 mM $CaCl_2$, 0.8 mM $MgSO_4$, and 11.1 mM dextrose, pH 7.4) or commercially available cell culture media such as L-15 or M199 Hanks' salt (Life Technologies, Carlsbad, CA) (*see* **Note 6**).

2. Ligands for the receptor under study as well as inhibitors for signaling pathways downstream molecules under investigation.

3. Glass microscope slides are purchased from Fisher Scientific (Fisherfinest Premium Plain Glass Microscope Slides, BK7 glass, $n = 1.515$, $3'' \times 1'' \times 1$ mm).

3 Methods

3.1 Preparation of Gold Surface for SPR Measurements

This section describes the preparation of SPR sensor chips for cell culture. As mentioned above, we use a custom-built SPR system and we opted to prepare the SPR chips using our clean room facilities. However, it should be noted that commercial chips suitable for cell culture with similar characteristics can be purchased (*see* **Note 7**).

1. Prepare a 1 % detergent solution (Hellmanex II, Hellma GmbH & Co. KG, Germany) and gently rub glass slides in the solution to mechanically remove residues.

2. Transfer glass slides into microscope slide staining dishes (Ted Pella, Inc., USA) for further processing.

3. Immerse slides in fresh detergent solution (*see* **step 2**) followed by 3 min in a sonication bath.

4. Rinse three times with deionized (DI) water followed by 3 min in a sonication bath after last washing step.

5. Prepare piranha solution by mixing 3:1 concentrated sulfuric acid and fresh 30 % hydrogen peroxide solution (*see* **Note 8**).

6. Immerse slide rack in Piranha solution for 12 min, followed by three rinsing steps with DI water, and then 3 min in a sonication bath in DI water.

7. Transfer slide rack in 2-propanol followed by 3 min in a sonication bath.

8. Dry glass slides under nitrogen flow.

9. Place three glass slides in an e-beam evaporator (BOC Edwards evaporator, model: AUTO 306) for a homogeneous metal deposition.

10. Start evaporation when the pressure in the chamber is less than $3–4 \times 10^{-7}$ Torr.

11. Deposit metal layers.

    (a) Deposit a chromium layer of 3 nm (deposition rate: 0.05 nm/s) on the glass slides (*see* **Note 9**).

    (b) Deposit sequentially another 48 nm gold layer (deposition rate: 0.35 nm/s) on the glass slides (*see* **Note 10**).

12. After evaporation, cut microscope slides into samples of approx. 12×12 mm squares using a diamond glass cutter (*see* **Note 11**).

13. Place sensor chips in glass Petri dishes and autoclave prior to cell culture. The sensor chips can be stored in a sealed autoclave bag until use (*see* **Note 12**).

3.2 Cell Culture

This section describes how to culture cells onto the SPR sensor chips. In general, typical cell culture technique can be directly adopted (*see* **Note 13**).

1. Transfer the gold substrates into individual 35 mm cell culture dishes using a pair of tweezers sterilized with ethanol and fire.

2. Add the extracellular matrix (ECM) coating on the gold-coated slides.

    (a) Fibronectin/gelatin coating: Cover the gold substrate with 2 ml of solution and incubate for at least 1 h at room temperature. Remove the solution when ready to proceed to **step 3**.

    (b) Poly-lysine coating: Cover the substrate and incubate for at least 1 h at room temperature. Then, rinse twice with sterile water when ready to proceed to **step 3**.

3. Seed each Petri dish with the desired cell suspension dilution and complete with your culture medium to 3 ml. Allow 48–72 h for cell adhesion and growth to confluence (*see* **Note 14**).

3.3 SPR Experiments

This section describes a general protocol to investigate the biased agonism of GPCR ligands. SPR allows for the real-time monitoring of GPCR ligand-induced phenotypic modifications of the cell monolayer. In a typical experiment, the reflectance signal, measured at a fixed angular position, is monitored as a function of time. Once acquired, the sensorgram is analyzed in terms of various dynamical parameters. Pharmacological inhibitors may have a different impact on these parameters obtained for various ligands targeting the same GPCR, therefore revealing the bias for one or more signaling pathways.

1. Set the temperature of the SPR chamber at 37 °C (*see* **Note 5**).

2. Prepare the experimental buffer. If a commercially available buffer is used, proceed to **step 3**.

3. Reserve a 50 ml tube of the experimental buffer solution and place it in a temperature-controlled bath at 37 °C. It will be used as the vehicle in the experiments and in the next step for stabilization.

4. Remove culture medium, wash once, and replace it with the assay buffer kept at 37 °C. Place the Petri dish in the SPR chamber for stabilization for at least 30 min prior to the experiment (*see* **Note 15**).

5. Add one drop of the index-matching fluid at the center of the prism (*see* **Note 16**).

6. Remove the gold substrate of the Petri dish with tweezers and wipe the assay buffer underneath the substrate with an absorbent paper (*see* **Note 17**).

7. Place the gold substrate on the drop of index-matching fluid. This operation requires the use of a plastic tweezers in order to prevent scratching the SPR prism.

8. Install the fluidic chamber (*see* **Notes 17** and **18**).

9. Add assay buffer (around 400 μL) (*see* **Notes 19** and **20**).

10. Start an angular scan in order to determine the working angle and select the angle value at the center of the quasi-linear portion of the scan (Fig. 2). The working angle will be constant for the whole experiment, allowing the real-time monitoring of the reflectance variations (Fig. 3a, b) (*see* **Notes 21** and **22**).

11. Add the vehicle (assay buffer; **step 3**) once signal is stabilized. This step allows exclusion of effect on the signal due to mechanical stimulation of the cells by the media exchange (Fig. 3a). Allow the signal to stabilize again before proceeding to **step 12** (*see* **Note 23**).

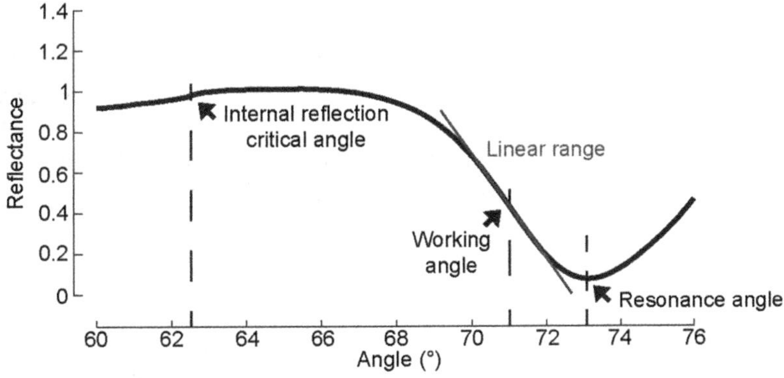

Fig. 2 Minimal reflectance at resonance angle. Typical scan of the reflectance as a function of the incident angle. Once the internal reflection critical angle is reached, the reflectance decreases to its lowest point, which is the resonance angle. The resonance angle represents the angle at which maximal surface plasmon coupling occurs, thus producing the most intense evanescent field. The working angle in the linear region is selected and kept constant for the duration of the experiment while reflectance is recorded vs. time.

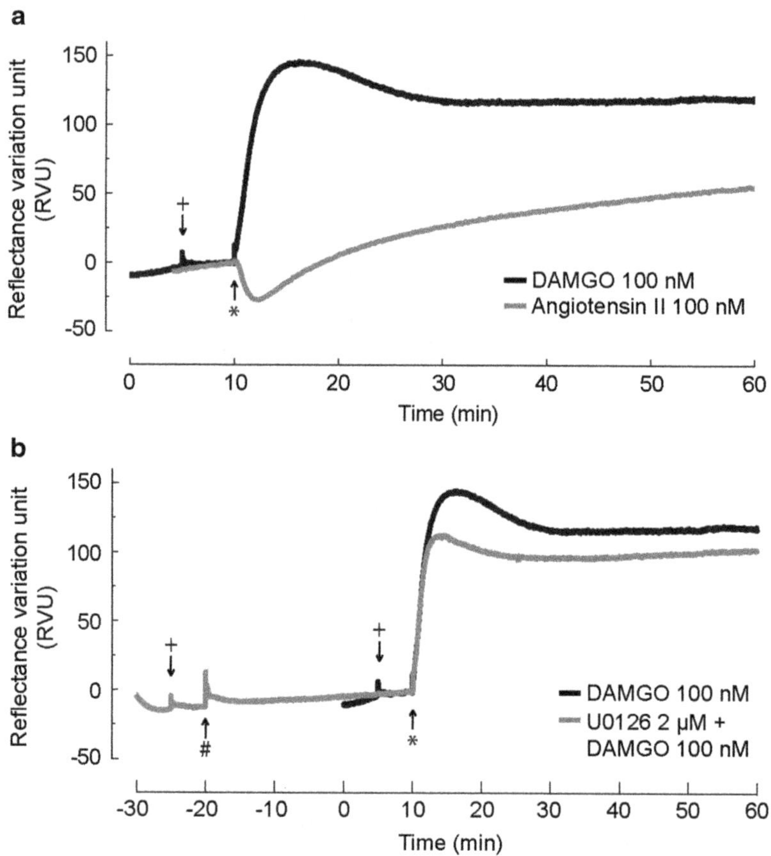

Fig. 3 SPR responses obtained following the stimulation of two G protein-coupled receptors. (**a**) The *black trace* is obtained following the stimulation with the agonist DAMGO on HEK cells stably expressing mu opioid receptor. The *grey trace* is obtained after the stimulation with AngII on HEK cells stably expressing angiotensin receptor type 1. (**b**) Pretreatment with the MEK inhibitor U0126 (*gray trace*) allows to evaluate whether the ERK1/2 signaling pathway is involved in the SPR response induced by DAMGO (*black trace*). Symbols: +: addition of vehicle; #: addition of U0126; *: addition of ligand. Data in (**b**) was reproduced from Ref. [9] with permission from ASPET

12. Cell signaling investigation:

    (a) Inhibitors are used to delineate the contribution of specific signaling pathways. Most pretreatments with pharmacological inhibitors can be performed inside the SPR chamber, revealing the effect of the inhibitor itself on the sensorgram (Fig. 3b) (*see* **Notes 24–26**).

    (b) Add the ligand of interest to activate signaling (Fig. 3a, b).

13. Analyze the SPR sensorgrams using a software such as Matlab (Mathworks, USA). As presented in Fig. 4, several different parameters can be extracted from the SPR sensorgrams such as:

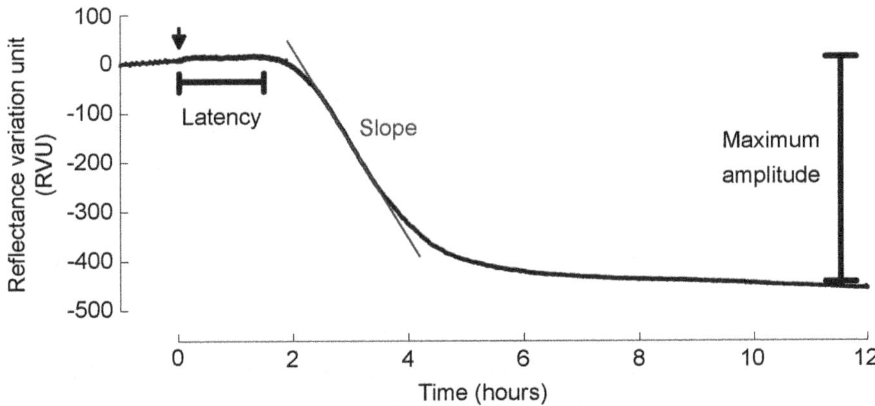

Fig. 4 Schematic representation of possible meaningful parameters in an SPR sensorgram. Coming from a typical experiment monitoring apoptosis: latency, representing the time lapse between stimulation and the beginning of the execution phase of apoptosis; slope, giving the rate of the execution phase of apoptosis; and maximal amplitude, illustrating the overall cell detachment, are represented. Data was reproduced from Ref. [8] with permission from Springer Science + Business Media

(a) Slope: informs about the rate of modification of cellular adhesion, cell shape, and cell loss/proliferation within the evanescent field.

(b) Amplitude: informs about the global change undergone by the cell monolayer within the evanescent field as compared to the beginning of the experiment.

(c) Latency: informs about the onset of the observed cellular responses (*see* **Notes 27** and **28**).

4   Notes

1. *Sine qua non* conditions for SPR experiment on cells are that the cells adhere unto the gold substrate and can form a confluent and regular monolayer.

2. Several kinds of transfection methods are available such as liposomes, electroporation, calcium phosphate, and dendrimers (i.e., polyethylenimine). Depending on the cell line, the optimal transfection conditions may vary. Although it is possible to use cells with a transitory expression, we recommend performing SPR experiments with cells stably expressing the protein of interest. The reason is that the SPR signal will ultimately represent the response from the whole-cell population within the evanescent field. Therefore, non-transfected cells will lower the overall response to a ligand and, by way of consequence, reduce the sensitivity of the method or produce experimental bias. Additionally, individual cells responding with different magnitudes will be convoluted as a broad SPR response profile.

3. Cell culture media and composition are selected according to the cell line under investigation.

4. Depending on the cell line, the extracellular matrix added on the SPR chips can differ. In addition, certain cell lines can adhere on gold without pre-coating. Therefore, we strongly recommend performing cell adhesion tests with the different ECM presented to identify the best conditions for the cell line under study.

5. For most cell lines, the temperature of the fluid chamber should be set to 37 °C. Temperature should be kept constant because variations in temperature have an impact on the resonance angle as well as on the cell metabolism. In fact, a temperature increase is associated with a decrease in resonance angle [14]. When possible, the overall SPR system is placed in a temperature-controlled chamber, which we have found to be very efficient in minimizing drift in the SPR signal often caused by thermal instability. In this configuration, it should be noted that stable temperature is normally reached after several hours.

6. CO_2 control can be realized either in the environmental chamber or by using buffered media designed for atmospheric equilibration. If inappropriate for the required experimental conditions, HEPES can be generally added to stabilize pH throughout the experiment.

7. If a commercial SPR apparatus is used, SPR sensor chips from the same company should be purchased to avoid instrument compatibility problems.

8. Piranha solution is a strong oxidizing agent and reacts strongly with organic matter. Further, the mixing is exothermic and the solution will become hot bearing the risk of breaking the glass container. Handle with care and use appropriate personal safety equipment.

9. This layer acts as an adhesion layer and other metals such as titanium are possible.

10. This thickness is optimized for 660 nm excitation wavelength and should therefore be optimized for the SPR system using different wavelengths.

11. Gold-coated slides should be cut in an appropriate size to fit conventional cell culture material.

12. Alternatively ethanol sterilization is possible. For this sterilization method, the samples are immersed in 100 % ethanol under a biological safety bench and dried prior to cell culture.

13. All steps in this section should be performed under a biological safety bench to avoid cell contamination.

14. Confluence is an important parameter during SPR experiments since the signal will ultimately depend on the biomolecular density within the evanescent field. Thus, cells should be dispersed homogeneously in the Petri dish since we observed that direct seeding of the gold substrate was associated with irregular surface covering.

15. In some instances, detachment of the cells from the gold substrate may occur during this step. If this situation happens repeatedly, we suggest considering doing this step inside the SPR chamber, which therefore implies to perform **steps 3–7** before the stabilization of 30 min and then continue the protocol from **step 8**.

16. The refractive index of the oil must match that of the prism, to limit refraction of the laser beam.

17. Presence of the assay buffer between the sensor chip and the prism will cause reflectance and scattering of the incoming light beam and therefore perturb the signal. Attention should be given that the fluidic chamber is tightly fixed, fully sealing the surface to ensure no buffer leaking.

18. In our system, the fluidic chamber is composed by a Teflon® cell fixed by screws. For commercial systems, the user should refer to the owner guide of the apparatus.

19. As opposed to most SPR systems, our version is not equipped with a peristaltic pump to assure a continuous flow in the chamber. Therefore, each reagent is added manually using pipettes of 100 or 1,000 μl. This step should be performed carefully to avoid cell detachment.

20. **Steps 6–9** in Section 3.3 should be performed as quickly as possible to prevent drying of the cells on the SPR chip.

21. If a point outside of this region is selected, non-linear effects and saturation will impact the sensorgram. Moreover, depending on the experiment at hand (i.e., monitoring apoptosis), cells can generate large shifts in θ_{SPR}. In such experiments an angle on top/bottom of the linear portion of the angular scan is chosen.

22. It is also possible to run SPR experiments by performing sequential angular scans to monitor the minimum of reflectance.

23. Signal usually stabilizes within 5 min. However, depending on the experimental conditions and cell types, the stabilization time may vary.

24. For experiments of long duration (i.e., few hours to days), the fluidic chamber should be sealed to prevent evaporation of the assay buffer. In our system, we use vacuum grease and a 25 mm coverslip to seal the fluidic chamber. If a commercial system

with an open configuration is used, the user should verify if a cover is available for that purpose. Evaporation increases the salt concentration in the buffer resulting in an alteration of cell morphology and in an augmentation of the refractive index in the sensing region [15]. In such experiments an antibiotic is often added to the assay buffer to prevent contamination.

25. Pretreatments for a period of time over 1 h, such as pretreatments with toxins to evaluate G protein coupling properties or transfection with siRNA, are generally performed outside the SPR chamber.

26. If possible, non-aqueous solvents in experiments should be avoided in the SPR chamber since they could perturb the refractive index of the sample buffer and impact the SPR sensorgram. Therefore, non-aqueous buffers such as dimethyl sulfoxide (DMSO) should be used at the lowest final concentration possible. It is possible to correct for this instantaneous change in the refractive index. Proper control experiments using this vehicle should always be done.

27. Depending on the cellular response probed in the SPR sensorgrams, other meaningful parameters could also be extracted.

28. For the particular purpose of studying GPCR functional selectivity, the analysis of several different parameters can lead to the identification of biased agonists for a specific signaling cascade because agonists, even if they target the same receptor, can differently regulate cell signaling. In that case, one or more SPR parameters may be affected after treatments with various inhibitors, therefore revealing the bias towards specific pathways.

References

1. Ward LD, Howlett GJ, Hammacher A, Weinstock J, Yasukawa K, Simpson RJ, Winzor DJ (1995) Use of a biosensor with surface plasmon resonance detection for the determination of binding constants: measurement of interleukin-6 binding to the soluble interleukin-6 receptor. Biochemistry 34(9):2901–2907

2. Navratilova I, Besnard J, Hopkins AL (2011) Screening for GPCR ligands using surface plasmon resonance. ACS Med Chem Lett 2(7):549–554. doi:10.1021/ml2000017

3. Fagerstam LG, Frostell A, Karlsson R, Kullman M, Larsson A, Malmqvist M, Butt H (1990) Detection of antigen-antibody interactions by surface plasmon resonance. Application to epitope mapping. J Mol Recognit 3(5–6): 208–214. doi:10.1002/jmr.300030507

4. Hide M, Tsutsui T, Sato H, Nishimura T, Morimoto K, Yamamoto S, Yoshizato K (2002) Real-time analysis of ligand-induced cell surface and intracellular reactions of living mast cells using a surface plasmon resonance-based biosensor. Anal Biochem 302(1):28–37. doi:10.1006/abio.2001.5535

5. Yanase Y, Suzuki H, Tsutsui T, Hiragun T, Kameyoshi Y, Hide M (2007) The SPR signal in living cells reflects changes other than the area of adhesion and the formation of cell constructions. Biosens Bioelectron 22(6):1081–1086. doi:10.1016/j.bios.2006.03.011

6. Cuerrier CM, Chabot V, Vigneux S, Aimez V, Escher E, Gobeil F, Charette PG, Grandbois M (2008) Surface plasmon resonance monitoring of cell monolayer integrity: implication of signaling pathways involved in actin-driven morphological remodeling. Cell Mol Bioeng 1(4):229–239. doi:10.1007/s12195-008-0028-4

7. Chabot V, Cuerrier CM, Escher E, Aimez V, Grandbois M, Charette PG (2009) Biosensing based on surface plasmon resonance and living cells. Biosens Bioelectron 24(6):1667–1673. doi:10.1016/j.bios.2008.08.025

8. Maltais JS, Denault JB, Gendron L, Grandbois M (2012) Label-free monitoring of apoptosis by surface plasmon resonance detection of morphological changes. Apoptosis 17(8):916–925. doi:10.1007/s10495-012-0737-y

9. Bourassa P, Tudashki HB, Pineyro G, Grandbois M, Gendron L (2014) Label-free monitoring of mu-opioid receptor-mediated signaling. Mol Pharmacol 86(2):138–149. doi:10.1124/mol.114.093450

10. Urban JD, Clarke WP, von Zastrow M, Nichols DE, Kobilka B, Weinstein H, Javitch JA, Roth BL, Christopoulos A, Sexton PM, Miller KJ, Spedding M, Mailman RB (2007) Functional selectivity and classical concepts of quantitative pharmacology. J Pharmacol Exp Ther 320(1):1–13. doi:10.1124/jpet.106.104463

11. Cunningham BT, Li P, Schulz S, Lin B, Baird C, Gerstenmaier J, Genick C, Wang F, Fine E, Laing L (2004) Label-free assays on the BIND system. J Biomol Screen 9(6):481–490. doi:10.1177/1087057104267604

12. Schroder R, Schmidt J, Blattermann S, Peters L, Janssen N, Grundmann M, Seemann W, Kaufel D, Merten N, Drewke C, Gomeza J, Milligan G, Mohr K, Kostenis E (2011) Applying label-free dynamic mass redistribution technology to frame signaling of G protein-coupled receptors noninvasively in living cells. Nat Protoc 6(11):1748–1760. doi:10.1038/nprot.2011.386

13. Arima Y, Teramura Y, Takiguchi H, Kawano K, Kotera H, Iwata H (2009) Surface plasmon resonance and surface plasmon field-enhanced fluorescence spectroscopy for sensitive detection of tumor markers. Methods Mol Biol 503:3–20. doi:10.1007/978-1-60327-567-5_1

14. Moreira CS, Lima AMN, Neff H, Thirstrup C (2008) Temperature-dependent sensitivity of surface plasmon resonance sensors at the gold-water interface. Sens Actuators B Chem 134:854–862. doi:10.1016/j.snb.2008.06.045

15. Robelek R, Wegener J (2010) Label-free and time-resolved measurements of cell volume changes by surface plasmon resonance (SPR) spectroscopy. Biosens Bioelectron 25(5):1221–1224. doi:10.1016/j.bios.2009.09.016

Chapter 11

Triple-Addition Label-Free Assays for High-Throughput Screening of Muscarinic M$_1$ Receptor Agonists, Antagonists, and Allosteric Modulators

Hannah J. Gitschier, Audrey B. Bergeron, David H. Randle, Caryn E. Bacon, Melvyn Baez, Peiyi Yang, Lisa M. Broad, Paul J. Goldsmith, Christian C. Felder, and Douglas A. Schober

Abstract

Label-free optical biosensor technology measures phenotypic responses in cell-based assays. Here, we describe a triple-addition cellular assay for simultaneously screening for agonists, allosteric potentiators, and antagonists of the muscarinic M$_1$ receptor. The assay validation, high-throughput screening (HTS), and hit confirmation assays all consisted of three sequential addition steps; the application of test compounds, followed by EC$_{20}$ and then EC$_{80}$ doses of the non-selective, orthosteric muscarinic receptor agonist, acetylcholine. The label-free data was also compared to those from screening using FLIPR. Results support that label-free technology is a valid and robust orthogonal approach for HTS applications that can be used for identifying multiple pharmacological classes of active compounds in one simple platform.

Key words Cell-based assays, Drug discovery, Dynamic mass redistribution, High-throughput screening, Label-free, Muscarinic M1 receptor, Optical biosensor, Phenotypic assays, Signal transduction pathways

1 Introduction

Muscarinic acetylcholine receptors belong to the super family of G protein-coupled receptors (GPCRs). GPCRs are integral membrane proteins that transduce extracellular binding of neurotransmitters into intracellular signaling events. The muscarinic receptor family has five members (M$_1$–M$_5$) which regulate the peripheral and central parasympathetic nervous system [1]. M$_1$, M$_3$, and M$_5$ receptors signal primarily through G$_q$ coupling to phospholipase C and calcium mobilization. The M$_2$ and M$_4$ subtypes signal primarily through G$_i$ coupling and regulate the second messenger cAMP. The M$_1$, M$_3$, and M$_5$ receptors are primarily localized to post synaptic terminals, while the M$_2$ and M$_4$ receptors primarily

Ye Fang (ed.), *Label-Free Biosensor Methods in Drug Discovery*, Methods in Pharmacology and Toxicology, DOI 10.1007/978-1-4939-2617-6_11, © Springer Science+Business Media New York 2015

to presynaptic terminals. Neural regulation is mediated by these receptors through modulation of neurotransmitter release, changes in membrane potential through modulation of ion channels, or regulation of a number of intracellular enzymes including phospholipases, kinases, and phosphatases. The M_1 receptor is highly expressed in the central nervous system, particularly in the cortex and hippocampus where it plays a key role in cognition and memory [2]. It is considered a promising target to help manage the memory loss and amyloid neural pathology associated with Alzheimer's disease.

Early phase drug discovery efforts involve screening chemical libraries for active samples. High-throughput screening (HTS) has traditionally been target-based, where the effect of compounds on a specific target protein or molecule is measured through the use of labels (i.e., fluorescent, luminescent, radiolabeled, etc.). These conventional assay technologies rely on the use of engineered and/or immortalized cell systems that focus on a single component or cellular event in a complex biological system. Target-based drug discovery requires testing of a specific molecular hypothesis with detailed knowledge of the targeted cell signaling pathway prior to screening. While this approach can provide ample information for numerous compounds and molecular targets, it is limited in predicting phenotypic outcome, mainly due to the clinically relevant polypharmacology of many compounds. Alternatively, HTS can be phenotype-based, where molecular target and signaling pathway-unbiased assays are used to examine the effect of compounds on a specific phenotypic outcome in complex biological systems. These phenotypic drug discovery strategies can complement traditional target-based approaches, and alleviate target validation issues and the high rate of late stage clinical failures, which are major contributors to the challenges that the pharmaceutical industry is currently facing.

Label-free optical biosensor technology for phenotypic drug discovery provides a versatile platform with assay design flexibility and HTS capabilities. Optical biosensors, such as resonant waveguide grating (RWG) biosensor in microplates (e.g., Corning Epic® Technology), can be used to measure drug-induced dynamic mass redistribution (DMR) responses in cells. DMR responses measure refractive index alterations within a 150 nm sensing region proximal to an embedded optical biosensor found in each well of the microplate. These information-rich real-time kinetic profiles represent an integrated cellular response that is dependent on receptor activation and downstream signaling pathways, namely, signaling molecule translocation and cytoskeletal reorganization [3]. Label-free screening of chemical libraries has been used to identify agonists, as well as antagonists of endogenous receptors in a high-throughput single assay format [4].

In this chapter, we describe a triple-addition label-free assay for the identification of agonists, antagonists and allosteric modulators for M_1 receptor in the same HTS campaign. The goals of this project were to (1) enable a validated HTS triple-addition assay utilizing Epic Technology and a set of commercially available ligands with known activity on the M_1 receptor, and (2) screen a library of approximately 180,000 compounds for M_1 activity. Using both a recombinant cell line stably expressing M_1 receptor and the parental cell line, DMR responses were evaluated upon stimulation with a panel of known test compounds in agonist mode, as well as for potentiator and antagonist activity using acetylcholine as the reference agonist (positive control compound). Assay conditions were optimized so the DMR profile was measured at fixed time points after compound addition, instead of reading continuously in kinetic mode. This HTS campaign allows for interleaving of assay plates and to rapidly screen a large number of compounds. Upon successful assay development, compounds were screened in single point concentration using the HTS strategy. Results showed that in agonist mode, out of the approximately 180,000 compounds screened, 0.6 % were identified as hits with greater than 20 % activity; of those, 90 % were DMR unique. In potentiator mode, 0.05 % of compounds initially screened were identified as hits with greater than 10 % activity; and in antagonist mode, 3 % of compounds initially screened were identified as hits with greater than 80 % inhibition. A subset of hits were confirmed again in single point concentration and tested for M_1 specificity by counter screening against parental cells. Following hit confirmation, concentration–response curves (CRCs) were performed for potency and efficacy.

2 Compound Source Plate Preparation

Chemical libraries prepared in 384-well or 1,536-well storage microplates are ideal for HTS using label-free optical biosensor technology. As these microplates are typically spotted with nano-liter volumes of compounds at high concentration in dimethyl sulfoxide (DMSO), these compounds can easily be reconstituted in an assay buffer so that the final DMSO content is minimal (0.5–1 %). Most compound library screens are designed so that the final concentration of compound experienced by the cells is in the 1–10 µM range.

1. Spot 384-well storage microplates with stock solutions of compounds in DMSO in single point concentration.

2. Dilute with assay buffer so the final concentration of compound in each well is 50 µM and 0.5 % DMSO. The assay buffer is 1× Hank's balanced salt solution (HBSS) containing

20 mM HEPES, 0.05 % bovine serum albumin (BSA), and 0.5 % DMSO. Preparing the compound plates in this manner allows for a fivefold dilution upon 10 μL addition to the Epic microplate containing cells in 40 μL of assay buffer, resulting in a final effective concentration of 10 μM for each compound tested (*see* **Note 1**).

3 Cell Culture and Cell Assay Microplate Preparation

Epic Technology can be used to study receptors that are endogenously expressed in cell lines, or primary cells, as well as for cell lines that have been engineered to express a receptor of interest if an endogenous system is not available or unknown. In addition to the cells of interest, appropriate cell culture medium is also required to culture cells in microplates. As cells can be plated freshly from culture or from frozen stocks, scaling cells up to sufficient quantities for HTS may involve cell culture vessels for large scale expansion. For all adherent cell-based assay applications, seeding the cells in complete growth media is recommended to allow for initial attachment and spreading at the bottom of the microplate. Seeding in a serum-free medium or incorporating subsequent serum-starvation steps after cell attachment may also be employed.

1. Harvest cells from fresh culture, or thaw cryopreserved cells from liquid nitrogen storage in a 37 °C water bath just until ice is no longer visible. For triple-addition HTS, a recombinant cell line stably expressing M_1 receptor and the parental cell line are used.

2. Centrifuge cells at $260 \times g$ for 5 min and aspirate off harvest or cryopreservation medium.

3. Resuspend cell pellet in complete cell culture medium (or seeding medium if different from growth medium) and determine cell density and viability. For triple-addition HTS, UltraCHO medium (Lonza, Cat. # 12-724Q) containing 1× penicillin–streptomycin in a volume of 40 μL per well is used.

4. Seed the cells into 384-well fibronectin-coated Corning® Epic® Microplates (Corning, Cat. # 5042) at appropriate seeding density to yield confluent monolayer after 18–22 h in a 37 °C, 5 % CO_2, humidified incubator (*see* **Note 2**).

5. Allow the cells to settle in the Epic microplate for approximately 30 min prior to incubation.

6. Culture the cells in the Epic microplate for 18–22 h in a 37 °C, 5 % CO_2, humidified incubator.

4   Label-Free Assay

4.1   Assay Buffer Exchange

Once cells have reached the desired level of confluence for optimal cellular responsiveness, growth medium should be removed from the microplate and replaced with assay buffer. Typical assay buffer is HBSS containing HEPES to control pH, with or without DMSO. It is necessary to include DMSO in the assay buffer if the chemical libraries used for screening contain compounds dissolved in DMSO, as they commonly do. DMSO mismatch between assay buffer and compounds will mask phenotypic responses in optical label-free assays due to index of refraction differences between the two solutions; therefore the DMSO concentration must be matched.

1. Once a confluent monolayer of cells is obtained, perform buffer exchange by removing cell culture medium and washing the microplate three times with assay buffer, leaving a final volume of 40 µL per well.

2. Allow the cells to recover from the buffer exchange process for 1–2 h prior to beginning the label-free assay. As thermal equilibration is critical to assay performance, equilibrate the microplate at the temperature of the label-free reader for at least 30 min prior to performing baseline measurements.

4.2   HTS Optimization

Prior to initiation of a high-throughput screen, label-free assay optimization is necessary. These optimization steps can be used to determine ideal conditions for maximal positive control compound responses, end read timing, and throughput rate. Using a subset of commercially available compounds of known M_1 activity, assay optimization for the M_1 screen was completed in the engineered cell line (Table 1). For these assays, a baseline read was obtained for 5 min, followed by the addition of 10 µL of compound from a source plate containing the test compounds; including control wells. Negative control wells received assay buffer and positive control wells received various concentrations of acetylcholine. A summary of the 384-well plate layout can be seen in Fig. 1. Compounds were added in the first addition, followed by a brief mixing, and then the microplate was returned to the label-free reader for end read measurements. For assay optimization, the end read was collected continuously for 60 min to obtain full kinetic profiles in agonist mode.

Upon completion of the agonist mode end read, a concentration of acetylcholine that produces 20 % activity (EC_{20}) was applied to all wells that previously received compound. Additional wells were designated to receive assay buffer (negative control), effective EC_{20} or maximally stimulating (EC_{100}) dose of acetylcholine (positive controls). A second end read was then collected in kinetic mode.

Table 1
Results of test compounds used in assay validation

Compound	Pharmacological classification	Agonist EC50 (nM)	Potentiator EC50 (nM)	Antagonist IC50 (nM)
VU-0255035	M1-selective orthosteric antagonist	–	–	1408.2 ± 750.2
Carbachol	Non-selective orthosteric agonist	653.5 ± 231	–	–
LY593093	M1-selective partial orthosteric agonist	35.4 ± 12.7	–	–
BuTAC	Partial M2/M4 orthosteric agonist	2.7 ± 1.2	–	–
McN-A-343	Partial M1 orthosteric agonist	1149.9 ± 217	–	–
Scopolamine	Non-selective orthosteric antagonist	–	–	31.1 ± 10.8
VU-10010	M4-selective PAM	–	–	–
TBPB	M1-allosteric agonist	101	–	–
LuAE51090	M1-selective allosteric agonist	595	–	–
BQCA	M1-selective PAM	–	133.3 ± 13.8	–
ML071	M1-selective allosteric agonist	1553.5 ± 403.8	–	–
PQCA	M1-selective PAM	–	45.1	–
Xanomeline	Partial M1/M4 orthosteric agonist	131.3 ± 48	–	–
Atropine	Non-selective orthosteric antagonist	–	–	35.2 ± 12.8
Pilocarpine	Non-selective orthosteric agonist	1809.6 ± 583.5	–	–
AFDX-384	M2/M4 antagonist	–	–	1898.3 ± 642.9
Acetylcholine	Non-selective orthosteric agonist	53.1 ± 18	–	–
Oxotremorine-M	Non-selective orthosteric agonist	40.9 ± 15.7	–	–
GSK	M1-selective allosteric agonist	43.3 ± 13.2	–	–
LY2033298	M4-selective PAM	–	–	–

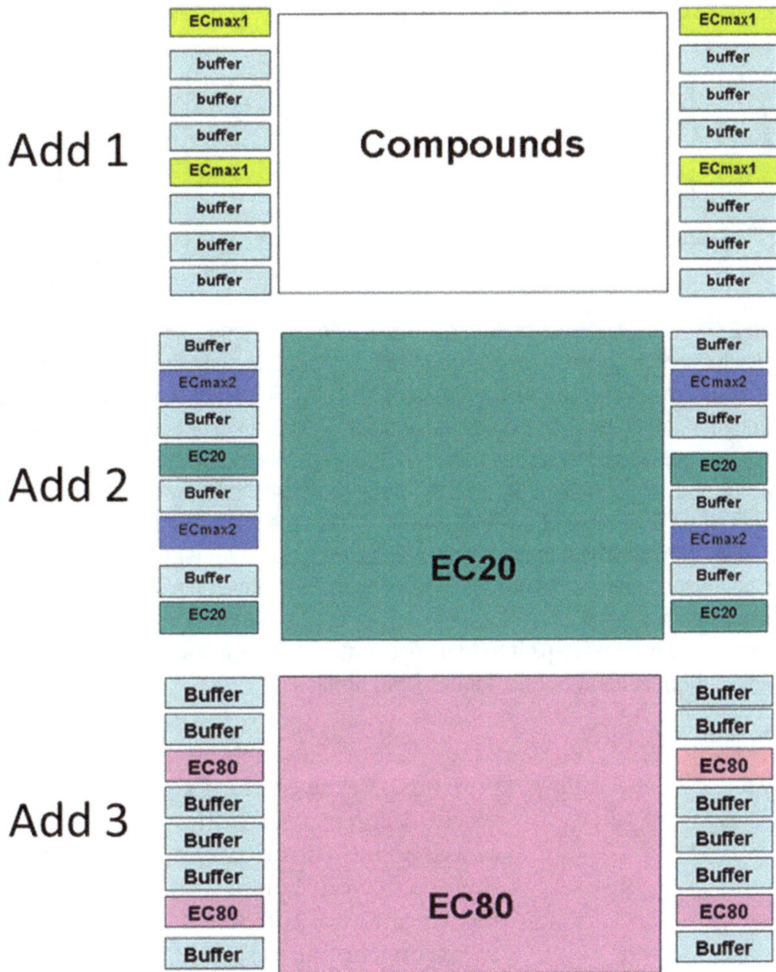

Fig. 1 Microplate template for triple mode addition. Representative template includes compounds assayed in single-point concentration (Compounds), as well as assay buffer (buffer) and positive control wells consisting of acetylcholine at an EC_{80} concentration (ECmax1) in the first addition (Add 1). In the second addition (Add 2), an EC_{20} concentration of acetylcholine (EC20) was added to all wells that previously received compound in the first addition. Additionally, assay buffer (Buffer) and positive control wells consisting of acetylcholine at EC_{20} (EC20) and EC_{100} (ECmax2) concentrations were also included. Finally, in the third addition (Add 3), all wells that received an EC_{20} concentration in Add 2, receive an EC_{80} concentration of acetylcholine (EC80). Negative control assay buffer wells (Buffer) and positive control wells containing an EC_{80} concentration of acetylcholine (EC80) were also included

This second addition allows for the identification of compounds that significantly potentiate the acetylcholine response, such as the potentiator control compound, BQCA (Table 1).

Finally, in a third addition, a concentration of acetylcholine that produces 80 % activity (EC_{80}) was applied to all wells that

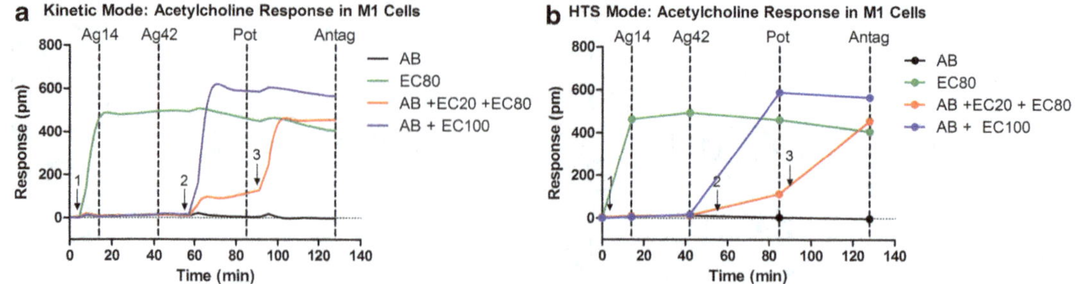

Fig. 2 DMR responses of triple mode screening collected in kinetic and HTS mode. (**a**) DMR responses were collected in kinetic mode for approximately 2 h continuously. In the first addition (Add 1), an EC_{80} dose of acetylcholine resulted in a peak response at 14 min (Ag14), followed by a plateaued response that persisted through 42 min (Ag42). In the second addition (Add 2), EC_{20} or EC_{100} doses of acetylcholine were added to wells that previously received assay buffer (AB), with peak responses persisting through 30 min after addition (Pot). In the third addition (Add 3), an EC_{80} dose of acetylcholine was added into the same wells that previously received an EC_{20} dose of acetylcholine in Add 2, resulting in a response that persisted through 30 min after addition (Antag). The negative control DMR response to AB was also collected. (**b**) DMR responses are plotted at optimized time points for HTS screening. Five time points were determined from kinetic mode, with responses measured for the baseline, Ag14, Ag42, potentiator, and antagonist end reads. The data collected at these time points were plotted to demonstrate how the triple mode screening data collection method in HTS mode is representative of the kinetic DMR profiles

previously received the EC_{20} dose of acetylcholine. Control wells received either assay buffer (negative control) or an EC_{80} dose of acetylcholine (positive control). A third and final end read was then collected kinetically. This third addition allows for the identification of antagonist compounds that significantly attenuate the acetylcholine response in the engineered M_1 cell line. The DMR responses collected in kinetic mode for all three additions are shown in Fig. 2a. Collecting full kinetic profiles continuously for each microplate provides rich information, but is not ideal for HTS. Therefore, the kinetic profiles can be simplified by collecting end reads at chosen time points after compound addition, instead of continuously monitoring the DMR responses. Based on these particular kinetic profiles in a recombinant cell line stably expressing M_1, it was determined that data collection at 14 and 42 min after compound addition was ideal for agonist mode analysis (Ag14 and Ag42), while data collection 30 min after Add 2 was optimal for potentiator mode comparison, and collection at 30 min after Add 3 was optimal for antagonist mode comparison. The DMR profiles shown in Fig. 2b display only the data recorded at the chosen HTS end read time points. As can be seen, the DMR profiles generated using this HTS campaign are very similar to those obtained in full kinetic mode, but now enable much greater throughput. For this M_1 screen, the timing for HTS profiling was determined based on the activity of the control compound acetylcholine. While this approach could easily be applied to a new target, the timing would need to be empirically determined. Once the HTS optimization is complete, it is straightforward to move into assay robustness testing and chemical library screening.

1. Once compound and cell assay plates are ready, initiate HTS platform for screening in triple-mode with the following method parameters (*see* **Note 3**):

   Baseline Read: Single point read.

   Add 1: Addition of compounds, assay buffer, or positive controls to cells in assay buffer.

   Agonist Read 1: Single point read at optimized time point.

   Agonist Read 2: Single point read at optimized time point.

   Add 2: Addition of EC_{20} dose of positive control on top of wells that previously received compound in Add 1. Also include EC_{20} dose of positive control on top of buffer wells, EC_{100} dose of positive control on top of buffer wells, and assay buffer on top of buffer wells.

   Allosteric Modulator Read: Single point read at optimized time point.

   Add 3: Addition of EC_{80} dose of positive control on top of wells that previously received EC_{20} dose in Add 2. Also includes assay buffer on top of buffer wells as negative control.

   Antagonist Read: Single point read at optimized time point.

2. Perform HTS assay in triple-mode with maximum number of plates determined during assay validation.

3. Analyze data for each compound tested (Section 5).

4.3 Assay Robustness

Using the HTS approach with single- or dual-point end reads after each addition, cellular responsiveness upon exposure to appropriate positive controls can be tested for robustness and reproducibility. This ensures that the potency of the positive control compound, as well as the thresholds set for data analysis and hit identification will continue to hold throughout the duration of the screen. Further, as cells are typically seeded in batch mode from one stock solution, rigorously testing microplates run over the course of an entire day can help determine if edge effect issues or cell density issues may arise during the screen.

Assay validation for the M_1 screen required running plate uniformity (PUNgent) studies and replicate-experiment studies prior to the DMR triple-addition assay being considered validated. Plate uniformity studies were run over the course of 3 days to assess uniformity and separation of signals. Variability was measured on two types of signals: (1) Max signals, which measures the maximum signal. For agonist mode this would be the maximal response of an agonist control (acetylcholine); for potentiator mode this would be the effect of pretreatment with a standard potentiator (BQCA) on an EC_{20} concentration of acetylcholine. For antagonist assays this would be the response to an EC_{80} concentration of acetylcholine. (2) Min signals, which measures background noise. In agonist mode this is the basal signal of assay buffer. For potentiator mode, this is an EC_{20} concentration of acetylcholine. For antagonist mode, this is the effect of pretreatment with a maximally inhibiting concentration of a standard antagonist (atropine) on an EC_{80} concentration of acetylcholine. The mean (AVG), standard deviation (SD), and coefficient of variance CV is just SD/AVG were computed for each signal (max and min) on each plate. Acceptance criterion included CV for each signal to be less than or equal to 20 %. It is also important to compute a Z factor (Z') for each plate using the following equation [5]:

$$Z = 1 - \left(\left(3SD_{max} + 3SD_{min} \right) / \text{absolute value of} \left(AVG_{max} - AVG_{max} \right) \right)$$

The recommended acceptance criterion is a $Z' \geq 0.4$ [6].

In addition to the PUNgent studies, replicate-experiment studies were also conducted to evaluate the within-run assay variability. This allows a preliminary assessment of the overall or between-run assay variability. For this screen, muscarinic reference compounds that have potencies covering the concentration range being tested were selected. Compounds were run in 8-point concentration–response curves (CRCs) and tested over the course of 2 days. The Minimum Significant Ratio (MSR) was then computed. This is the smallest potency ratio between two compounds that is statistically significant, and should be less than 3.0. Figure 3 highlights the results of PUNgent and replicate-experiment studies. In summary, for agonist mode the min on CRC1-1 and CRC1-2 fail the criterion $SD_{min} < SD_{max}$ because of one observation on each plate. All of the max and min data points have a number of extreme observations with no pattern, however all Z' (0.5), CV (<20 %) and MSR (1.45) criteria were met. In potentiator mode, the min on CRC1-2 failed the criterion $SD_{min} < SD_{max}$ because of four observations on the right side of the plate, and the min plates fail the CV criteria because of one or two extreme observations. However, both the Z' (0.4) and MSR (1.99) met criteria. For the antagonist response, min SD on CRC1-1 failed the criterion $SD_{min} < SD_{max}$ but there was a discernible pattern that might explain the excessive variation. Further, MSR (2.42) and Z' (0.5) criteria were met.

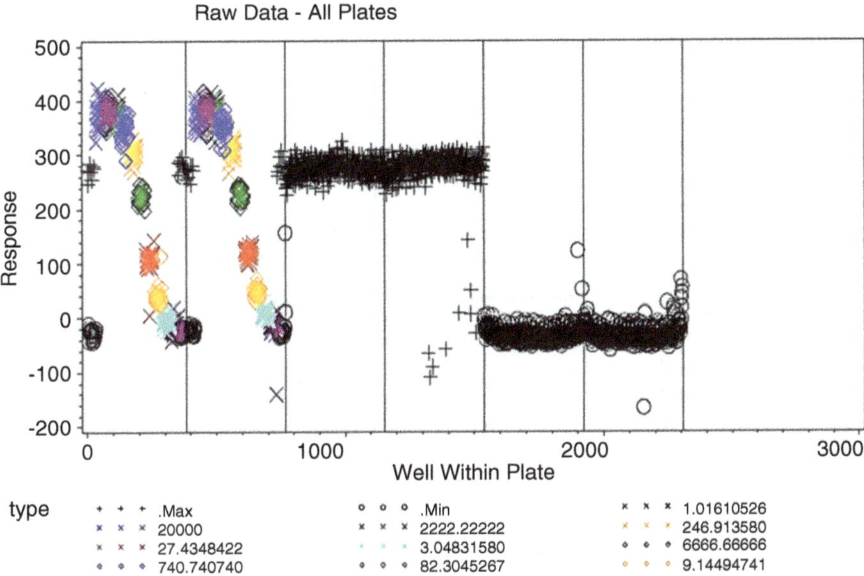

Fig. 3 Results from PUNgent and replicate experiment studies. Representative data from the first day of testing is shown. Concentration–response curves (CRC), maximum (MAX), and minimum (MIN) doses of the positive control compound, acetylcholine, were evaluated. From these data, Z' values, coefficient of variance (CV) and MSR values were calculated to assess overall reproducibility and robustness of assay design

4.4 HTS Screen

Once assay validation is complete, screening large chemical libraries in HTS mode is relatively straightforward. Using the optimized HTS schedule for a recombinant cell line stably expressing M_1, a library of approximately 180,000 compounds was screened in single point concentration. The triple mode assay format was applied for each microplate, resulting in the collection of five separate data points for every compound tested: a baseline read, agonist reads at 14 min (Ag14) and 42 min (Ag42), a potentiator read (Pot), and an antagonist read (Antag). DMR activity at each time point could then be assessed for the identification of hits in agonist, potentiator, and antagonist modes, by comparing individual well activity to that of the positive control, acetylcholine. For example, in Fig. 4a, representative agonist hits are displayed at the Ag14 and Ag42 time points compared to the HTS DMR profile of an EC_{80} concentration of acetylcholine and negative control assay buffer response. The responses are plotted as percent activity, relative to acetylcholine for the agonist and potentiator time points, or as percent inhibition of the EC_{80} activity of acetylcholine for the antagonist time point (for details on this conversion, please *see* Section 5.1). In addition to the identification of hits that are similar in activity to the positive control, hits with unique agonist activity profiles can also be identified. As can be seen for this M_1 screen, hits that display late activity or negative agonist activity were also identified. Positive allosteric modulators can be identified by comparing the percent activity of each compound after experiencing an EC_{20}

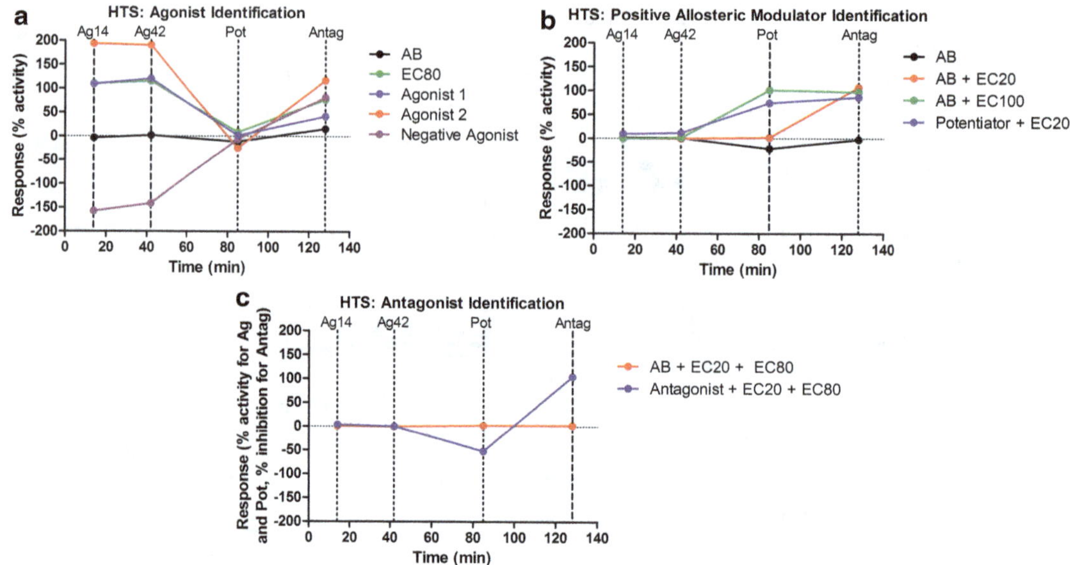

Fig. 4 DMR profiles of representative agonist, potentiator, and antagonist hits. (**a**) Percent activity of representative agonist hits are displayed at the Ag14 and Ag42 end reads compared to the DMR profile of the positive control EC_{80} concentration of acetylcholine (EC80) and assay buffer (AB). A hit identified with similar activity to the positive control is shown (Agonist 1), as well as hits that displayed late agonist activity (Agonist 2) or negative agonist activity (Negative Agonist). (**b**) A positive allosteric modulator (Potentiator + EC20) hit was identified when the EC_{20} percent activity of acetylcholine $\left(AB + EC20\right)$ was potentiated after Add 2 to a response that was comparable to the EC_{100} percent activity of acetylcholine $\left(AB + EC100\right)$. (**c**) An antagonist hit was identified $\left(\text{Antagonist} + EC20 + EC80\right)$ as having high percent inhibition of the EC_{80} response of acetylcholine $\left(AB + EC20 + EC80\right)$ after Add 3

concentration of acetylcholine to that of an EC_{100} concentration of acetylcholine. In Fig. 4b, a positive allosteric modulator hit is identified that potentiates the EC_{20} activity of acetylcholine after Add 2 to a response that is comparable to the EC_{100} activity of acetylcholine. Finally, in Fig. 4c, an antagonist hit is identified as it attenuates the EC_{80} activity of acetylcholine at the final end read obtained after Add 3. Here, the percent inhibition is relative to the response from an EC_{80} dose of acetylcholine in a recombinant cell line stably expressing M_1. As shown, an antagonist hit has a high percent inhibition of the EC_{80} activity of acetylcholine in the final data point collected. Using defined cut-off criteria for hit selection (Section 5.1), a subset of approximately 1,000 compounds were identified to pursue for agonist (hit rate of 0.6 %) activity, approximately 100 compounds were identified to pursue for potentiator (hit rate of 0.05 %) activity, and approximately 6,000 compounds were identified to pursue for antagonist (hit rate of 3 %) mode inhibition.

4.5   Hit Confirmation   Hit confirmation is useful to ensure that all active compounds identified during the chemical library screen are indeed active and not outliers. When the initial screen is completed in an engineered cell line, hit confirmation can also be used to determine the specificity of the elicited response to the receptor of interest by also screening the identified hits in the parental cell line. Here a subset of compounds identified as hits in either agonist, potentiator, or antagonist mode from the initial 180,000 compound screen were run in single point concentration in both the recombinant M_1 stably expressing cell line and the parental cell line. The same triple mode assay format was used as in HTS optimization, assay validation and the initial screen. By comparing the HTS DMR profiles of compounds in the recombinant cell line to the profiles in the parental cell line, M1 selective agonists (Fig. 5a), potentiators (Fig. 5b), and antagonists (Fig. 5c) were confirmed. As shown, compounds that previously exhibited agonist, potentiator, or antagonist activity during the initial screen were confirmed when tested again in single-point concentration. Further, these compounds did not show activity in the parental cell line, highlighting the selectivity for the M_1 receptor. Of note, as the parental cell line does not display acetylcholine agonist activity to begin with, the

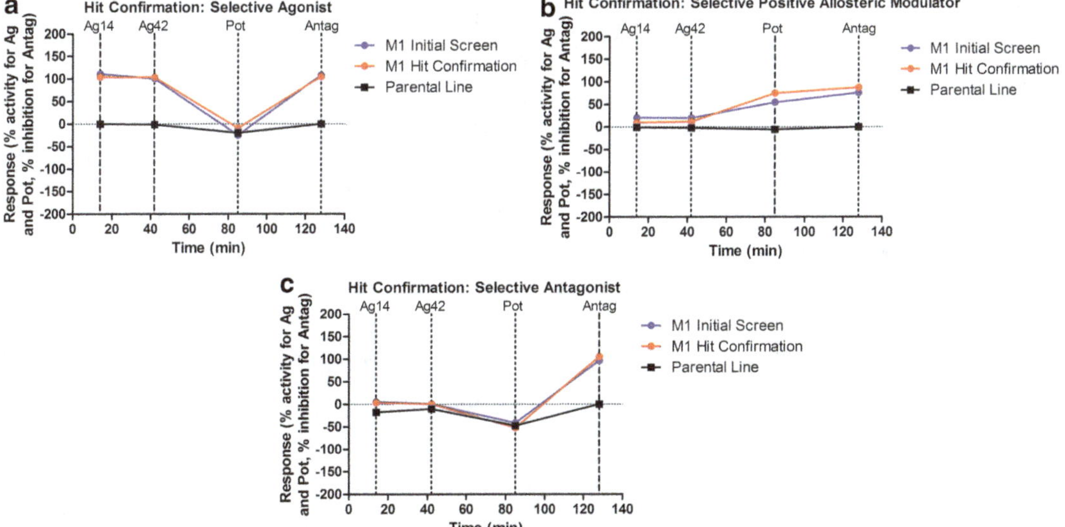

Fig. 5 DMR profiles of a representative agonist, potentiator, and antagonist identified in the initial screen were confirmed during hit confirmation. (**a**) An agonist hit repeats during hit confirmation testing (M1 Hit Confirmation) compared to the initial 180,000 compound screen (M1 Initial Screen), and displays selective activity in M1 cells without showing activity in parental cells (Parental Line) at both the Ag14 and Ag42 end reads. (**b**) A positive allosteric modulator displays the ability to potentiate the EC_{20} activity of acetylcholine in M1 cells, but does not display activity in parental cells. (**c**) A representative antagonist displays high percent inhibition of the EC_{80} response of acetylcholine in M1 cells, while the parental cells do not show this antagonist effect

antagonist mode percent inhibition of the EC_{80} acetylcholine response is irrelevant. Based on the hit confirmation results in agonist and potentiator modes, 63 % of those compounds tested were pursued for CRC testing. Further, for antagonist hits, 89 % of those hits identified in the initial 180,000 compound screen repeated in the single-point hit confirmation follow-up assays.

4.6 CRC Testing

Finally, to determine the potency and efficacy of the confirmed hits, CRC testing is necessary. By testing a dilution series of the confirmed hits against both the engineered and parental lines, the pharmacology of selective active compounds can be measured. To test a dose series of each confirmed hit, compounds were provided in 384-well storage microplates in a ten-point dilution series. These compounds were diluted using the same method as for the initial screen and hit confirmation studies, resulting in CRCs with an effective top concentration of 10 µM. Once added to the cells, the same triple mode assay format was used for detecting agonist, potentiator, and antagonist activity in both cell types. CRC testing is useful as promiscuous compounds can be readily identified by showing similar unsaturable activity in both cell types, as well as for providing EC_{50} and IC_{50} details. M_1 agonist (Fig. 6a), potentiator

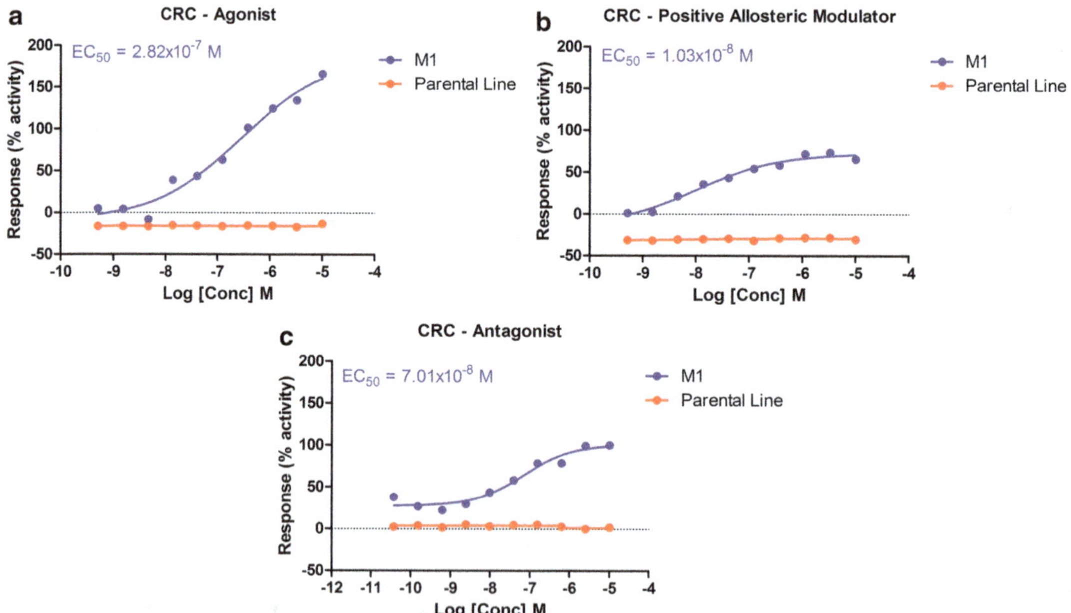

Fig. 6 Concentration–response curves (CRCs) of representative agonist, potentiator, and antagonist hits. A ten-point dilution series of each confirmed hit was tested against the engineered M1 cell line and the parental line. (**a**) An agonist elicits a dose-dependent response in the M1 cell line $\left(EC_{50} = 2.82 \times 10^{-7}\,M \right)$ with an absence of a response in the parental line. (**b**) A positive allosteric modulator elicits a dose-dependent potentiation of the EC_{20} acetylcholine response in the M1 cell line $\left(EC_{50} = 1.03 \times 10^{-8}\,M \right)$ with an absence of potentiation in the parental line. (**c**) An antagonist inhibits the EC_{80} acetylcholine response in a dose-dependent manner in the M1 cell line $\left(IC_{50} = 7.01 \times 10^{-8}\,M \right)$ but shows no inhibition activity in the parental line

(Fig. 6b), and antagonist (Fig. 6c) CRC DMR responses are compared to the parental cell line. As can be seen, the CRC profiles are dose-dependent and M_1 specific, providing useful potency data with percent activity relative to the positive control compound, acetylcholine. To analyze these curves for pharmacological values, please *see* (Section 5.2). Of the agonist and potentiator his examined during hit confirmation studies, 675 were CRC confirmed. Of the 675 CRC confirmed agonists, 579 were active at the Ag14 end read and 467 were active at the Ag42 end read. Of those, 208 were Ag14 unique hits, while 96 were Ag42 unique hits. For potentiator hits, 45 active compounds were CRC confirmed.

---

5 Data Analysis

5.1 Hit Identification

As DMR data was collected by recording a baseline read, followed by four end-read time points, percent activity in each mode of the triple-addition assay were evaluated. To collect an early agonist response using DMR, data points were collected at 14 min following the baseline read and are referred to as Ag 14. The differences in wavelength shift (pm response) between Ag 14 and baseline were copied into a Microsoft Excel template to generate percent activity calculations and Z' values. Data collected at 42 min post compound addition to measure late agonist responders are referred to as Ag 42. To generate percent activity calculations and Z' values for Ag 42, the difference in wavelength shift between Ag 42 and baseline were then pasted into the template. To generate data for Potentiator mode, the difference in wavelength shift between the third data point collected following baseline from the Ag 42 time point was calculated, and pasted in the template to generate percent activity calculations and Z' values. For Antagonist mode, the difference between the fourth data point following baseline and the third data point (the potentiator time point) were used to generate percent activity calculations and Z' values. The template selects each data point and calculates an activity fraction, followed by a percent activity from the fraction. The formulas for calculating activity fractions are as follows:

For Agonist time points:

$$\frac{\left(X - \mathrm{AVG}_{\mathrm{Buf}}\right)}{\left(\mathrm{AVG}_{\mathrm{EC80}} - \mathrm{AVG}_{\mathrm{Buf}}\right)}$$

For Potentiator time point:

$$\frac{\left(X - \mathrm{AVG}_{\mathrm{EC20}}\right)}{\left(\mathrm{AVG}_{\mathrm{EC100}} - \mathrm{AVG}_{\mathrm{EC20}}\right)}$$

For Antagonist time point:

$$\frac{\left(X - \mathrm{AVG}_{\mathrm{EC80}}\right)}{\left(\mathrm{AVG}_{\mathrm{Buf}} - \mathrm{AVG}_{\mathrm{EC80}}\right)}$$

Where X is the raw data point, $\mathrm{AVG}_{\mathrm{Buf}}$ is the mean of the buffer wells, $\mathrm{AVG}_{\mathrm{EC80}}$ is the mean of the response from EC_{80} acetylcholine wells, $\mathrm{AVG}_{\mathrm{EC20}}$ is the mean of the response from EC_{20} acetylcholine wells, and $\mathrm{AVG}_{\mathrm{EC100}}$ is the mean of the response from EC_{100} acetylcholine wells. To calculate percent activity from these fractions, the values were multiplied by 100. For this M_1 screen, hits were identified in agonist mode based on having >20 % activity relative to the positive control acetylcholine response at either the Ag14 or Ag42 time points. Additionally, hits were identified in potentiator mode based on having >10 % activity relative to the difference between the EC_{20} and EC_{100} doses of acetylcholine after Add 2. Finally, hits were identified in antagonist mode based on having >80 % inhibition with regards to the EC_{80} dose of acetylcholine response. For hit confirmation analysis, the same templates were used for the recombinant cell line stably expressing M_1; however, for the parental cell line several modifications were made, as these cells do not display positive control compound (acetylcholine) activity. Therefore, for the parental cell line, agonist and potentiator mode activity was compared to the activity of control compound SFLLR (PAR1 agonist). In antagonist mode, percent activity could not be calculated as these parental cells did not display agonist activity which could be inhibited with M_1 antagonist compounds.

5.2 CRC Analysis

For concentration–response curve (CRC) analysis, the same Microsoft Excel template described in Section 5.1 was used to determine percent activity for all compounds at each concentration tested. Using GraphPad Prism, the percent activity at each concentration was imported to generate EC_{50} or IC_{50}, Hillslope, and Top and Bottom percent activity values. These values were then used in the appropriate assay validation templates to evaluate compounds with confirmed, potent, and selective M_1 activity.

6 Notes

1. For the model screen, compound stock solutions were provided in 384-well storage plates at a concentration of 10 mM in 100 % DMSO. For the first addition, compounds were diluted in a ratio of 1:200 to a concentration of 50 µM in assay buffer with 0.5 % DMSO, which was the concentration used in the 5× source plates. Positive control wells containing an EC_{80} dose of acetylcholine at a 5× final concentration, as well as negative control wells containing assay buffer, were also included in the 5× source plates. For the second addition, positive controls,

EC_{20} and EC_{100} doses of acetylcholine, were prepared at a 6×
final concentration in assay buffer. For the third addition, positive control wells containing an EC_{80} dose of acetylcholine were
prepared at 7× final concentration in assay buffer.

2. Typical cell seeding density for adherent cell lines is between
2,500 and 25,000 cells per well in a 384-well Epic microplate;
however, optimal cell seeding density should be determined
experimentally. For the triple-addition HTS assays described,
optimal cell seeding densities were determined by cellular
responsiveness to control compounds; acetylcholine (muscarinic agonist) for the engineered cell line, and SFLLR (PAR-1
agonist) for the parental cell line.

3. As the protocols provided detail the use of label-free optical biosensor technology, such as Epic Technology, to enable users to
evaluate chemical libraries in HTS mode using a triple-addition
assay format for phenotypic screening, the DMR traces collected
can also be used to provide detailed information about underlying signal transduction pathways that comprise the DMR
response profiles. Alternative protocols focusing on eliciting
DMR profiles in cell lines and primary cells have previously been
developed [7]. Additional methodologies can be employed to
determine the significance of hits identified in phenotypic-based
screens. For example, a subset of agonist mode identified hits
were also tested in a FLIPR calcium mobilization assay to assess
whether utilizing a phenotypic rather than a specific signaling
pathway assay could yield novel SAR diversity (Fig. 7). Of the
657 agonists CRC confirmed by DMR, 66 of those were also
FLIPR active. Subsequently, the DMR unique active compounds were narrowed down to 28, which displayed M_1 specificity through pirenzipine inhibition. Of those, 13 were identified
that also displayed G_q inhibition. Thus, through phenotypic
screening, M_1 selective compounds that appear to signal through
G_q were identified, but were missed during FLIPR screening.
Therefore, this triple-addition assay format for phenotypic
screening is a useful tool for the evaluation of chemical libraries
in HTS mode, providing end users with the ability to confirm
active compounds detected by conventional technologies, as
well as to detect DMR unique compounds.

Glossary

HTS	High-throughput screening
DMSO	Dimethyl sulfoxide
HBSS	Hank's balanced salt solution
FBS	Fetal bovine serum
CRC	Concentration–response curve

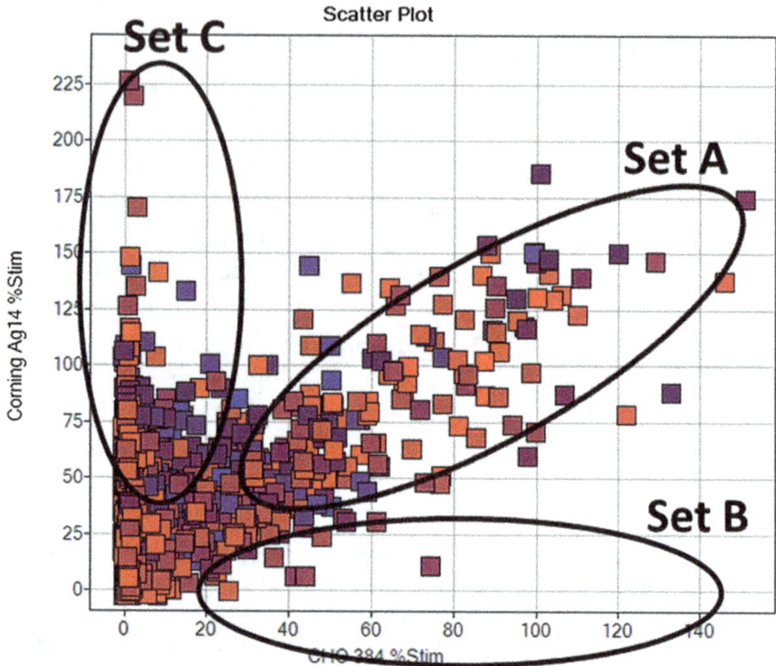

Fig. 7 Plot of percentage stimulation for compounds tested in agonist mode in both label-free optical biosensor (DMR) and FLIPR assays. Each point represents an individual compound. Set A represents compounds active in both technologies (>30 % stimulation) and Set C represents compounds active only in DMR (>30 % stimulation). Set B represents a small number of compounds that were FLIPR active and DMR inactive

References

1. Wess J (1996) Molecular biology of muscarinic acetylcholine receptors. Crit Rev Neurobiol 10(1):69–99

2. Wess J, Duttaroy A, Zhang W, Gomeza J, Cui Y, Miyakawa T, Bymaster FP, McKinzie L, Felder CC, Lamping KG et al (2003) M1-M5 muscarinic receptor knockout mice as novel tools to study the physiological roles of the muscarinic cholinergic system. Receptors Channels 9(4):279–290

3. Fang Y (2006) Label-free cell-based assays with optical biosensors in drug discovery. Assay Drug Dev Technol 4(5):583–595. doi:10.1089/adt.2006.4.583

4. Tran E, Fang Y (2008) Duplexed label-free G protein-coupled receptor assays for high-throughput screening. J Biomol Screen 13(10):975–985. doi:10.1177/1087057108326141

5. Zhang J, Chung TDY, Oldenburg KR (1999) A simple statistical parameter for use in evaluation and validation of high throughput screening assays. J Biomol Screen 4(2):67–73. doi:10.1177/108705719900400206

6. Iversen PW, Beck B, Chen YF et al (2012) HTS assay validation. In: Sittampalam GS, Gal-Edd N, Arkin M et al (eds) Assay guidance manual (internet). Eli Lilly and Company and the National Center for Advancing Translational Sciences, Bethesda, MD, http://www.ncbi.nlm.nih.gov/books/NBK83783/

7. Gitschier HJ, Bergeron AB, Randle DH (2014) Label-free cell-based dynamic mass redistribution assays. Curr Prot Chem Biol 6(1):39–51. doi:10.1002/9780470559277.ch130205

Multiplexing Label-Free and Fluorescence-Based Methods for Pharmacological Characterization of GPCR Ligands

Huailing Zhong, Xinyan Huang, and Dario Doller

Abstract

Cell-based assays are essential to drug discovery and biomedical research. Most cell-based assays have been targeting specific components of signaling pathways with considerable mechanistic significance. G protein-coupled receptors (GPCRs) represent a major class of drug targets. In addition to G protein-dependent pathways, G protein-independent signaling mechanisms such as β-arrestin pathways, allosteric modulation of receptor function, and receptor oligomerization are among currently active research areas. High-throughput calcium- and membrane potential-based assays have been widely used as efficient screening platforms. The Hamamatsu FDSS7000 instrument is capable of simultaneous compound addition and fluorescence monitoring in 96- or 384-wells for fluorescence-based calcium or membrane potential assays. However, phenotypic or holistic cellular measurements of combined effects contributed by multiple signaling pathways may also be required to complement label-based assays that target specific signaling events. For this purpose, the effects mediated by GPCRs may be measured by dynamic mass redistribution (DMR) through Resonant Waveguide Grating (RWG) biosensors embedded in 384-well plates using a Corning EPIC BT label-free assay system. Herein, we describe experimental protocol for profiling ADX88178, a potent and selective positive allosteric modulator (PAM) of the metabotropic glutamate 4 receptor (mGluR4) using both Ca^{2+} and DMR phenotypic readouts, and discuss the complementary features of each assay type. Further, we demonstrate, for the first time, a unique integrated procedure multiplexing FDSS calcium mobilization and EPIC label-free assays using a single set of cell/compound plates.

Key words Dynamic mass redistribution, Functional drug screening system, G protein-coupled receptor, Label-free, Resonant waveguide grating

1 Introduction

G protein-coupled receptors (GPCRs) constitute of the largest member of membrane proteins and host one of the major mechanistic targets for therapeutic drugs in clinical use [1, 2]. Among the approximately 800 possible GPCR genes, there are at least 120 orphan GPCRs which do not have identified endogenous ligands and are potential targets for novel drug discovery [2]. The activation of GPCRs by their ligands and modulators can be quantified

Ye Fang (ed.), *Label-Free Biosensor Methods in Drug Discovery*, Methods in Pharmacology and Toxicology, DOI 10.1007/978-1-4939-2617-6_12, © Springer Science+Business Media New York 2015

by changes in the functions of downstream signaling proteins. These functional changes are demonstrated by various G protein-dependent measurements; for instance, the production of second messenger molecules such as cAMP, cGMP, diacylglycerol, inositol (1, 4, 5)-trisphosphate (IP3), phosphatidyl inositol (3, 4, 5)-trisphosphate (PIP3), and ions like Ca^{2+} [3]. G protein-independent effectors such as β-arrestins have been well characterized [4]. An important role of β-arrestins is their involvement in the desensitization, sequestration, and vesicular trafficking of activated GPCRs [5, 6]. β-arrestins are thought to function as mediators of G-protein-independent modulation of kinases and GTPases, leading to further cellular changes such as cell migration and actin reorganization [7, 8]. This differential coupling of GPCRs to G protein-dependent versus G protein-independent pathways is known as ligand-directed or biased signaling, and demonstrates the complex nature of GPCR signaling mechanisms [9, 10]. Studies of the interplay between these G protein- and β-arrestin-mediated functions suggest the therapeutic potential of selectively targeting β-arrestin pathways involved in disease states [11]. Novel drug screening methods have been also developed for assessing β-arrestin mediated pathways and phenotypic readouts [12].

In addition to classical orthosteric ligands, the use of allosteric mechanisms is a growing design strategy to affect the receptor signal transduction by pharmacological agents [13–15]. Various selective allosteric compounds without orthosteric site activities have been discovered as valuable tool compounds for pharmacological interventions, which have aided the understanding of the physiological and pathophysiological roles of GPCRs. For example, a large number of positive allosteric modulators (PAMs) and negative allosteric modulators (NAMs) have been reported for the metabotropic glutamate receptors and muscarinic acetylcholine receptors [16, 17]. Allosteric interactions are also common for non-GPCR targets, such as the nicotinic acetylcholine ion channels including the α4β2 and α7 subtypes [18–20], as well as the serotonin transporter [21, 22]. Allosteric modulators with potential therapeutic benefits for various targets have been described in many central nervous system (CNS) diseases such as pain, Alzheimer's disease, schizophrenia, and depression [20–25].

The screening of GPCR-targeted orthosteric and allosteric compounds has largely aimed at specific signaling events and depended on methods utilizing labels, mostly being fluorescent, chemiluminescent, or colorimetric [26, 27]. However, signaling event-specific and label-based assays have met challenges, such as predictability of disease states, correlation to polypharmacology, and label-specific artifacts [28]. To overcome these challenges, label-free methods, including electrical impedance, surface plasmon resonance (SPR), optical resonant waveguide grating (RWG), and mass spectrometry for detecting biochemical and cellular activities have experienced significant development, including new applications, in recent years [28–33]. Label-free assays provide advantages including less artifact and noninvasiveness, and offer the capability of detecting polypharmacology and cellular phenotypic responses which have gained renewed interest in modern drug discovery [28, 34, 35]. For label-free cellular assays especially with GPCRs, optical RWG and electrical impedance are two main methodologies and offer real-time activity kinetics, high-throughput capability, as well as multi-pathway, holistic, and phenotypic measurements of drug responses [28, 36]. The optical RWG biosensor, consisting of a substrate layer, a waveguide film embedding a grating structure, a medium, and a surface layer, employs surface-bound evanescent waves generated by resonant coupling of light into the waveguide by diffraction grating for cell sensing [37]. A change in the amount of protein mass within the detection range of the surface is correlated with change in refractive index detected by the biosensor and is reported as a shift in resonant wavelength [38].

The optical RWG biosensor measures protein mass changes associated with GPCR- and other target-mediated signaling events, a phenomenon which is known as dynamic mass redistribution (DMR) [37]. It is recognized that GPCR signaling commonly results in receptor trafficking [39], protein relocalization [40], and cytoskeletal dynamics [38, 41]. Moreover, a large number of GPCR-interacting proteins (GIPs), which have important functions on their own, may be involved in GPCR translocation and trafficking by assembling into large functional complexes called "receptosomes" [42]. DMR changes associated with receptor activation are natural downstream effects, and the measurement of ligand impact on the system phenotype does not rely on exogenously engineered proteins [43–45]. This is also true with other label-free cellular analysis including impedance-based detection [46–48]. For non-$G\alpha_q$-coupled GPCRs, high-throughput screening with calcium mobilization requires promiscuous or engineered $G\alpha$ [49–51]. However, such unnatural $G\alpha$ coupling may lead to altered agonist specificity, such as agonist EC_{50}-ranking [52, 53]. Thus label-free methods such as optical RWG that measure phenotypic and sometimes morphological responses mediated through target receptor activation can serve as complementary assay applications to label-based readouts.

This chapter describes a unique multiplexing assay protocol for measuring cellular Ca^{2+} mobilization using functional drug screening system (FDSS) platform and DMR phenotypic responses using EPIC BT system with a single set of cell/compound plates.

2   Materials

2.1   Tissue Culture Medium and Cell Line

1. CHO-M_1 cell line. The muscarinic acetylcholine M_1 receptor was cloned and stably expressed in Chinese hamster ovary (CHO) cells.

2. BHK-mGluR4 cell line. The $mGluR_4$ receptor was cloned and stably expressed in Baby hamster kidney (BHK) cells.

3. BHK-mGluR4-$G\alpha_{15}$ cell line. A co-stable cell line was made expressing mGluR4 and $G\alpha_{15}$.

4. Dulbecco's modified Eagle's medium (DMEM) (Life Technologies, Carlsbad, CA, USA).

5. F-12 HAM media (Life Technologies).

6. Regular and dialyzed fetal bovine serum (FBS) (Life Technologies).

7. Antibiotic P/S solution 100×: 10,000 units/ml penicillin, 10,000 μg/ml streptomycin.

8. Trypsin–ethylenediaminetetraacetic acid (EDTA) solution 10×: 2.5 % Trypsin, 0.2 % $4Na^+$-EDTA.

2.2   Reagents and Consumables

1. GlutaMAX, sodium pyruvate (Life Technologies).

2. Fluo-8 NW no wash calcium assay dye (Cat # UPL-36315 or UPL-36316) (U-Pharm Laboratories, Parsippany, NJ, USA).

3. Poly-D-Lysine (PDL) coated 384-well assay plates (Corning # 7244) (Corning Incorporated, Corning, NY, USA).

4. Fibronectin-coated Epic 384-well cell assay plates (Corning # 5042) (Corning Incorporated).

5. Corning 384-well polypropylene compound storage plate.

6. 1× HBSS: Hank's Balanced Salt Solution (138 mM NaCl, 5 mM KCl, 1.3 mM $CaCl_2$, 0.5 mM $MgCl_2$, 0.4 mM $MgSO_4$, 0.3 mM KH_2PO_4, 0.3 mM Na_2HPO_4, 5.6 mM glucose).

2.3   Instruments and Software

1. Epic® BT system (Corning Incorporated) (Fig. 1a, b).

2. FDSS7000 (Hamamatsu Corporation, Bridgewater, NJ, USA) (Fig. 1c).

3. BioTek cell plate washer ELx405 (BioTek Instruments Inc., Winooski, VT, USA).

4. GraphPad Prism 5 (GraphPad, San Diego, CA, USA).

3   Methods

3.1   General Cell Culture

This section describes different media conditions to culture different cell lines, as well as general culture protocol to prepare cell assay plates for multiplexing Ca^{2+} and DMR assays. The biosensor

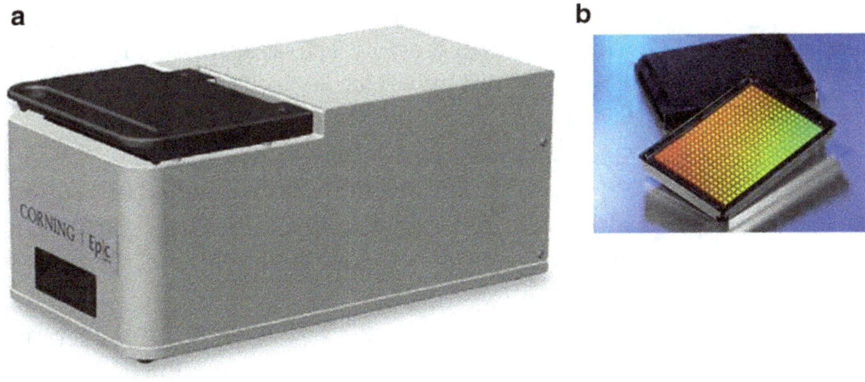

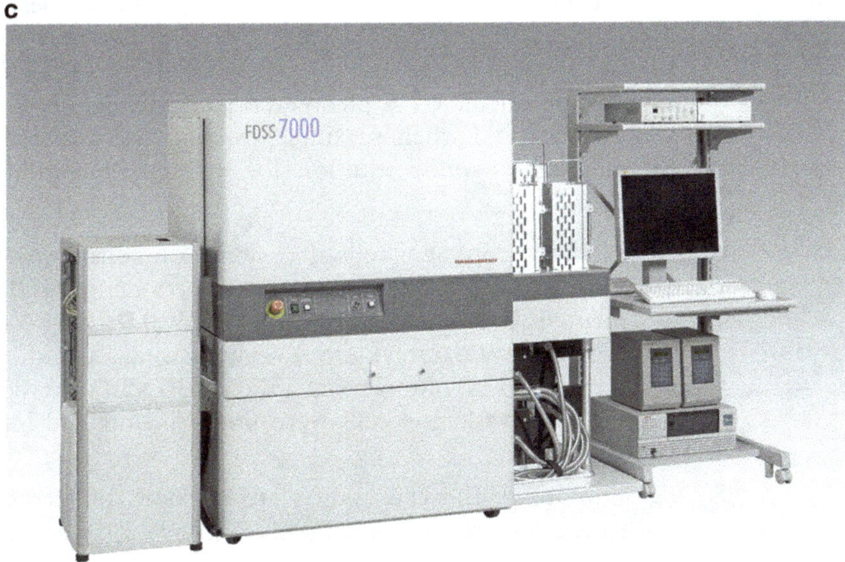

Fig. 1 Epic BT label-free and FDSS7000 used for multiplexed cell based assays. (**a**) Epic BT label-free system. (**b**) Epic 384 cell assay plates. (**c**) FDSS7000 high-throughput screening system

microplate is ready for culture and is directly used. For different cell lines the culture protocol can be optimized by altering cell culture medium and duration, initial cell seeding numbers, cell synchronization, and coating of biosensor surfaces.

1. Culture CHO in F-12 HAM medium supplemented with 10 % FBS, 4 mM L-glutamine, 1× antibiotic P/S solution.

2. Culture CHO-M1 cells in F-12 HAM medium supplemented with 10 % FBS, 4 mM L-glutamine, 1× antibiotic P/S solution, and 0.5 mg/ml G418 (geneticin) at 37 °C, 5 % CO_2.

3. Culture BHK cells in DMEM medium supplemented with 10 % dialyzed and heat-inactivated FBS, 1 % GlutaMAX, 1 mM sodium pyruvate, 1× antibiotic P/S solution at 37 °C, 5 % CO_2.

4. Culture BHK-mGluR4 cells in DMEM medium supplemented with 10 % dialyzed and heat-inactivated FBS, 1 % GlutaMAX, 1 mM sodium pyruvate, 1× antibiotic P/S solution. 1 mg/ml G418 at 37 °C, 5 % CO_2.

5. Seed the cells into fibronectin-coated 384-well Epic plates at a density of 12,000–15,000 cells per well. The seeding was done with a cell seeder or manual multichannel pipet with sufficient dispensing speed to avoid air bubbles at the bottom of wells (*see* **Note 1**).

6. Culture overnight at 37 °C, 5 % CO_2. After overnight culture, the cells become confluent with a confluency of ~95 %.

3.2 Label-Free Assay on Epic BT

This section describes the protocol to perform label-free DMR assays using the Epic BT system. All label-free assays were performed at room temperature. DMR measurements from label-free assays were calculated as picometer (pm) wavelength shifts for all well at the time when maximal response was reached, typically 50 min after agonist addition for both the mGluR4 and M1 receptors.

1. Wash the confluent cells after overnight culture in the biosensor microplate using the assay buffer containing HBSS supplemented with 20 mM HEPES, pH 7.4, 0.05 % BSA, and 0.5 % dimethyl sulfoxide (DMSO). The washing was done for five times at 60 µl volume using a BioTek ELx50 strip washer. After the final wash, the cells were finally maintained in 40 µl the assay buffer.

2. Equilibrate the cell assay plate at room temperature for at least 2 h.

3. Prepare compound source plate by diluting compound solutions to the desired concentrations using the same assay buffer containing 0.5 % DMSO. This is to eliminate the effect of DMSO mismatch during compound addition.

4. Place the cell assay plate on the Epic BT reader. Each plate must be aligned before assays. If the plates need to be switched during assays, plate alignment needs to be done for each plate before reading. The following parameters were chosen for plate alignment: 384-well, 2 mm cell.

5. Establish the baseline reading for at least 5 min.

6. Pause the reader.

7. Transfer the compound solutions from the compound source plate to the cell assay plate using liquid handing instrument.

8. Restart the reader. For typical DMR reading, the settings of 2 mm cell and 900 data points with four scanning averages per data point were applied. In modulator assays, PAM compounds were added first and measured for 30 min, followed by the

addition of an agonist and at least 60 min continuous recording.

9. Analyze the DMR results using Microsoft Excel, and Epic Viewer.

10. Calculate dose response curves using GraphPad Prism 5 (*see* **Note 2**).

3.3 Calcium Mobilization Assay on FDSS7000

This section describes how to perform calcium mobilization assay using FDSS7000 system. Before preparing for this assay, cell plates, especially the fibronectin-coated Epic plates, must be calibrated on FDSS for each detection method and plate type, and calibration was done as follows for Microplate Mapping, Auto Fluorescence, and Shading.

3.3.1 System Setup and Preparation

1. Start the system including hardware and software.

2. Select a fluorescent method and an assay plate type.

3. Choose supervisory mode for calibration.

4. Choose calibration selections in Setup option.

5. For the assay plate type to be calibrated, use an empty plate to view its live images in "Manual Control" mode, with correct filter wavelengths (Excitation 490 nm/Emission 525 nM for Fluo-3, 4, and 8), and a proper sensitivity level.

6. Prepare a fluorescence plate by adding 40 µl of culture media (DMEM or other types) to each well of a clean plate to be used for Plate Mapping and Shading Calibration.

7. Prepare a water plate by adding 40 µl of water (double-distilled or mini-Q) to each well of another clean plate to be used for Auto Fluorescence Calibration.

3.3.2 Plate Mapping Calibration

1. Under Microplate Mapping option, load the fluorescence plate.

2. Set a proper sensitivity level, acquire the data to preview the image of the plate. When the numbers of "Size" and "Real Well Size" were made to be the same, perform and save the calculation so that all wells in the plate image had the best overlap with digital wells (white boxes).

3.3.3 Auto Fluorescence Calibration

1. Determine Auto Fluorescence calibration for each of the available exposure levels on FDSS for use as background subtraction of autofluorescence by the plate itself. Before each calibration, choose each exposure time under Manual Control.

2. Under Auto Fluorescence setup, load the water plate and make a pre-acquisition to ensure a clean image of the plate displayed. Acquire the final calibration data ("Acquire Data") and save the data.

3.3.4 Shading Calibration

Shading calibration for each method was necessary since factors such as light, camera sensitivity and well-to-well optical inconsistencies affect spatial uniformity of a plate type.

1. Under Shading Calibration setup, load the fluorescence plate and make pre-acquisition while adjusting exposure time and sensitivity level so that the pre-acquired image of the plate was in the yellow/orange pseudo color range.

2. Acquire the final data ("Acquire Data") and save the data. Shading calibration might need to be repeated so that a plate read for the fluorescence plate resulted in a coefficient of variation (CV) of less than 2 %.

3.3.5 Calcium Mobilization Assays

1. Seed the cells into 384-well PDL-coated or fibronectin-coated Epic plates at a density of 15,000 cells per well and incubate overnight at 37 °C, 5 % CO_2. After overnight culture, the cells typically reach ~95 % confluency.

2. Decant and replace the culture medium with 20 μl the HBSS assay buffer as mentioned in **Step 1** of Section 3.2.

3. Add Fluo-8 calcium dye at 20 μl per well to achieve 2 μM final concentration and then incubate at 37 °C for 30 min followed by incubation at room temperature for an additional 30 min.

4. Monitor the basal fluorescence in FDSS7000 using optical filters with a peak excitation wavelength of 490 nm and a peak emission 525 nm.

5. For agonist only experiments, stimulate the cells at room temperature with an agonist and measure the fluorescence at 1.5 s intervals over a period of 3 min.

6. For modulation experiments, add a PAM and read the fluorescence at 1.5 s intervals over a period of 3 min. Incubate at room temperature for 20 min, add an agonist and read the fluorescence again.

7. Analyze the data. Analyze concentration response results using GraphPad Prism 5. Ca^{2+} mobilization data from FDSS were expressed as either peak fluorescent changes or ratios over background.

3.4 Multiplexed Calcium and Label-Free Assays

This section describes the protocol to perform multiplexing calcium and label-free assays on the same Epic plate with the same compound additions (Fig. 2a). Epic DMR reading is made immediately after calcium measurement (Fig. 2b). The ability to perform dual detection using the same set of cells and compounds is due to different kinetics of calcium and DMR signals triggered by the activation of a receptor (Fig. 2c) (*see* **Note 2**). Both M1 and mGluR4 are used as model systems to demonstrate the duplexing assays. Drug discovery efforts for mGluR receptors have been

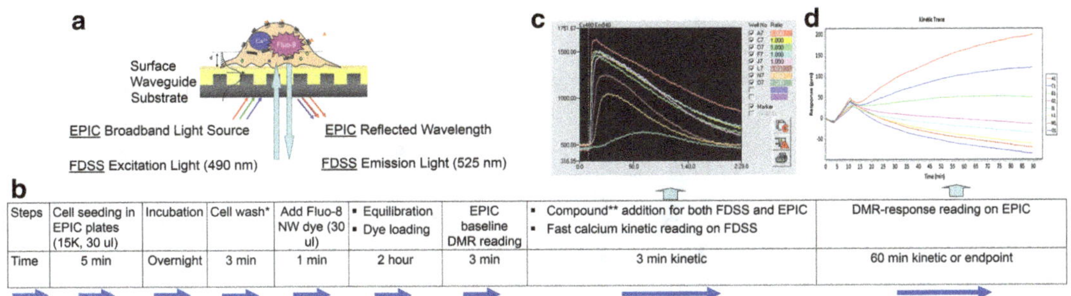

Fig. 2 An integrated assay procedure for measuring cellular responses on FDSS and Epic platforms using a single set of cell/compound plates. (**a**) Mechanistic diagram of integrated measurements of cellular calcium and DMR responses. (**b**) Assay work flow of multiplexing Epic label-free and FDSS calcium assays. * Cells in EPIC plates were washed with assay buffer containing HBSS, 0.05 % BSA, 0.5 % DMSO using a BioTek ELX50 strip washer; ** Compound: ACh dose response (0.3 nM to 1 μM). (**c**) Sample kinetic traces of calcium mobilization by M1-CHO on FDSS. (**d**) Sample kinetic traces of label-free DMR measurement on Epic BT

mainly reported with specific G protein-mediated assays in primary screens [54–58]. However, β-arrestin pathways tend to be ubiquitous in non-G protein-mediated GPCR signaling [4]. In fact, mGluR1 and mGluR7 receptors have been reported to involve β-arrestin signaling [59, 60]. Thus, label-free assays such as DMR measurements as phenotypic tests may need to be utilized to bolster the characterization of mGluR compounds before in vivo testing. Results showed that in the Ca^{+2} flux assay with BHK-mGluR4-$G\alpha_{15}$ cells using FDSS7000, the potent and selective mGluR4 PAM chemical probe ADX88178 [61] was found to progressively shift glutamate dose-response curve to the left, with the EC_{50} of glutamate changing up to 100-fold from ~10,000 nM in the absence of this PAM to 100 nM in the presence of this PAM at 1,000 nM (Fig. 3a). This PAM also increased the maximal response of glutamate by ~100 % (Fig. 3a). In label-free assays with the same cell plate and compound set using Epic BT, glutamate gave rise to a dose-dependent response with an EC_{50} of ~30,000 nM, slightly higher than that in the Ca^{+2} flux assay (Fig. 3b). This PAM also progressively shifted glutamate dose-response curve to the left with a tenfold increase in EC_{50}, as evidenced by the EC_{50} of glutamate that was found to be ~3,000 nM at the highest [PAM] tested (1,000 nM) (Fig. 3b). The different modulatory potency of the PAM molecule obtained may help interpret differences when evaluating in vivo efficacy of PAM effects or guide experimental planning for in vivo studies. To our best knowledge, the investigation of functional mGluR4 receptor activation by either orthosteric or allosteric mechanisms in label-free assays has not been reported.

To achieve an optimal procedure for specific GPCR targets and signaling pathways, modifications of procedures such as assay buffer, cell washing, and assay timing may be necessary (*see* **Note 3**).

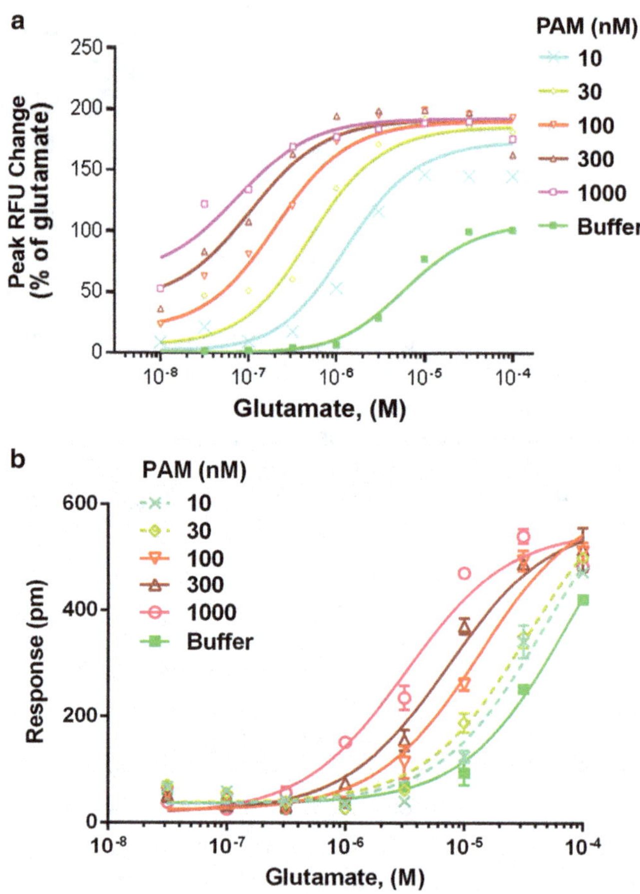

Fig. 3 Comparison of agonist and PAM ADX88178 functional activities at the mGluR4 receptor, Ca^{2+} versus DMR. (**a**) PAM activities with Ca^{2+} readout for mGluR4-$G\alpha_{15}$-BHK. (**b**) PAM activities with DMR label-free readout for mGluR4-BHK

Our methods and results show that the activities of agonist as well as positive allosteric modulator (PAM) compounds for the mGluR4 receptor can be measured using both Ca^{2+} and DMR phenotypic readouts with complementary features of each assay type. We also demonstrated a unique integrated assay procedure multiplexing FDSS calcium mobilization and EPIC label-free platforms to generate both assay readouts using a single set of cell and compound plates. This facilitates the interrogation of mutually complementary cellular responses with greatly reduced cell/compound plate variations, turnaround time, as well as material and operational costs.

1. Seed the cells into fibronectin-coated 384-well Epic plates at a density of 12,000–15,000 cells per well.

2. Culture the cells overnight.

3. Wash the cells using the assay buffer containing 0.5 % DMSO.

4. Add Fluo-8 dye (at the same final concentration as mentioned earlier) to achieve 30 µl final volume for modulation assays, or 40 µl final volume for agonist-only experiment.

5. Incubate the cells at room temperature for 2 h to allow for simultaneous dye-loading and DMR equilibration.

6. Read the baseline DMR reading on Epic BT for 3 min after plate alignment.

7. Remove and transfer the plate to FDSS7000.

8. Add agonist and perform calcium assay.

9. Immediately after calcium reading, transfer the cell plate back to Epic BT to monitor for 60 min. For modulation assays, first addition on FDSS7000 was with PAM compounds followed by Epic DMR reading for 20 min. Then, the cell plate was moved to FDSS7000 for agonist calcium assay (3 min), immediately followed by DMR reading on Epic BT for a final 60 min.

4 Notes

1. It is important to eliminate any air bubbles in the biosensor microplate. Epic plate wells tend to be hydrophobic and air bubbles may form inside the wells. If this happens, spin down the plate using a plate centrifuge at ~500 rpm for 30 s to 1 min. Check under the microscope to make sure the cells are not concentrated in one side. Set the plate at room temperate for 15 min before placing in the incubator.

2. Calcium mobilization and DMR signals often display significantly different kinetics. For example, by using the promiscuous $G\alpha_{15}$ protein in BHK-mGluR4-$G\alpha_{15}$ cells, the activation of mGluR4 receptors results in both calcium mobilization and DMR signals. The calcium trace obtained is similar to that of a typical G_q-coupled receptor and displays fast kinetics (that is, usually peaks at ~40 s) (Fig. 2c). Owing to its fast kinetics, calcium assay is generally considered to be as running under nonthermodynamic equilibrium conditions [62, 63]. Some pharmacological characterizations require equilibration between drugs and target of investigation, such as Schild regression [64, 65]. With the Epic label-free system, DMR measurements delineated natural receptor-mediated signaling without exogenous G proteins. Furthermore, Epic DMR readout often displays much slower kinetics than calcium kinetics (Fig. 2d) and thus may mimic equilibration more closely.

3. Given the different features of calcium mobilization and label-free DMR assays (Table 1), performing duplexed assays in a single Epic plate may require optimization. We exemplify an integrated work flow using a G_q-coupled muscarinic M1 receptor in

Table 1
Comparison of Epic label-free and FDSS calcium assays

	Epic label-free assay	FDSS calcium assay
Label	No	Fluorescence
Optical	Visible broadband	Ex 490 nm/Em 525 nm
Measurement	DMR	Calcium mobilization
Measurement type	Phenotypic, holistic	Specific to signaling molecules
Require promiscuous or chimeric G protein	Not needed	Yes for Gi/o or Gs-coupled receptors
Can assay endogenous receptor	Yes	Limited
Equilibrium reaction	Equilibrium	Semi-equilibrium
Assay kinetics	15–60 min	2–3 min
End-point read?	Yes, suitable	Not suitable
Throughput	Medium to high	High

The features of Epic label-free and FDSS calcium assays are summarized and compared. Multiplexed assays of the two platforms integrate complementary benefits of each type

CHO-M1 cells (Fig. 2). The original assays for individual calcium and Epic label-free involved different washing, loading and compound addition operations, thus we tested the effects of several perturbations of one assay on the other. For calcium assays, after successful plate calibration, the Epic cell plate did not generate autofluorescent interference, and produced robust response upon agonist acetylcholine (ACh) addition (Fig. 4a), with nanomolar EC_{50}. Fluo-8 dye gave similar responses with or without media removal or buffer washing (Fig. 4a). In Epic label-free assays, CHO-M1 cells also generated a robust dose response with EC_{50} of ~100 nM (Fig. 4b, solid squares). EC_{50} values determined using the label-free DMR assay seemed to be significantly weaker than those from Ca^{+2} flux assays, probably for reasons related to factors such as different effector efficiency, equilibration time, etc. When cells were not washed before Fluo-8 dye loading, the Epic label-free signal was very small, as expected, probably due to suppression by serum in culture media (Fig. 4b, open squares). In addition, if the cell washing step used only HBSS buffer without DMSO, the effect of ACh was similar, suggesting 0.5 % DMSO during the 2 h incubation period had no adverse effect on assay signal. Furthermore, the presence of Fluo-8 dye in the 2 h incubation period did not significantly affect agonist concentration response curves in the label-free measurement either (Fig. 4b). Lastly, ACh agonist was usually

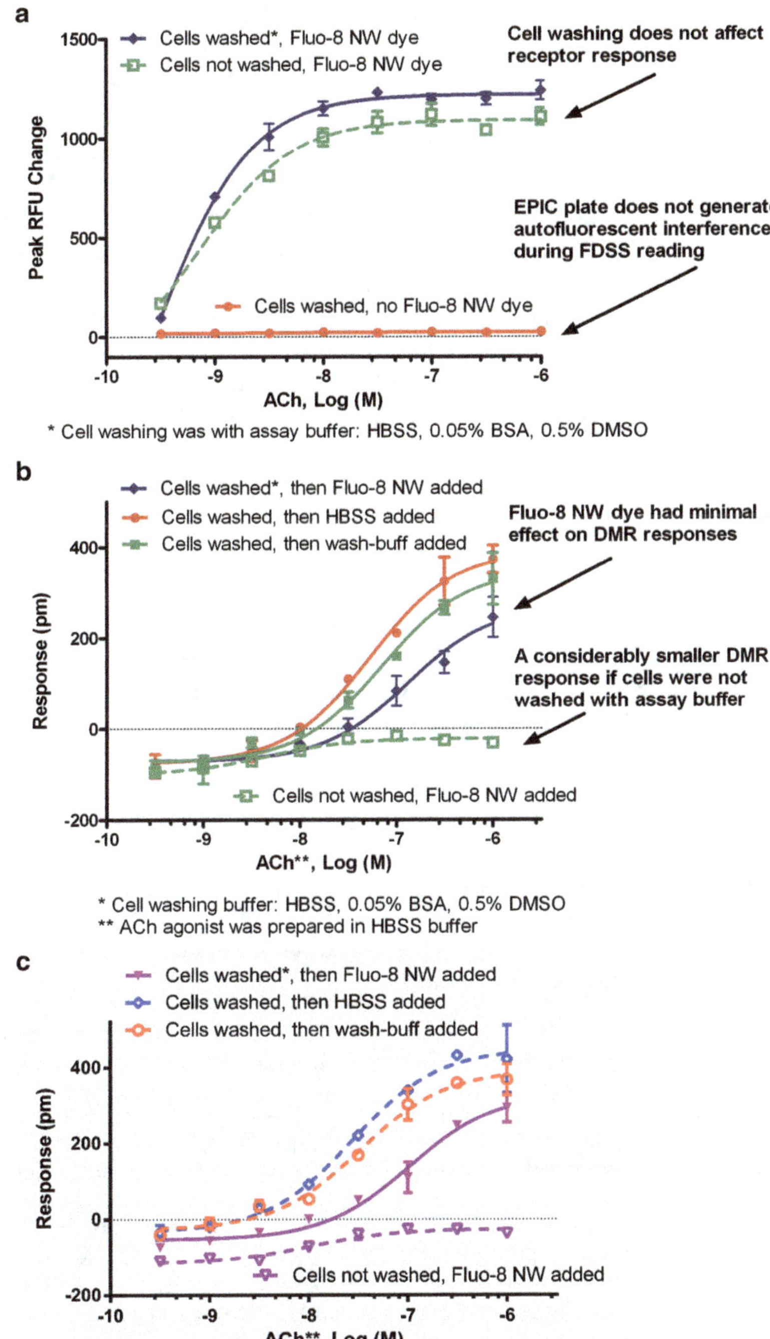

Fig. 4 Suitability of multiplexing label-free and FDSS assays using a single Epic test plate. (**a**) FDSS is capable of measuring calcium kinetics using EPIC optical plates (with proper calibration). (**b**) Cell tested for calcium on FDSS7000 yielded meaningful DMR responses on EPIC BT label-free system. (**c**) Agonist compound produced similar DMR response profiles when prepared in wash buffer containing DMSO

made in HBSS buffer, and in a typical Epic label-free assay, compounds were made in wash buffer containing DMSO. To rule out any effect by 0.5 % DMSO, we also prepared ACh in wash buffer containing 0.5 % DMSO, and found that its activity profiles at all the test conditions were similar to its effects at corresponding conditions described above (Fig. 4c). These results demonstrated that the assay conditions and perturbations in Ca^{2+} flux and label-free screens can be modified to accommodate each other. This strongly indicates the suitability of multiplexing Epic label-free measurement immediately after calcium assay on FDSS7000. Of note, muscarinic acetylcholine receptors such as M2 and M3 have been reported using label-free assays recently [43, 66, 67].

Acknowledgements

The authors thank Drs. Shouming Du, Yiwen Wang, Alex Sanchez, and Al McGrath of Hamamatsu Corporation, and Drs. Hung Cuong Louie Tran and Ye Fang of Corning Incorprated for technical assistance. We are also grateful to Mr. Michael Collins and Noel J. Boyle for technical support.

References

1. Flower DR (1999) Modelling G-protein-coupled receptors for drug design. Biochim Biophys Acta 1422:207–234. doi:10.1016/S0304-4157(99)00006-4

2. Lagerstrom MC, Schioth HB (2008) Structural diversity of G protein-coupled receptors and significance for drug discovery. Nat Rev Drug Discov 7:339–357. doi:10.1038/nrd2518

3. Marinissen MJ, Gutkind JS (2001) G-protein-coupled receptors and signaling networks: emerging paradigms. Trends Pharmacol Sci 22:368–376. doi:10.1016/S0165-6147(00)01678-3

4. Lefkowitz RJ, Whalen EJ (2004) Beta-arrestins: traffic cops of cell signaling. Curr Opin Cell Biol 16:162–168. doi:10.1016/j.ceb.2004.01.001

5. Tian X, Kang DS, Benovic JL (2014) Beta-arrestins and G protein-coupled receptor trafficking. Handb Exp Pharmacol 219:173–186. doi:10.1007/978-3-642-41199-1_9

6. Walther C, Ferguson SS (2013) Arrestins: role in the desensitization, sequestration, and vesicular trafficking of G protein-coupled receptors. Prog Mol Biol Transl Sci 118:93–113. doi:10.1016/B978-0-12-394440-5.00004-8

7. Dewire SM, Ahn S, Lefkowitz RJ et al (2007) Beta-arrestins and cell signaling. Annu Rev Physiol 69:483–510. doi:10.1146/annurev.physiol.69.022405.154749

8. Luttrell LM, Gesty-Palmer D (2010) Beyond desensitization: physiological relevance of arrestin-dependent signaling. Pharmacol Rev 62:305–330. doi:10.1124/pr.109.002436

9. Kenakin T (2007) Functional selectivity through protean and biased agonism: who steers the ship? Mol Pharmacol 72:1393–1401. doi:10.1124/mol.107.040352

10. Violin JD, Lefkowitz RJ (2007) Beta-arrestin-biased ligands at seven-transmembrane receptors. Trends Pharmacol Sci 28:416–422. doi:10.1016/j.tips.2007.06.006

11. Michel MC, Seifert R, Bond RA (2014) Dynamic bias and its implications for GPCR drug discovery. Nat Rev Drug Discov 13:869. doi:10.1038/nrd3954-c3

12. Chen L, Jin L, Zhou N (2012) An update of novel screening methods for GPCR in drug discovery. Exp Opin Drug Discov 7:791–806. doi:10.1517/17460441.2012.699036

13. Changeux JP, Edelstein SJ (2005) Allosteric mechanisms of signal transduction. Science 308:1424–1428. doi:10.1126/science.1108595

14. Kenakin T (2007) Collateral efficacy in drug discovery: taking advantage of the good

(allosteric) nature of 7TM receptors. Trends Pharmacol Sci 28:407–415. doi:10.1016/j.tips.2007.06.009

15. Gao ZG, Jacobson KA (2006) Keynote review: allosterism in membrane receptors. Drug Discov Today 11:191–202. doi:10.1016/S1359-6446(05)03689-5

16. Conn PJ, Christopoulos A, Lindsley CW (2009) Allosteric modulators of GPCRs: a novel approach for the treatment of CNS disorders. Nat Rev Drug Discov 8:41–54. doi:10.1038/nrd2760

17. Keov P, Sexton PM, Christopoulos A (2011) Allosteric modulation of G protein-coupled receptors: a pharmacological perspective. Neuropharmacology 60:24–35. doi:10.1016/j.neuropharm.2010.07.010

18. Arneric SP, Holladay M, Williams M (2007) Neuronal nicotinic receptors: a perspective on two decades of drug discovery research. Biochem Pharmacol 74:1092–1101. doi:10.1016/j.bcp.2007.06.033

19. Pandya A, Yakel JL (2011) Allosteric modulators of the $\alpha_4\beta_2$ subtype of neuronal nicotinic acetylcholine receptors. Biochem Pharmacol 82:952–958. doi:10.1016/j.bcp.2011.04.020

20. Wallace TL, Porter RH (2011) Targeting the nicotinic alpha7 acetylcholine receptor to enhance cognition in disease. Biochem Pharmacol 82:891–903. doi:10.1016/j.bcp.2011.06.034

21. Zhong H, Haddjeri N, Sanchez C (2012) Escitalopram, an antidepressant with an allosteric effect at the serotonin transporter-a review of current understanding of its mechanism of action. Psychopharmacology (Berl) 219:1–13. doi:10.1007/s00213-011-2463-5

22. Zhong H, Sanchez C, Caron MG (2012) Consideration of allosterism and interacting proteins in the physiological functions of the serotonin transporter. Biochem Pharmacol 83:435–442. doi:10.1016/j.bcp.2011.09.020

23. Kenakin T (2013) Allosteric drugs and seven transmembrane receptors. Curr Top Med Chem 13:5–13.doi:10.2174/1568026611313010003

24. Kenakin TP (2012) Biased signalling and allosteric machines: new vistas and challenges for drug discovery. Br J Pharmacol 165:1659–1669.doi:10.1111/j.1476-5381.2011.01749.x

25. Conn PJ, Lindsley CW, Meiler J et al (2014) Opportunities and challenges in the discovery of allosteric modulators of GPCRs for treating CNS disorders. Nat Rev Drug Discov 13:692–708. doi:10.1038/nrd4308

26. Thomsen W, Frazer J, Unett D (2005) Functional assays for screening GPCR targets. Curr Opin Biotechnol 16:655–665. doi:10.1016/j.copbio.2005.10.008

27. Eglen RM (2005) Functional G protein-coupled receptor assays for primary and secondary screening. Comb Chem High Throughput Screen 8:311–318. doi:10.2174/1386207054020813

28. Fang Y (2014) Label-free drug discovery. Front Pharmacol 5:52. doi:10.3389/fphar.2014.00052

29. Rask-Andersen M, Almen MS, Schioth HB (2011) Trends in the exploitation of novel drug targets. Nat Rev Drug Discov 10:579–590. doi:10.1038/nrd3478

30. Halai R, Cooper MA (2012) Using label-free screening technology to improve efficiency in drug discovery. Exp Opin Drug Discov 7:123–131. doi:10.1517/17460441.2012.651121

31. Citartan M, Gopinath SC, Tominaga J et al (2013) Label-free methods of reporting biomolecular interactions by optical biosensors. Analyst 138:3576–3592. doi:10.1039/C3AN36828A

32. Lunn CA (2010) Label-free screening assays: a strategy for finding better drug candidates. Future Med Chem 2:1703–1716. doi:10.4155/fmc.10.246

33. Wong JW, Cagney G (2010) An overview of label-free quantitation methods in proteomics by mass spectrometry. Methods Mol Biol 604:273–283. doi:10.1007/978-1-60761-444-9_18

34. Eggert US (2013) The why and how of phenotypic small-molecule screens. Nat Chem Biol 9:206–209. doi:10.1038/nchembio.1206

35. Lee JA, Uhlik MT, Moxham CM et al (2012) Modern phenotypic drug discovery is a viable, neoclassic pharma strategy. J Med Chem 55:4527–4538. doi:10.1021/jm201649s

36. Fang Y (2013) Troubleshooting and deconvoluting label-free cell phenotypic assays in drug discovery. J Pharmacol Toxicol Methods 67:69–81. doi:10.1016/j.vascn.2013.01.004

37. Fang Y, Ferrie AM, Fontaine NH et al (2006) Resonant waveguide grating biosensor for living cell sensing. Biophys J 91:1925–1940. doi:10.1529/biophysj.105.077818

38. Fang Y, Ferrie AM, Li G (2005) Probing cytoskeleton modulation by optical biosensors. FEBS Lett 579:4175–4180. doi:10.1016/j.febslet.2005.06.050

39. Tan CM, Brady AE, Nickols HH et al (2004) Membrane trafficking of G protein-coupled receptors. Annu Rev Pharmacol Toxicol 44:559–609. doi:10.1146/annurev.pharmtox.44.101802.121558

40. Wehrman TS, Casipit CL, Gewertz NM et al (2005) Enzymatic detection of protein translocation. Nat Methods 2:521–527. doi:10.1038/nmeth771

41. Garbison KE, Heinz BA, Lajiness ME et al (2004) Impedance-based technologies. In: Sittampalam GS, Gal-Edd N, Arkin M, Auld D, Austin C, Bejcek B, Glicksman M, Inglese J, Lemmon V, Li Z, McGee J, McManus O, Minor L, Napper A, Riss T, Trask OJ, Weidner J (eds) Assay guidance manual. Eli Lilly & Company and the National Center for Advancing Translational Sciences, Bethesda, MD

42. Bockaert J, Fagni L, Dumuis A et al (2004) GPCR interacting proteins (GIP). Pharmacol Ther 103:203–221. doi:10.1016/j.pharmthera.2004.06.004

43. Deng H, Sun H, Fang Y (2013) Label-free cell phenotypic assessment of the biased agonism and efficacy of agonists at the endogenous muscarinic M3 receptors. J Pharmacol Toxicol Methods 68:323–333. doi:10.1016/j.vascn.2013.07.005

44. Sun H, Wei Y, Deng H et al (2014) Label-free cell phenotypic profiling decodes the composition and signaling of an endogenous ATP-sensitive potassium channel. Sci Rep 4:4934. doi:10.1038/srep04934

45. Carter RL, Grisanti LA, Yu JE, Repas AA, Woodall M, Ibetti J, Koch WJ, Jacobson MA, Tilley DG (2014) Dynamic mass redistribution analysis of endogenous β-adrenergic receptor signaling in neonatal rat cardiac fibroblasts. Pharmacol Res Perspect 2:24. doi:10.1002/prp2.24

46. Watts AO, Scholten DJ, Heitman LH et al (2012) Label-free impedance responses of endogenous and synthetic chemokine receptor CXCR3 agonists correlate with Gi-protein pathway activation. Biochem Biophys Res Commun 419:412–418. doi:10.1016/j.bbrc.2012.02.036

47. Verdonk E, Johnson K, Mcguinness R et al (2006) Cellular dielectric spectroscopy: a label-free comprehensive platform for functional evaluation of endogenous receptors. Assay Drug Dev Technol 4:609–619. doi:10.1016/j.jala.2005.06.002

48. Geetha T, Langlais P, Luo M et al (2011) Label-free proteomic identification of endogenous, insulin-stimulated interaction partners of insulin receptor substrate-1. J Am Soc Mass Spectrom 22:457–466. doi:10.1007/s13361-010-0051-2

49. Zhu T, Fang LY, Xie X (2008) Development of a universal high-throughput calcium assay for G-protein-coupled receptors with promiscuous G-protein Galpha15/16. Acta Pharmacol Sin 29:507–516. doi:10.1111/j.1745-7254.2008.00775.x

50. Walker MW, Jones KA, Tamm J et al (2005) Use of Caenorhabditis elegans Gαq chimeras to detect G-protein-coupled receptor signals. J Biomol Screen 10:127–136. doi:10.1177/1087057104272006

51. New DC, Wong YH (2004) Characterization of CHO cells stably expressing a G alpha 16/z chimera for high throughput screening of GPCRs. Assay Drug Dev Technol 2:269–280. doi:10.1089/1540658041410641

52. Shirokova E, Schmiedeberg K, Bedner P et al (2005) Identification of specific ligands for orphan olfactory receptors. G protein-dependent agonism and antagonism of odorants. J Biol Chem 280:11807–11815. doi:10.1074/jbc.M411508200

53. Krueger KM, Witte DG, Ireland-Denny L et al (2005) G protein-dependent pharmacology of histamine H3 receptor ligands: evidence for heterogeneous active state receptor conformations. J Pharmacol Exp Ther 314:271–281. doi:10.1124/jpet.104.078865

54. Niswender CM, Johnson KA, Weaver CD et al (2008) Discovery, characterization, and anti-parkinsonian effect of novel positive allosteric modulators of metabotropic glutamate receptor 4. Mol Pharmacol 74:1345–1358. doi:10.1124/mol.108.049551

55. Dhanya RP, Sheffler DJ, Dahl R et al (2014) Design and synthesis of systemically active metabotropic glutamate subtype-2 and -3 (mGlu2/3) receptor positive allosteric modulators (PAMs): pharmacological characterization and assessment in a rat model of cocaine dependence. J Med Chem 57:4154–4172. doi:10.1021/jm5000563

56. Monn JA, Valli MJ, Massey SM et al (2013) Synthesis and pharmacological characterization of 4-substituted-2-aminobicyclo[3.1.0]hexane-2,6-dicarboxylates: identification of new potent and selective metabotropic glutamate 2/3 receptor agonists. J Med Chem 56:4442–4455. doi:10.1021/jm4000165

57. Wenthur CJ, Morrison RD, Daniels JS et al (2014) Synthesis and SAR of substituted pyrazolo[1,5-a]quinazolines as dual mGlu(2)/mGlu(3) NAMs. Bioorg Med Chem Lett 24:2693–2698. doi:10.1016/j.bmcl.2014.04.051

58. Hammond AS, Rodriguez AL, Townsend SD et al (2010) Discovery of a novel chemical class of mGlu(5) allosteric ligands with distinct modes of pharmacology. ACS Chem Neurosci 1:702–716. doi:10.1021/cn100051m

59. Iacovelli L, Felicioni M, Nistico R et al (2014) Selective regulation of recombinantly expressed mGlu7 metabotropic glutamate receptors by G protein-coupled receptor kinases and arrestins. Neuropharmacology 77:303–312. doi:10.1016/j.neuropharm.2013.10.013

60. Iacovelli L, Salvatore L, Capobianco L et al (2003) Role of G protein-coupled receptor kinase 4 and beta-arrestin 1 in agonist-stimulated metabotropic glutamate receptor 1 internalization and activation of mitogen-activated protein kinases. J Biol Chem 278:12433–12442. doi:10.1074/jbc.M203992200

61. Le Poul E, Bolea C, Girard F et al (2012) A potent and selective metabotropic glutamate receptor 4 positive allosteric modulator improves movement in rodent models of Parkinson's disease. J Pharmacol Exp Ther 343:167–177. doi:10.1124/jpet.112.196063

62. Perdona E, Faggioni F, Buson A et al (2011) Pharmacological characterization of the ghrelin receptor antagonist, GSK1614343 in rat RC-4B/C cells natively expressing GHS type 1a receptors. Eur J Pharmacol 650:178–183. doi:10.1016/j.ejphar.2010.10.042

63. Miller TR, Witte DG, Ireland LM et al (1999) Analysis of apparent noncompetitive responses to competitive H1-histamine receptor antagonists in fluorescent imaging plate reader-based calcium assays. J Biomol Screen 4:249–258. doi:10.1177/108705719900400506

64. Arunlakshana O, Schild HO (1959) Some quantitative uses of drug antagonists. Br J Pharmacol Chemother 14:48–58

65. Kenakin T (2004) Principles: receptor theory in pharmacology. Trends Pharmacol Sci 25:186–192. doi:10.1016/j.tips.2004.02.012

66. Schrage R, Seemann WK, Klockner J et al (2013) Agonists with supraphysiological efficacy at the muscarinic M2 ACh receptor. Br J Pharmacol 169:357–370. doi:10.1111/bph.12003

67. Deng H, Wang C, Su M et al (2012) Probing biochemical mechanisms of action of muscarinic M3 receptor antagonists with label-free whole cell assays. Anal Chem 84:8232–8239. doi:10.1021/ac301495n

Chapter 13

Label-Free Cell Phenotypic Identification of Active Compounds in Traditional Chinese Medicines

Xinmiao Liang, Jixia Wang, Xiuli Zhang, and Ye Fang

Abstract

Traditional Chinese medicines (TCMs) have been used in clinic for thousands of years. These TCMs display reliable therapeutic efficacy and are important resources for drug discovery. Elucidating mechanisms of action (MOAs) of active compounds is essential to the development and clarification of TCMs. As one of new generation pharmacological assays, label-free cell phenotypic assays can provide a holistic view of ligand–receptor interactions in living cells with wide pathway coverage, high throughput, and high temporal resolution, thus enabling effectively elucidating the MOAs of TCMs. For identifying active compounds from TCMs, effective separation and purification methods are indispensable since TCMs usually contain hundreds or even thousands of compounds. This chapter provides a general protocol of preparative techniques and label-free cell phenotypic assays to determine the target engagement of active TCM fractions and compounds.

Key words Active compounds, Label-free cell phenotypic assay, Separation and purification, Traditional Chinese medicines

1 Introduction

Traditional Chinese medicines (TCMs), mainly referring to Chinese herbal medicines (CHMs) in this chapter, have been long receiving considerable attention owing to their reliable clinical efficacy [1–3]. They are important resources for lead compounds or drugs [4]. Clinically used natural product drugs include paclitaxel (anticancer), artemisinin (antimalarial), morphine (analgesic), rapamycin (immunosuppression), and reserpine (antihypertensive), to name a few. Recent analysis showed that almost half of drugs approved by the US Food and Drug Administration (FDA) were based on natural products [5], and 18 first-in-class small-molecule drugs originated from natural products between 1994 and 2008 [6]. Given the complex chemical compositions of TCMs and the importance to identify pharmacologically active constituents in TCMs and elucidate their mechanisms of action (MOAs), it is

Ye Fang (ed.), *Label-Free Biosensor Methods in Drug Discovery*, Methods in Pharmacology and Toxicology, DOI 10.1007/978-1-4939-2617-6_13, © Springer Science+Business Media New York 2015

233

prerequisite to develop effective screening and purification methods for the discovery of active compounds in TCMs.

Pharmacological assays generally divide into two types, molecular assays and phenotypic assays [6]. Molecular assays often use artificial systems and are biased to a specific MOA to determine drug effects, often resulting in poor correlation of the in vitro results with in vivo therapeutic impacts [7]. Phenotypic assays directly examine drug activity in native cells, tissues, or animals. The results obtained may be related to the therapeutic effect for a given disease state [8, 9]. Label-free cell phenotypic assays represent one of the promising phenotypic assays for drug discovery [10–13], owing to their ability to provide a holistic view of ligand–receptor interactions in living cells and mirror the innate complexity of drug actions [14–17]. Furthermore, these assays can be performed using flexible formats with high throughput, thus enabling mechanistic elucidation [18–21]. These unique characteristics give label-free assays a great potential in identifying active compounds of TCMs.

On the other hand, effective separation and purification methods are also important for obtaining active compounds from TCMs, given that a TCM generally contain a large number of compounds with great differences in category, polarity and concentration. High-performance liquid chromatography (HPLC) is the most widely used technique for the separation and purification of compounds from TCMs [22–24]. One-dimensional liquid chromatography (1D-LC) often fails to provide sufficient separation power to purify the targeted compounds in TCMs. Two-dimensional liquid chromatography (2D-LC) has been shown to be able to improve peak capacity and reduce sample complexity to an acceptable level [25]. HPLC can be operated using different modes, such as reversed-phase liquid chromatography (RPLC), hydrophilic interaction liquid chromatography (HILIC), and ion-exchange chromatography (IEX). To date, various 2D-LC systems have been successfully developed and used for the separation of TCMs, including RPLC×RPLC [26–28], RPLC×HILIC [29–32], HILIC×HILIC [33, 34], and RPLC×IEX [35].

Given the clinical efficacy and complexity of TCMs, we describe in detail how to effectively discover active compounds and clarify their MOAs in TCMs using label-free cell phenotypic assays.

2   Label-Free Cell Phenotypic Assays

2.1   Label-Free Biosensors

Resonant waveguide grating (RWG) and electric biosensors are widely used in label-free cell phenotypic assays mostly due to their high throughput. RWG biosensor uses the resonant coupling of light into a waveguide via grating diffraction, leading to a characteristic resonant wavelength, which is a function of the local refractive index near or at the sensor surface. The refractive index is proportional to local mass density. Thus, RWG biosensor can noninvasively track in real-time the dynamic redistribution of cellular constituents within ~150 nm of the biosensor surface upon stimulation with a ligand, leading to a dynamic mass redistribution (DMR) signal, which is often recorded as a shift in resonant wavelength in picometer (pm) [11, 36–38]. The DMR signal represents a cell phenotypic response, which is a holistic view of the functional consequence of ligand–receptor interactions in live cells. Furthermore, since it is noninvasive, DMR assay can be performed using flexible formats and permits intervention with probe molecules, thus enabling mechanistic elucidation of receptor biology [18, 19, 39] and drug pharmacology [40–42]. On the other hand, electric biosensor utilizes a microelectrode array with sinusoidal voltages that sweep in a continuous wave mode within a range of frequencies [16, 17]. It converts cell responses into impedance signals. Compared to RWG biosensor, electric biosensor has a relative deeper sensing range. Nevertheless, electric biosensor has minimal invasiveness to sense cells and the impedance signal is sensitive to cell morphological changes and its ionic redistribution. Electric biosensor has been widely used to investigate cell spreading [17], cell growth [43], and stem cell differentiation [44] and to identify bioactive natural products [12]. In this chapter, we use RWG biosensor-based cellular assay as an example to illustrate how TCM fractions and compounds should be screened.

2.2 Key Considerations in Label-Free Phenotypic Assays

In label-free phenotypic assays, there are many important factors that need to be considered, including cell culture conditions, probe molecules against targets and key enzymes in pathway, and the surrounding environment.

First, to obtain robust and reproducible cellular signals, it is very important to optimize cell culture conditions. Generally, the optimal cell density is that cells on the surface of biosensor form a monolayer after culture. Because cells cultured onto the biosensor surface undergo a dynamic and multistep process from cell adhesion to cell spreading and cell proliferation, each phase giving rise to distinct background signals. When cells reach high confluency, the biosensor often accompanies with a steady background signal [13, 45]. Concurrently, the optimal culture time equals to its doubling time for most proliferative cell lines. For instance, A431 and HT-29 cells are often cultured in the biosensor microplates for ~20 h, and SH-SY5Y cells are often cultured for ~48 h. In addition, cell starvation using serum-free medium may also impact assay results. Certain cell lines generate stronger response signals after pretreatment with serum-free medium, which can improve assay robustness. An example is that A431 cells are often starved overnight with serum-free medium when receptors (e.g., epidermal growth factor receptor, EGFR) whose signaling is known to be sensitive to cellular status are examined.

Second, given that the DMR signal is an integrated response, appropriate probe molecules should be selected to intervene receptor signaling, an important step for determining target engagement. In general, one target needs 3–5 probe molecules, including agonists, antagonists, and pathway modulators. The selection of probe molecules can refer to databases established in Sigma (http://www.sigmaaldrich.com), Tocris Bioscience (http://www.tocris.com/), Selleckchem (http://www.selleckchem.com/), Drugbank (http://beta.drugbank.ca/), and so on.

Third, environmental factors including assay temperature and solvents such as dimethyl sulfoxide (DMSO) commonly used for compound storage should also be considered. It is necessary to minimize temperature fluctuations throughout the whole experiment, temperature mismatch between cell solution and compound solution, as well as the mismatch in bulk index between different solutions. Of note, the bulk index mismatch induced by DMSO can be subtracted out in most cases by using intra-plate negative controls, that is, wells treated with the buffer solution containing equal amount of DMSO.

2.3 High-Throughput Screening of Active Compounds

With the increasing number of compounds and druggable targets, high-throughput screening (HTS) is crucial for drug discovery and development [46, 47]. Owing to the wide pathway coverage and the use of high density microplate formats such as 384- or 1,536-well microplates, label-free biosensor holds a great potential in HTS [48]. Based on the DMR kinetic profile, an end-point assay is easily developed by selecting a specific time point, often the maximal DMR response post stimulation, as the readout. Using this method, Dodgson et al. screened 100 K compounds to identify antagonists of the muscarinic M3 receptor. They identified a number of active compounds that were not found using a classical Ca^{2+} flux based HTS, suggesting that label-free offered an attractive approach for screening [49]. More importantly, label-free biosensor enables multiplexed screening against multiple targets. An example is screening 1,280 compounds in the Library of Pharmaceutically Active Compounds from Sigma against two endogenous receptors, the G_s-coupled β_2-adrenergic receptor (β_2AR) and the G_q-coupled histamine H_1 receptor in A431 cells. The agonist screening correctly identified all full agonists for both receptors and the succeeding antagonist screening identified 77 antagonists for the β_2AR and 51 antagonists for the H_1 receptor [50].

3   Label-Free Cell Phenotypic Assays for Discovering Active Compounds in TCMs

TCMs are important resources for drugs or lead compounds. Label-free cell phenotypic assay is suitable for identifying active compounds in TCMs, owing to its wide pathway coverage and high throughput.

3.1   General Protocol for Development and Clarification of TCMs

To effectively screen active compounds in TCMs using label-free cell phenotypic assay, a general protocol was proposed (Fig. 1). Here, the major research points are to clarify the composition, structure, and function of TCMs, to elucidate possible MOA(s) of

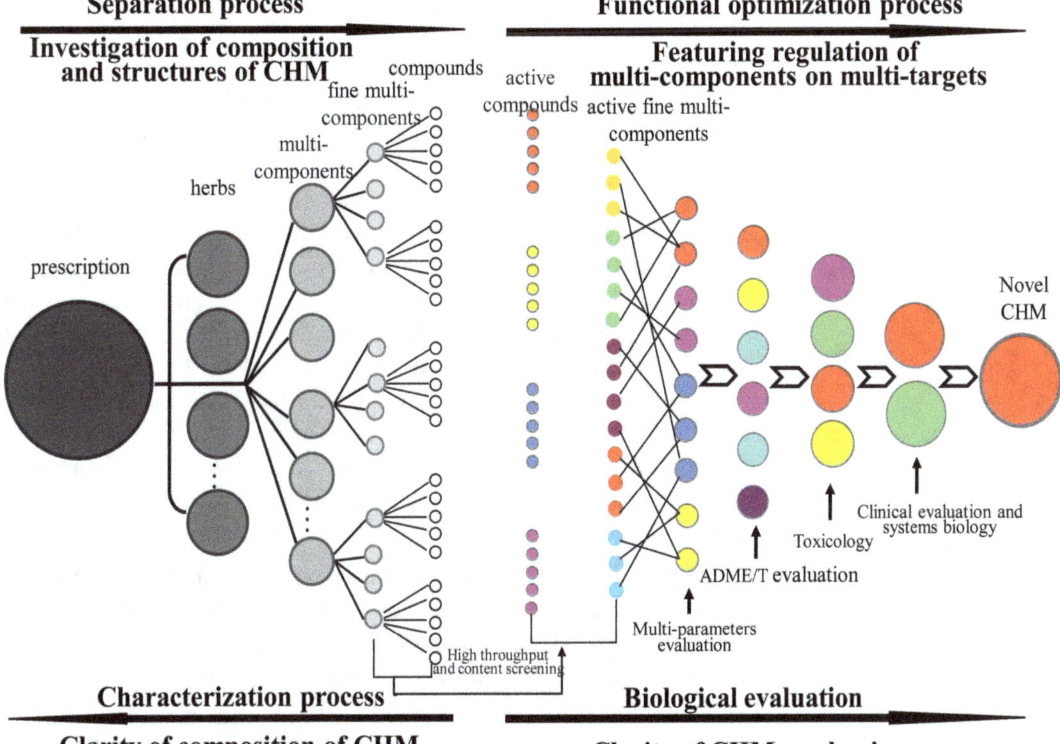

Fig. 1 A general protocol for the discovery of active compounds in TCMs. A clinical prescription was considered as one objective and its effective herbs could be obtained, which were separated into multicomponent fractions. These multicomponent fractions were further separated into fine multicomponent fractions. Compounds can be purified from these fine multicomponent fractions. This process was a separation and characterization process, which investigated the composition and structures of TCMs. The fractions and compounds were screened using label-free cell phenotypic assays in high throughput and high content to discovery active fractions and compounds. The active fractions and compounds were evaluated in terms of ADME/Tox, system biology and clinic to obtain a novel candidate drug. This process was a functional optimization and biological evaluation process, which elucidated and clarified the molecular mechanisms of TCMs (adapted from Ref. [77] with permission)

active compounds and interpret synergistic and complementary mechanism of multicomponents on multi-targets. The detailed steps of this protocol are as follows:

1. Select a clinically effective TCM. The primary principle for selecting a TCM is based on clinical indications and documents such as *Shen Nong Ben Cao Jing* and *Ben Cao Gang Mu*. For a specific disease, a clinical prescription is acquired, and its effective herbs are then obtained.

2. Separate and prepare fine multicomponent fractions. This is to reduce the typical complexity of a TCM. The prescription is separated into a set of mixtures, named "multicomponent fractions." These multicomponent fractions are continually subdivided into a series of simple mixtures using HPLC. These simple mixtures are called "fine multicomponents (FMCs)," together of which should contain all components in the prescription.

3. Perform high throughput/content screening using label-free cell phenotypic assays. These FCMs are screened in a set of cell lines using label-free cell phenotypic assay. Ideally, these cell lines are linked to diseases treated with the TCMs of interest. The more information on receptor biology in the cell lines is, the easier the MOAs of TCMs can be inferred and determined. Generally, the DMR signal obtained in a single cell line is not sufficient to infer MOAs. At least three kinds of cell lines with their own sets of expressed receptors are used to improve the differentiation power of the assay. After screening, similarity analysis such as the one using Ward hierarchical clustering algorithm and Euclidean distance metrics is performed to develop the relationship among different biological response, ascertain active FCMs and predict their targets.

4. Purify and confirm the active compounds. Generally, it is difficult to further separate active FCMs because compounds within a FCM may be similar in chemical characteristics. To successfully separate each compound within a given FCM, the second dimensional liquid chromatography with good orthogonality to the first dimensional liquid chromatography in Step 2 should be developed. After purification, the compounds should be characterized by ultraviolet (UV), mass spectrometry (MS), nuclear magnetic resonance (NMR), single X-ray crystallography, and so on to determine their actual identity and structures. Follow-up confirmation should be carried out using label-free cell assay. If the pharmacological activity of purified compound(s) is consistent with that of the FCM, we can assure that this compound is responsible for the activity of FCM. Of note, sometimes we cannot purify compounds from active FCMs. In this case, we would separate the active FCMs into simpler FCMs, screen their activities, and finally purify active compounds.

5. Determine possible MOA(s) of active compounds. The chemical structure and screening results in Step 4 are useful for the identification of potential targets. The expression of receptors in respective cell line can be ascertained by quantitative real time PCR (qRT-PCR) and gene manipulation techniques. The MOAs of active compounds can be determined using pharmacological tools (e.g., agonists, antagonists, and modulators) together with multiple label-free assay formats and conventional assays.

6. Determine the effect of active compound combinations. Given that a specific disease is generally linked to multi-targets, it is important to optimize the combination of active compounds. After combination, they are considered as one object and their targets and pathways need to be revalidated.

7. Evaluate ADME/Tox and clinical effects. Active compounds and their effective combination should be evaluated in terms of absorption, distribution, metabolism, excretion, and toxicity (ADME/Tox) before becoming a candidate drug.

3.2 An Example of Label-Free Cell Phenotypic Assays for TCMs

According to the abovementioned protocol, we demonstrated how to identify active compounds from *Paederia scandens* (Lour.) Merri. and *Millettia pachyloba* Drake [51].

First, 320 FCMs, 160 from each TCM, were separated in the first dimension and were assayed against three cell lines including A431, A549, and HT-29. The DMR signal for each fraction was then translated into a multidimensional coordinate to perform similarity analysis. A heat map of 320 FCMs in three cell lines was obtained (Fig. 2). The agonism assay identified 57 active FCMs from *Millettia pachyloba* Drake extract and 12 active FCMs from *Paederia scandens* extract.

Second, FCM hits are selected and further purified and validated. Here, a two-step DMR desensitization assay was first used to examine the activities of these FCMs against GPR35. Results showed that both TCMs contained GPR35 agonists. Interestingly, the FCM JST-003 itself triggered a robust DMR signal in A431 cells, but little DMR in HT29, and had no effect on the GPR35 activation mediated DMR. Thus, we focused on elucidating this active FCM. This active FCM was further prepared to obtain enough amounts for purifying compounds using a 2D HILIC× RPLC orthogonal system (Fig. 3). JST-003-#1–5 were successfully purified from JST-003 using a Click XIon column in the first dimension (Fig. 3a). These fractions were reassayed using label-free biosensor. It was found that only JST-003-#1 gave rise to a DMR signal similar to that in the initial screen (Fig. 3b, c). Therefore, JST-003-#1 were further separated, and JST-003-#1-C1 and JST-003-#1-C2 compounds were purified using a XAqua column in the second dimension (Fig. 3d). DMR agonist assay confirmed that only JST-003-#1-C2 triggered almost identical DMR signal. The JST-003-#1-C2 compound was thus further

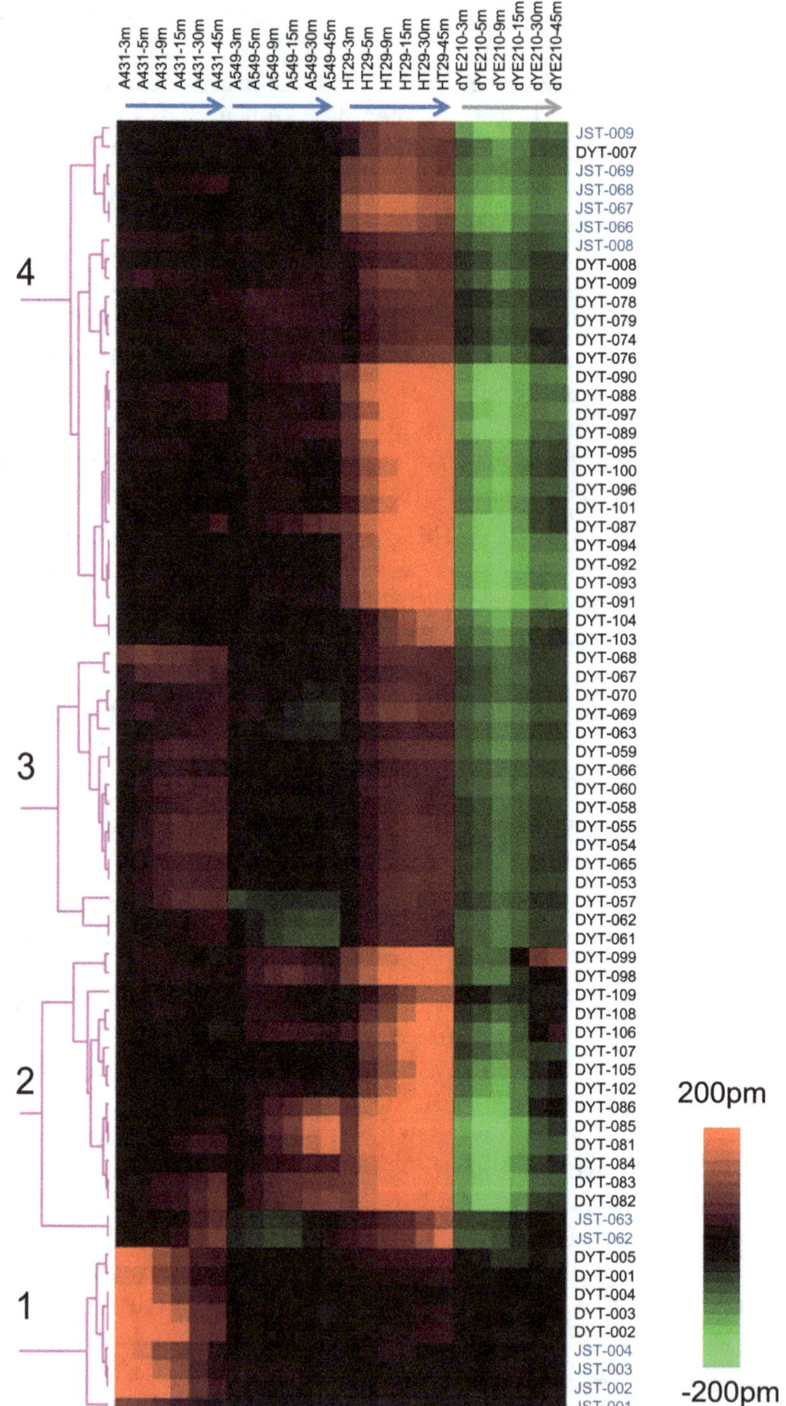

Fig. 2 A heat map of 320 FCMs from two TCMs in A431, A549, and HT-29 cells. This heat map was obtained using similarity analysis of the DMR signals of the fractions in the three cell lines, and the net change of the DMR of the GPR35 agonist YE210 at 1 µM in HT29 induced by the pretreatment with a specific fraction. For each agonist profile, the real amplitudes at 3, 5, 9, 15, 30, and 45 min post stimulation were used and color coded—*green*: negative; *red*: positive; *black*: zero response. For the DMR of 1 µM YE210 in HT29, the net difference between the fraction-pretreated cells and the buffer-pretreated cells was used and also color coded—*green*: suppression; *red*: potentiation; *black*: no change. False color scale bar is included to assist the data visualization (adapted from Ref. [51] with permission)

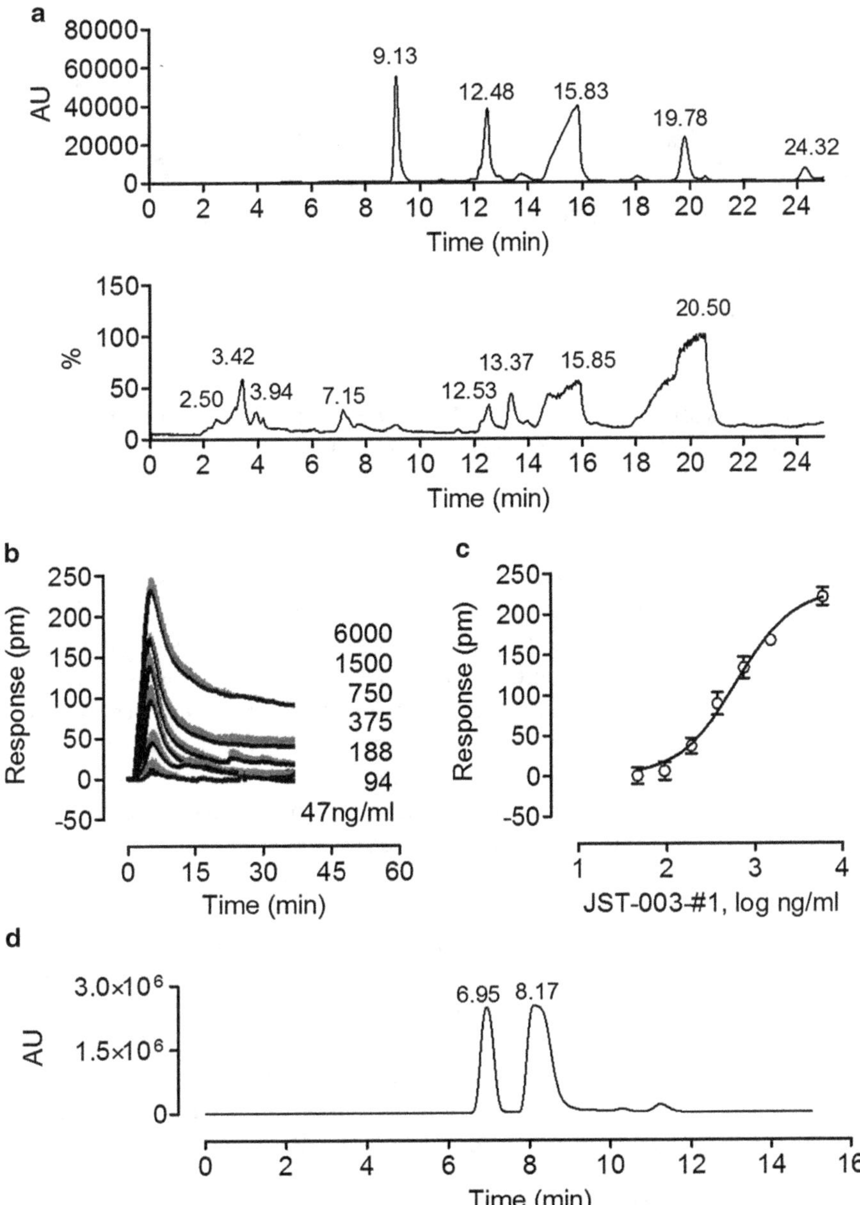

Fig. 3 Analysis of the fraction JST-003. (**a**) UV (260 nm, *top*) and total ion (positive ESI mode, *bottom*) MS chromatograms of JST-003 in the first dimension using a Click Xlon column. Mobile phase A was 0.1 % (v) formic acid in water and B was 0.1 % (v) formic acid in methanol. The gradient of separations was 0 min (3 %, phase B)—15 min (25 %, phase B)—20 min (95 %, phase B). The flow rate was 1 mL/min. (**b**) Real-time dose response of JST-003-#1 in A431. (**c**) The maximal DMR amplitudes as a function of JST-003-#1 dose. Data represents mean ± s.d. (*n* = 4). (**d**) Purification of C1 and C2 from JST-003-#1 under UV chromatograms at 260 nm in the second dimension using an XAqua column. 0.1 % (v) formic acid in water was used as mobile phase during 15 min separation. The flow rate was 1 mL/min (adapted from Ref. [51] with permission)

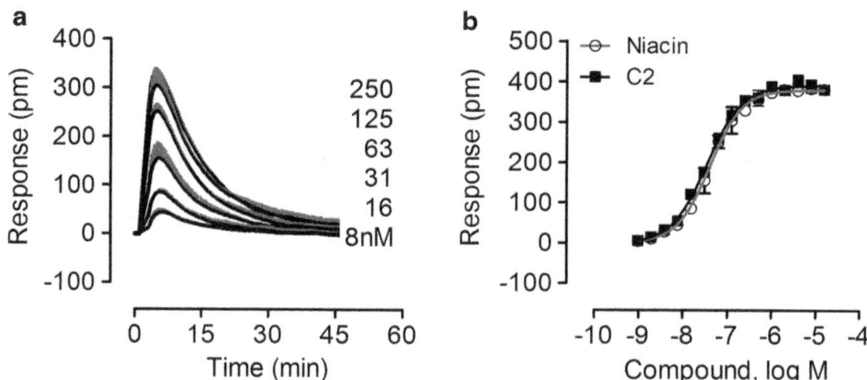

Fig. 4 DMR dose responses of compounds in A431 cell line. (**a**) Real-time dose response of niacin in A431; (**b**) the maximal DMR amplitudes as a function of compound doses. Data represents mean ± s.d. ($n = 4$) (adapted from Ref. [51] with permission)

characterized using MS and NMR. Results showed that the JST-003-#1-C2 compound was niacin. The finding of niacin in *Paederia scandens* (Lour.) Merri. and *Millettia pachyloba* Drake would be helpful for elucidating their antihyperlipidemic effect observed in clinic. These results demonstrated the great potential of label-free cell phenotypic assays for the discovery of active compounds in TCMs.

Third, the target engagement of active compounds identified is assessed using multiple techniques. First, quantitative RT-PCR is used to ascertain the receptor expression [52] and gene manipulation techniques (e.g., gene transfection, RNA interference and gene deletion) can be further employed to validate the target [53]. For the discovery of active compounds in *Paederia scandens* (Lour.) Merri. and *Millettia pachyloba* Drake, qRT-PCR of hydroxyl carboxylic acid receptor-2 (HCA-2) and HCA-3 in A431, A549, and HT-29 cells was performed. It was found that mRNAs for both receptors were at high level in A431 cells but at moderate level in HT-29, and at low level in A549 cells. Second, the noninvasive and manipulation-free feature of label-free phenotypic assay provides a powerful means to determine MOAs of active compounds in TCMs [15]. Various assay formats mainly contain agonism, desensitization, antagonism, and pathway deconvolution assays [19, 39, 54, 55]. The agonism assay was used to detect the DMR signal triggered by the active compound. By comparing DMR profiles between the active compound and the known agonists, the more similar the DMR profiles are, the more possible the active compound acts on the same receptor. Results showed that the purified JST-003-#1-C2 behaved almost identically to niacin, a known HCA2 agonist [56], both triggering identical dose responses with log EC_{50} of -7.46 ± 0.03 and -7.39 ± 0.02 (Fig. 4). Thus, it can be inferred that JST-003-#1-C2 was also an agonist for HCA2. Desensitization and antagonism assays can also be performed to identify the specificity of the active compound-induced DMR to the receptor. The desensitization assay is performed to confirm the desensitization of the receptor to the repeat stimulation with known agonists and the antagonism assay is used to examine the DMR signal of the active compound after pretreatment with the receptor antagonists. Using the desensitization assay, we found that niacin and JST-003-#1-C2 dose-dependently desensitized the niacin-induced DMR signal with log IC_{50} of -6.95 ± 0.03 and -7.14 ± 0.05. These results indicated that JST-003-#1-C2 was indeed niacin. Lastly, the DMR pathway deconvolution assay can be used to deconvolute the pathway responsible for the active compound-induced DMR signal. The signaling pathway may contain various activator, effectors and enzymes, which can be intervened by probe molecules. For instance, pertussis toxin (PTx) binds to $G\alpha_i$, resulting in inhibition of $G\alpha_i$ [57]; cholera toxin (CTx) binds to $G\alpha_s$, resulting in activation of $G\alpha_s$ [58]; forskolin is a known activator of adenylyl cyclase [59]; U73122, U0126, SB202190, SP600125, LY294002, and 4,5,6,7-tetrabromo-benzotriazole are known kinase pathway inhibitors for PLC, MEK1/2, p38 MAPK, JNK, PI3K, and CK2, respectively [60–62]. To study the signaling of the niacin-induced DMR, we used PTx to pretreat A431 cells and found that PTx completely and dose-dependently suppressed the niacin-induced DMR, suggesting that the DMR signal induced by niacin originated from the $G\alpha_i$ pathway. Additionally, conventional assays can be employed to further validate targets and signaling pathways, including Ca^{2+} mobilization assay, cAMP assay, inositol phosphate assay, immunocapture GTPγS binding assay, Western blotting, and so on.

4   Separation and Purification of Active Compounds in TCMs

Effective separation and purification methods are critical for obtaining active FCMs or compounds identified by label-free cell phenotypic assay. Given that alkaloids, steroids, saponins, and flavonoids are the important and popular compounds in TCMs, specific separation and purification methods for each of them were developed. Based on these practices, a set of general methods for the separation and purification of active compounds in TCMs was developed and discussed.

4.1 Separation and Purification of Alkaloids

Alkaloids are one of the most important classes of natural products, which comprise ~15.6 % of the known natural products but nearly 50 % of the plant-derived pharmaceuticals [63]. The separation and purification of alkaloids remain a hotspot in the natural product research. Owing to peak tailing and overloading, it is a great challenge to separate and purify these basic compounds. Given that basic compounds have different sensitivities to the mobile phase pH, a RPLC-RPLC system has been developed [64]. Moderate and weak basic compounds, but not strong basic compounds, tend to give rise to good peak shape and high loading amount. This is probably because moderate and weak basic compounds are unionized in the mobile phase with high pH, while silanols on the surface of the stationary phase would be ionized and then interacted with strong basic compounds. To solve this problem, a positively charged stationary phase C18 has been synthesized and used to purify quaternary alkaloids from *Corydalis yanhusuo* W. T. Wang [65]. The good performance for basic compounds on this column could be explained using the multiple-site adsorption theory, in which the ionic repulsion would shield compounds from occupying high-energy sites in C18 deeper layer [66]. Using this column, 80 fractions of *Corydalis yanhusuo* W. T. were obtained, and then assayed for their ability to activate μ-opioid receptor. Results showed that only one fraction was able to trigger a reproducible and dose-dependent intracellular Ca^{2+} mobilization [67]. Due to the complexity of the active fraction, an orthogonal IEC×RPLC system was constructed to purify the active compound in this fraction. Fortunately, this active compound was successfully purified and identified as dehydrocorybulbine (DHCB) using UV, MS, NMR, and single X-ray crystallography. Further testing using selective pharmacological compounds and dopamine receptor knockout mice showed that the antinociceptive effect of DHCB was primarily due to its interaction with dopamine D2 receptor. Interestingly, we found that DHCB was effective to treat injury-induced neuropathic pain and inflammatory pain with no antinociceptive tolerance. These results suggested that DHCB was a different type of analgesic compound and would be a promising lead compound in pain management.

4.2 Separation and Purification of Steroids

Steroids are widely distributed in TCMs. Bufadienolides are an important type of steroids with cardiotonic, anesthetic, blood pressure-stimulating and antitumor bioactivities [68]. To systematically separate bufadienolides, an XTerra Prep C18 column and a Click β-CD column were used to construct an orthogonal isolation system [32]. The XTerra Prep C18 column was used in the first dimension and 75 fractions were prepared from the toad skin extract. After screening for their activities, two active fractions were selected for further purification in the second dimension using the Click β-CD column. As a result, seven compounds were successfully obtained at high purity, including four stereoisomers. Recently, we have used hydrophilic interaction liquid chromatography solid-phase extraction (HILIC-SPE) to separate amino acid-conjugated bufadienolides and amino acid-unconjugated bufadienolides, which co-eluted on C18 columns [69]. Using this strategy, eight bufadienolides were obtained from one active fraction. These efficient separation and purification methods would accelerate the process of discovery of active compounds from natural products.

4.3 Separation and Purification of Saponins

Saponins are made up of aglycones coupled to sugar chain units and used for the treatment of cardiovascular diseases in East Asia. Due to their complex chemical structures, it is very difficult to synthesize them. Purification from TCMs is an important source of saponins [70, 71]. RPLC is one of the most popular techniques for the separation of saponins. However, the separation selectivity for saponins is not always sufficient. Given that saponins had good retention in the HILIC mode and RPLC had good orthogonality to HILIC, a 2D-RPLC×HILIC system was developed to separate saponins from leaves of *Panax notoginseng* [30] (Fig. 5). Eight saponins were prepared and identified from three representative fractions, including two pairs of isomeric saponins and one novel saponin. These results indicated that this method was useful for the purification of low-content and novel active saponins from natural products. Furthermore, by selecting the optimal HILIC column and optimizing mobile phase components, we established another efficient method to separate isomeric saponins in the HILIC mode [72]. The method was applied to the purification of saponins from leaves of *Panax notoginseng*; eleven saponins were then identified, including three sets of isomeric saponins. This method was efficient for the separation and preparation of saponins, especially for isomeric saponins.

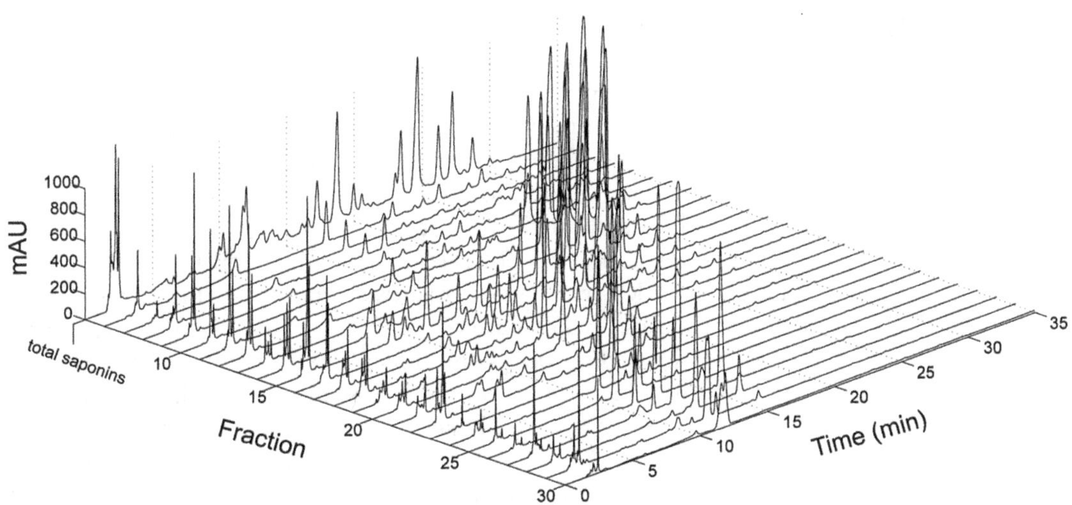

Fig. 5 A three-dimensional chromatogram for the 2-D RPLC/HILIC separation of extract from leaves of *Panax notoginseng*. In the first dimensional LC method, a 3.0 g of extract was loaded on an XUnion C18 (220 mm × 80 mm, 10 μm). A gradient program was according to 0–5 min, 20–32 % mobile phase B; 5–45 min, 32–68 % mobile phase B; 45–50 min, 68–95 % mobile phase B; 50–55 min, 95 % mobile phase B. Fractions were collected manually from 1 to 55 min with 1-min intervals. Fractions 6–30 were reanalyzed on an XAmide HILIC column (150 × 4.6 mm, 5 μm). The mobile phase gradient was as follows: 0–30 min, 5–26 % mobile phase A; 30–35 min, 26–40 % mobile phase A. Mobile phases A and B were water and ACN, respectively. The flow rate was 1 mL/min, the temperature was 30 °C, and UV detection was at 203 nm (adapted from Ref. [30] with permission)

4.4 Separation and Purification of Flavonoids

Flavonoids are a broad class of secondary plant phenolics with a chromane-type skeleton and a phenyl substituent in the C_2 or C_3 position [73]. They have significant antioxidant and chelating properties [74]. To efficiently separate them, different methods were developed. For isolation of flavonoids from licorice extract, a 2D RPLC×HILIC orthogonal system was used and 11 flavonoids were identified [75]. For preparation of flavonoids from *Lignum Dalbergiae Odoriferae*, a 2D RPLC×RPLC preparation method was established to realize an orthogonal separation at preparative level [27]. A Click oligo (ethylene glycol) column and a C18 column were used in the first and second dimension, respectively. In the first dimension, 7.2 g sample was separated into 11 fractions. In the second dimension, eight compounds in fraction 6 and two compounds in fraction 8 were obtained. For purification flavonoids from *Scutellaria barbata D. Don*, multichannel parallel preparative HPLC combined with pretreatment methods was adopted [76]. Twelve compounds were isolated, including three compounds that were first to be found from this plant. Overall, these results demonstrated that these methods were efficient for the isolation and purification of flavonoids from natural products and would be helpful for the discovery of active flavonoids.

4.5 Two-Dimensional Liquid Chromatography for Systematic Separation of TCMs

TCMs usually contain hundreds or even thousands of compounds, so the separation capacity of one-dimensional chromatography cannot meet the separation need. Generally, each fraction in the first dimension still contains many compounds. It is very necessary to develop 2D-LC to separate such a complex system. The principles for the development of 2D-LC are as follows: (1) each dimension should have high peak capacity and separation efficiency; (2) these two dimensions should have high orthogonality between each other. To meet these requirements, a general 2D-LC mode was proposed for systematic separation of TCMs [77] (Fig. 6).

For separation of polar components, an off-line 2D-HILIC× HILIC was designed. A click maltose column used in the first dimension and a click β-CD column (System I) or TSKgel Amide-80 column (System II) used in the second dimension were employed to separate polar compounds in *Carthamus tinctorius Linn.* [33]. Approximately 879 and 554 peaks were obtained by System I and System II, respectively, which suggested that this system had good orthogonality and efficient separation ability. Similarly, we used Atlantis HILIC Silica column and XAmide column to establish a 2D-HILIC×HILIC system for the analysis of polar fraction in *Scutellaria barbata D. Don* [34]. Sometimes normal-phase chromatography with nonaqueous mobile phases was used in the first dimension and HILIC mode was used in the second dimension. For separation of medium-polar components, we developed a 2D-RPLC×HILIC system. An Inertsil ODS-3 column and a click β-CD column were used in the first and second dimension to separate *Carthamus tinctorius Linn.* [29]. Results indicated that the orthogonality of this system was excellent. For

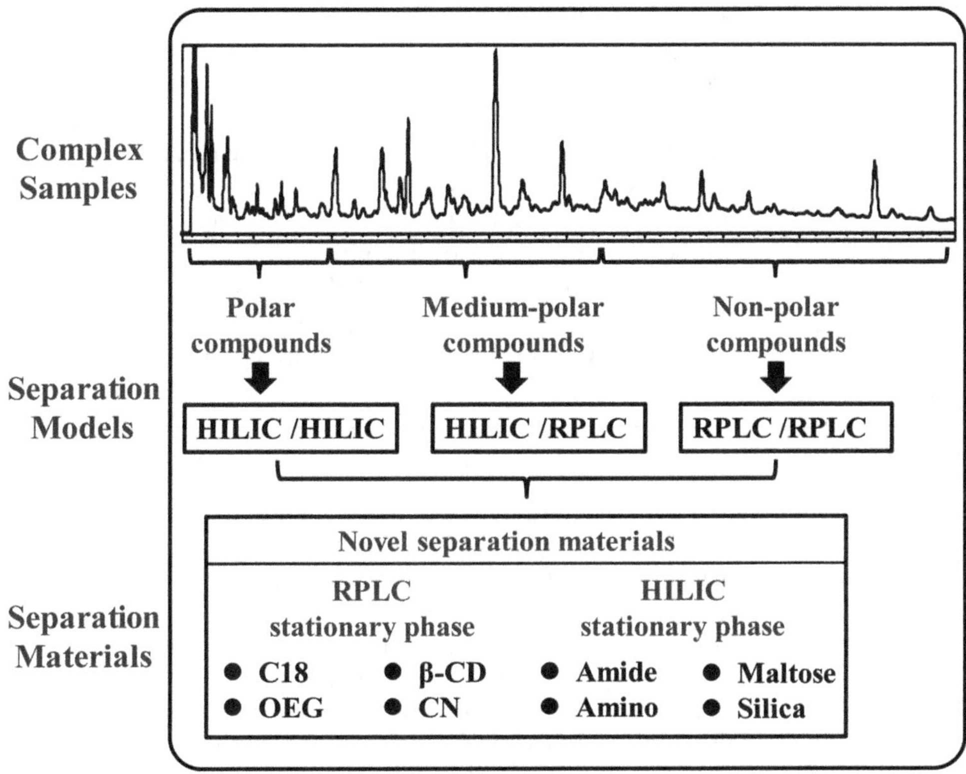

Fig. 6 2D-LC modes designed for systematic separation of TCMs. TCMs usually contain hundreds or even thousands of compounds. These compounds can be classified into polar, medium-polar, and nonpolar compounds. Their relative distribution was displayed in this figure when TCM was separated on a C18 column. For separation of polar, medium-polar, and nonpolar compounds, off-line 2D-HILIC × HILIC, HILIC × RPLC, and RPLC × RPLC were designed, respectively. The separation materials for RPLC included C18, OEG (oligo(ethylene glycol)), β-CD, and cyano bonded phases. The separation materials for HILIC contained amide, silica, amino, and maltose bonded phases (adapted from Ref. [77] with permission)

separation of nonpolar components, a 2D-RPLC×RPLC system was proposed. A novel click oligo(ethylene glycol) (Click OEG) stationary phase and a C18 column were employed to separate *Lignum Dalbergiae Odoriferae* [26]. Excellent separation performance validated the high orthogonality between these two columns in the separation of complex samples.

5   Future Prospects

Screening and purification of active compounds from TCMs is a long-term and difficult task. Fortunately, combining label-free cell phenotypic assay with advanced separation and purification methods offers an effective means for the discovery of active compounds in TCMs. Owing to its wide pathway coverage and high throughput screening, label-free phenotypic assay has a great potential in discovering active compounds in TCMs as well as elucidating their mechanisms of action. To improve efficiency of screening, varieties of orthogonal 2D-LC systems have been developed for separating alkaloids, steroids, saponins and flavonoids. In the future, three important aspects should be strengthened, including data analysis methods for deconvoluting the molecular mechanisms from biosensor signals, new biosensor technologies that can achieve duration and termination of stimulation for living cells, and effective purification methods for obtaining active compounds at the low-content level in TCMs. Nonetheless, label-free phenotypic assay, combining with separation and purification methods, can accelerate the process of drug discovery from TCMs.

6   Glossary

TCM	Traditional Chinese medicine
MOA	Mechanism of action
FDA	Food and Drug Administration
HPLC	High-performance liquid chromatography
2D-LC	Two-dimensional liquid chromatography
RPLC	Reversed-phase liquid chromatography
HILIC	Hydrophilic interaction liquid chromatography
IEX	Ion-exchange chromatography
FMCs	Fine multicomponents
ADME/Tox	Absorption, distribution, metabolism, excretion and toxicity
RWG	Resonant waveguide grating
DMR	Dynamic mass redistribution

References

1. Yuan R, Lin Y (2000) Traditional Chinese medicine: an approach to scientific proof and clinical validation. Pharmacol Ther 86(2):191–198. doi:10.1016/s0163-7258(00)00039-5

2. Wang JF, Wei DQ, Chou KC (2008) Drug candidates from traditional Chinese medicines. Curr Top Med Chem 8(18):1656–1665. doi:10.2174/156802608786786633

3. Ma HD, Deng YR, Tian ZG, Lian ZX (2013) Traditional Chinese medicine and immune regulation. Clin Rev Allergy Immunol 44(3):229–241. doi:10.1007/s12016-012-8332-0

4. Newman DJ, Cragg GM (2012) Natural products as sources of new drugs over the 30 years from 1981 to 2010. J Nat Prod 75(3):311–335. doi:10.1021/np200906s

5. Butler MS (2008) Natural products to drugs: natural product-derived compounds in clinical trials. Nat Prod Rep 25(3):475–516. doi:10.1039/b514294f

6. Swinney DC, Anthony J (2011) How were new medicines discovered? Nat Rev Drug Discov 10(7):507–519. doi:10.1038/nrd3480

7. Gleeson MP, Hersey A, Montanari D, Overington J (2011) Probing the links between in vitro potency, ADMET and physicochemical parameters. Nat Rev Drug Discov 10(3):197–208. doi:10.1038/nrd3367

8. Butcher EC (2005) Can cell systems biology rescue drug discovery? Nat Rev Drug Discov 4(6):461–467. doi:10.1038/nrd1754

9. Kepp O, Galluzzi L, Lipinski M, Yuan JY, Kroemer G (2011) Cell death assays for drug discovery. Nat Rev Drug Discov 10(3):221–237. doi:10.1038/nrd3373

10. Fang Y, Ferrie AM, Fontaine NH, Yuen PK (2005) Characteristics of dynamic mass redistribution of epidermal growth factor receptor signaling in living cells measured with label-free optical biosensors. Anal Chem 77(17):5720–5725. doi:10.1021/ac050887n

11. Fang Y (2007) Non-invasive optical biosensor for probing cell signaling. Sensors 7(10):2316–2329. doi:10.3390/s7102316

12. Fu HY, Fu WQ, Sun MJ, Shou QY, Zhai YY, Cheng HQ, Teng L, Mou XZ, Li YW, Wan SY, Zhang SS, Xu QQ, Zhang X, Wang JC, Zhu J, Wang XB, Xu X, Lv GY, Jin L, Guo WS, Ke YH (2011) Kinetic cellular phenotypic profiling: prediction, identification, and analysis of bioactive natural products. Anal Chem 83(17):6518–6526. doi:10.1021/ac201670e

13. Fang Y (2011) The development of label-free cellular assays for drug discovery. Expert Opin Drug Discov 6(12):1285–1298. doi:10.1517/17460441.2012.642360

14. Fang Y (2006) Label-free cell-based assays with optical biosensors in drug discovery. Assay Drug Dev Technol 4(5):583–595. doi:10.1089/adt.2006.4.583

15. Fang Y (2013) Troubleshooting and deconvoluting label-free cell phenotypic assays in drug discovery. J Pharmacol Toxicol Methods 67(2):69–81. doi:10.1016/j.vascn.2013.01.004

16. Giaever I, Keese CR (1993) A morphological biosensor for mammalian-cells. Nature 366 (6455):591–592. doi:10.1038/366591a0

17. Wegener J, Keese CR, Giaever I (2000) Electric cell-substrate impedance sensing (ECIS) as a noninvasive means to monitor the kinetics of cell spreading to artificial surfaces. Exp Cell Res 259(1):158–166. doi:10.1006/excr.2000.4919

18. Verrier F, An SO, Ferrie AM, Sun H, Kyoung M, Deng H, Fang Y, Benkovic SJ (2011) GPCRs regulate the assembly of a multienzyme complex for purine biosynthesis. Nat Chem Biol 7(12):909–915. doi:10.1038/nchembio.690

19. Schroder R, Janssen N, Schmidt J, Kebig A, Merten N, Hennen S, Muller A, Blattermann S, Mohr-Andra M, Zahn S, Wenzel J, Smith NJ, Gomeza J, Drewke C, Milligan G, Mohr K, Kostenis E (2010) Deconvolution of complex G protein-coupled receptor signaling in live cells using dynamic mass redistribution measurements. Nat Biotechnol 28(9):943–950. doi:10.1038/nbt.1671

20. Deng H, Wang C, Su M, Fang Y (2012) Probing biochemical mechanisms of action of muscarinic M3 receptor antagonists with label-free whole cell assays. Anal Chem 84(19):8232–8239. doi:10.1021/ac301495n

21. Schrage R, Seemann WK, Klockner J, Dallanoce C, Racke K, Kostenis E, De Amici M, Holzgrabe U, Mohr K (2013) Agonists with supraphysiological efficacy at the muscarinic M2 ACh receptor. Br J Pharmacol 169(2):357–370. doi:10.1111/bph.12003

22. Liang XM, Jin Y, Wang YP, Jin GW, Fu Q, Xiao YS (2009) Qualitative and quantitative analysis in quality control of traditional Chinese medicines. J Chromatogr A 1216(11):2033–2044. doi:10.1016/j.chroma.2008.07.026

23. Yang M, Sun JH, Lu ZQ, Chen GT, Guan SH, Liu X, Jiang BH, Ye M, Guo DA (2009) Phytochemical analysis of traditional Chinese medicine using liquid chromatography coupled with mass spectrometry. J Chromatogr A 1216(11):2045–2062. doi:10.1016/j.chroma.2008.08.097

24. Zhao HY, Jiang JG (2010) Application of chromatography technology in the separation of active components from nature derived drugs. Mini-Rev Med Chem 10(13):1223–1234

25. Gilar M, Olivova P, Daly AE, Gebler JC (2005) Orthogonality of separation in two-dimensional liquid chromatography. Anal Chem 77(19):6426–6434. doi:10.1021/ac050923i

26. Liu YM, Guo ZM, Jin Y, Xue XY, Xu Q, Zhang FF, Liang XM (2008) "Click oligo(ethylene glycol)": an excellent orthogonal stationary phase to C18 for two-dimensional reversed-phase/reversed-phase liquid chromatography. J Chromatogr A 1206(2):153–159. doi:10.1016/j.chroma.2008.08.013

27. Feng JT, Xiao YS, Guo ZM, Yu DH, Jin Y, Liang XM (2011) Purification of compounds from Lignum Dalbergia Odorifera using two-dimensional preparative chromatography with Click oligo (ethylene glycol) and C18 column. J Sep Sci 34(3):299–307. doi:10.1002/jssc.201000609

28. Jin GW, Dai YT, Feng JT, Qin XM, Xue XY, Zhang FF, Liang XM (2010) 2-D RP/RPLC method to separate components in Fructus schisandrae chinensis. J Sep Sci 33(4–5):564–569. doi:10.1002/jssc.200900563

29. Liu YM, Xue XY, Guo ZM, Xu Q, Zhang FF, Liang XM (2008) Novel two-dimensional reversed-phase liquid chromatography/hydrophilic interaction chromatography, an excellent orthogonal system for practical analysis. J Chromatogr A 1208(1–2):133–140. doi:10.1016/j.chroma.2008.08.079

30. Guo XJ, Zhang XL, Feng JT, Guo ZM, Xiao YS, Liang XM (2013) Purification of saponins from leaves of Panax notoginseng using preparative two-dimensional reversed-phase liquid chromatography/hydrophilic interaction chromatography. Anal Bioanal Chem 405(10):3413–3421. doi:10.1007/s00216-013-6721-8

31. Zhao YY, Guo ZM, Zhang XL, Liang XM, Zhang YK (2010) Off-line 2-D RPLC/RPLC method for separation of components in Dalbergia odorifera T. Chen. J Sep Sci 33(9): 1224–1230. doi:10.1002/jssc.200900778

32. Liu YF, Feng JT, Xiao YS, Guo ZM, Zhang J, Xue XY, Ding J, Zhang XL, Liang XM (2010) Purification of active bufadienolides from toad skin by preparative reversed-phase liquid chromatography coupled with hydrophilic interaction chromatography. J Sep Sci 33(10): 1487–1494. doi:10.1002/jssc.200900848

33. Liu YM, Guo ZM, Feng JT, Xue XY, Zhang FF, Xu Q, Liang XM (2009) Development of orthogonal two-dimensional hydrophilic interaction chromatography systems with the introduction of novel stationary phases. J Sep Sci 32(17):2871–2876. doi:10.1002/jssc.200900086

34. Liang Z, Li KY, Wang XL, Ke YX, Jin Y, Liang XM (2012) Combination of off-line two-dimensional hydrophilic interaction liquid chromatography for polar fraction and two-dimensional hydrophilic interaction liquid chromatography x reversed-phase liquid chromatography for medium-polar fraction in a traditional Chinese medicine. J Chromatogr A 1224:61–69. doi:10.1016/j.chroma.2011.12.046

35. Long Z, Guo ZM, Xue XY, Zhang XL, Liang XM (2013) Two-dimensional strong cation exchange/positively charged reversed-phase liquid chromatography for alkaloid analysis and purification. J Sep Sci 36(24):3845–3852. doi:10.1002/jssc.201300863

36. Fang Y (2012) Ligand-receptor interaction platforms and their applications for drug discovery. Expert Opin Drug Discov 7(10):969–988. doi:10.1517/17460441.2012.715631

37. Ferrie AM, Wu Q, Fang Y (2010) Resonant waveguide grating imager for live cell sensing. Appl Phys Lett 97(22):223704. doi:10.1063/1.3522894

38. Fang Y (2011) Label-free biosensors for cell biology. Intl J Electrochem 2011:460850. doi:10.4061/2011/460850

39. Schroder R, Schmidt J, Blattermann S, Peters L, Janssen N, Grundmann M, Seemann W, Kaufel D, Merten N, Drewke C, Gomeza J, Milligan G, Mohr K, Kostenis E (2011) Applying label-free dynamic mass redistribution technology to frame signaling of G protein-coupled receptors noninvasively in living cells. Nat Protoc 6(11):1748–1760. doi:10.1038/nprot.2011.386

40. Deng H, Hu H, Fang Y (2011) Tyrphostin analogs are GPR35 agonists. FEBS Lett 585(12):1957–1962. doi:10.1016/j.febslet.2011.05.026

41. Ferrie AM, Sun H, Fang Y (2011) Label-free integrative pharmacology on-target of drugs at the beta(2)-adrenergic receptor. Sci Rep 1:1–8. doi:10.1038/srep00033

42. Deng H, Sun H, Fang Y (2013) Label-free cell phenotypic assessment of the biased agonism and efficacy of agonists at the endogenous muscarinic M-3 receptors. J Pharmacol Toxicol Methods 68(3):323–333. doi:10.1016/j.vascn.2013.07.005

43. Xiao C, Luong JHT (2003) On-line monitoring of cell growth and cytotoxicity using electric cell-substrate impedance sensing (ECIS). Biotechnol Prog 19(3):1000–1005. doi:10.1021/bp025733x

44. Bagnaninchi PO, Drummond N (2011) Real-time label-free monitoring of adipose-derived stem cell differentiation with electric cell-substrate impedance sensing. Proc Natl Acad Sci U S A 108(16):6462–6467. doi:10.1073/pnas.1018260108

45. Fang Y, Ferrie AM, Fontaine NH, Mauro J, Balakrishnan J (2006) Resonant waveguide grating biosensor for living cell sensing. Biophys J 91(5):1925–1940. doi:10.1529/biophysj.105.077818

46. Inglese J, Johnson RL, Simeonov A, Xia MH, Zheng W, Austin CP, Auld DS (2007) High-throughput screening assays for the identification of chemical probes. Nat Chem Biol 3(8):466–479. doi:10.1038/nchembio.2007.17

47. Hertzberg RP, Pope AJ (2000) High-throughput screening: new technology for the 21st century. Curr Opin Chem Biol 4(4):445–451. doi:10.1016/s1367-5931(00)00110-1

48. Fang Y (2010) Live cell optical sensing for high throughput applications. Adv Biochem Eng Biotechnol 118:153–163. doi:10.1007/10_2009_4

49. Dodgson K, Gedge L, Murray DC, Coldwell M (2009) A 100K well screen for a muscarinic receptor using the Epic (R) label-free system – a reflection on the benefits of the label-free approach to screening seven-transmembrane receptors. J Recept Signal Transduct 29(3–4): 163–172. doi:10.1080/10799890903079844

50. Tran E, Fang Y (2008) Duplexed label-free G protein-coupled receptor assays for high-throughput screening. J Biomol Screen 13(10): 975–985. doi:10.1177/1087057108326141

51. Zhang XL, Deng H, Xiao YS, Xue XY, Ferrie AM, Tran E, Liang XM, Fang Y (2014) Label-free cell phenotypic profiling identifies pharmacologically active compounds in two traditional Chinese medicinal plants. RSC Adv 4(50): 26368–26377. doi:10.1039/c4ra03609c

52. Bustin SA, Benes V, Nolan T, Pfaffl MW (2005) Quantitative real-time RT-PCR – a perspective. J Mol Endocrinol 34(3):597–601. doi:10.1677/jme.1.01755

53. Lamb J, Crawford ED, Peck D, Modell JW, Blat IC, Wrobel MJ, Lerner J, Brunet JP, Subramanian A, Ross KN, Reich M, Hieronymus H, Wei G, Armstrong SA, Haggarty SJ, Clemons PA, Wei R, Carr SA, Lander ES, Golub TR (2006) The connectivity map: using gene-expression signatures to connect small molecules, genes, and disease. Science 313(5795):1929–1935. doi:10.1126/science.1132939

54. Hu H, Deng H, Fang Y (2012) Label-free phenotypic profiling identified D-luciferin as a GPR35 agonist. PLoS One 7(4):e34934. doi:10.1371/journal.pone.0034934

55. Tran E, Sun H, Fang Y (2012) Dynamic mass redistribution assays decode surface influence on signaling of endogenous purinergic P2Y receptors. Assay Drug Dev Technol 10(1):37–45. doi:10.1089/adt.2011.0392

56. Offermanns S, Colletti SL, Lovenberg TW, Semple G, Wise A, Ijzerman AP, International Union of Basic and Clinical Pharmacology (2011) LXXXII: nomenclature and classification of hydroxy-carboxylic acid receptors (GPR81, GPR109A, and GPR109B). Pharmacol Rev 63(2):269–290. doi:10.1124/pr.110.003301

57. Barbieri JT, Cortina G (1988) ADP-ribosyltransferase mutations in the catalytic s-1 subunit of pertussis toxin. Infect Immun 56(8):1934–1941

58. Gill DM, Meren R (1978) ADP-ribosylation of membrane proteins catalyzed by cholera toxin – basis of activation of adenylate-cyclase. Proc Natl Acad Sci U S A 75(7):3050–3054. doi:10.1073/pnas.75.7.3050

59. Tran E, Fang Y (2009) Label-free optical biosensor for probing integrative role of adenylyl cyclase in G protein-coupled receptor signaling. J Recept Signal Transduct 29(3–4):154–162. doi:10.1080/10799890903052544

60. Jin WZ, Lo TM, Loh HH, Thayer SA (1994) U73122 inhibits phospholipase c-dependent calcium mobilization in neuronal cells. Brain Res 642(1–2):237–243. doi:10.1016/0006-8993(94)90927-x

61. Davis MI, Hunt JP, Herrgard S, Ciceri P, Wodicka LM, Pallares G, Hocker M, Treiber DK, Zarrinkar PP (2011) Comprehensive analysis of kinase inhibitor selectivity. Nat Biotechnol 29(11):1046–U1124. doi:10.1038/nbt.1990

62. Karaman MW, Herrgard S, Treiber DK, Gallant P, Atteridge CE, Campbell BT, Chan KW, Ciceri P, Davis MI, Edeen PT, Faraoni R, Floyd M, Hunt JP, Lockhart DJ, Milanov ZV, Morrison MJ, Pallares G, Patel HK, Pritchard S, Wodicka LM, Zarrinkar PP (2008) A quantitative analysis of kinase inhibitor selectivity. Nat Biotechnol 26(1):127–132. doi:10.1038/nbt1358

63. Cordell GA, Quinn-Beattie ML, Farnsworth NR (2001) The potential of alkaloids in drug discovery. Phytother Res 15(3):183–205. doi:10.1002/ptr.890

64. Zhang J, Jin Y, Liu YF, Mao YS, Feng JT, Xue XY, Zhang XL, Liang XM (2009) Purification of alkaloids from Corydalis yanhusuo W.T. Wang using preparative 2-D HPLC. J Sep Sci 32(9):1401–1406. doi:10.1002/jssc.200800729

65. Wang CR, Guo ZM, Zhang J, Zeng J, Zhang XL, Liang XM (2011) High-performance purification of quaternary alkaloids from Corydalis yanhusuo W.T. Wang using a new polar-copolymerized stationary phase. J Sep Sci 34(1):53–58. doi:10.1002/jssc.201000625

66. Wang CR, Guo ZM, Long Z, Zhang XL, Liang XM (2013) Overloading study of basic compounds with a positively charged C18 column in liquid chromatography. J Chromatogr A 1281:60–66. doi:10.1016/j.chroma.2013.01.074

67. Zhang Y, Wang CR, Wang L, Parks GS, Zhang XL, Guo ZM, Ke YX, Li KW, Kim MK, Vo B, Borrelli E, Ge GB, Yang L, Wang ZW, Garcia-Fuster MJ, Luo ZD, Liang XM, Civelli O (2014) A novel analgesic isolated from a traditional Chinese medicine. Curr Biol 24(2):117–123. doi:10.1016/j.cub.2013.11.039

68. Steyn PS, van Heerden FR (1998) Bufadienolides of plant and animal origin. Nat Prod Rep 15(4):397–413

69. Li XL, Liu YF, Shen AJ, Wang CR, Yan JY, Zhao WJ, Liang XM (2014) Efficient purification of active bufadienolides by a class separation method based on hydrophilic solid-phase extraction and reversed-phase high performance liquid chromatography. J Pharm Biomed Anal 97:54–64. doi:10.1016/j.jpba.2014.04.015

70. Oleszek WA (2002) Chromatographic determination of plant saponins. J Chromatogr A 967(1):147–162. doi:10.1016/s0021-9673(01)01556-4

71. Oleszek W, Bialy Z (2006) Chromatographic determination of plant saponins – an update (2002–2005). J Chromatogr A 1112(1–2):78–91. doi:10.1016/j.chroma.2006.01.037

72. Guo XJ, Zhang XL, Guo ZM, Liu YF, Shen AJ, Jin GW, Liang XM (2014) Hydrophilic interaction chromatography for selective separation of isomeric saponins. J Chromatogr A 1325:121–128. doi:10.1016/j.chroma.2013.12.006

73. de Rijke E, Out P, Niessen WMA, Ariese F, Gooijer C, Brinkman UAT (2006) Analytical separation and detection methods for flavonoids. J Chromatogr A 1112(1–2):31–63. doi:10.1016/j.chroma.2006.01.019

74. Heim KE, Tagliaferro AR, Bobilya DJ (2002) Flavonoid antioxidants: chemistry, metabolism and structure-activity relationships. J Nutr Biochem 13(10):572–584. doi:10.1016/s0955-2863(02)00208-5

75. Zhang H, Guo ZM, Li W, Feng JT, Xiao YS, Zhang FF, Xue XY, Liang XM (2009) Purification of flavonoids and triterpene saponins from the licorice extract using preparative HPLC under RP and HILIC mode. J Sep Sci 32(4):526–535. doi:10.1002/jssc.200800526

76. Wang YP, Xue XY, Xiao YS, Zhang FF, Xu Q, Liang XM (2008) Purification and preparation of compounds from an extract of Scutellaria barbata D. Don using preparative parallel high performance liquid chromatography. J Sep Sci 31(10):1669–1676. doi:10.1002/jssc.200700609

77. Zhang XL, Liu YF, Guo ZM, Feng JT, Dong J, Fu Q, Wang CR, Xue XY, Xiao YS, Liang XM (2012) The herbalome-an attempt to globalize Chinese herbal medicine. Anal Bioanal Chem 402(2):573–581. doi:10.1007/s00216-011-5533-y

Chapter 14

Use of the Quartz Crystal Microbalance with Dissipation Monitoring for Pharmacological Evaluation of Cell Signaling Pathways Mediated by Epidermal Growth Factor Receptors

Jennifer Y. Chen, Marcela P. Garcia, Lynn S. Penn, and Jun Xi

Abstract

The quartz crystal microbalance with dissipation monitoring (QCM-D) is a highly sensitive, noninvasive, and label-free sensing device. This device is capable of providing real-time monitoring of the properties of complex biological systems, such as cells, in response to environmental stimuli. The unique dissipation monitoring function of the QCM-D has been shown to be able to profile the inhibition of signaling pathways mediated by epidermal growth factor receptors. The QCM-D method has the potential to become an effective sensing platform for drug screening.

Key words Cell adhesion, Cell-based assay, Drug discovery, Energy dissipation, EGFR signaling, Inhibitors, Inhibitor screening, Label-free, QCM-D

1 Introduction

1.1 EGFR-Mediated Cell De-adhesion

Epidermal growth factor receptor (EGFR) is a transmembrane receptor. When activated with the binding of epidermal growth factor (EGF), EGFR regulates cell growth, proliferation, motility, and differentiation through its downstream signaling pathways [1, 2] (Fig. 1), such as the mitogen-activated protein kinase/extracellular signal-regulated kinase (MAPK/ERK) pathway [3], the phosphoinositide 3-kinase (PI3K) pathway [4], and the phospholipase C (PLC) pathway [5]. It is known that overexpression and/or mutation of EGFR may deregulate these downstream signaling pathways and lead to the development of epithelial malignancies such as cancers [6, 7].

Cell de-adhesion, the reverse of cell adhesion, leads to a weaker adhesion of adherent cells to the underlying substrate [8]. The EGF-induced cell de-adhesion that often results from disassembly

Ye Fang (ed.), *Label-Free Biosensor Methods in Drug Discovery*, Methods in Pharmacology and Toxicology,
DOI 10.1007/978-1-4939-2617-6_14, © Springer Science+Business Media New York 2015

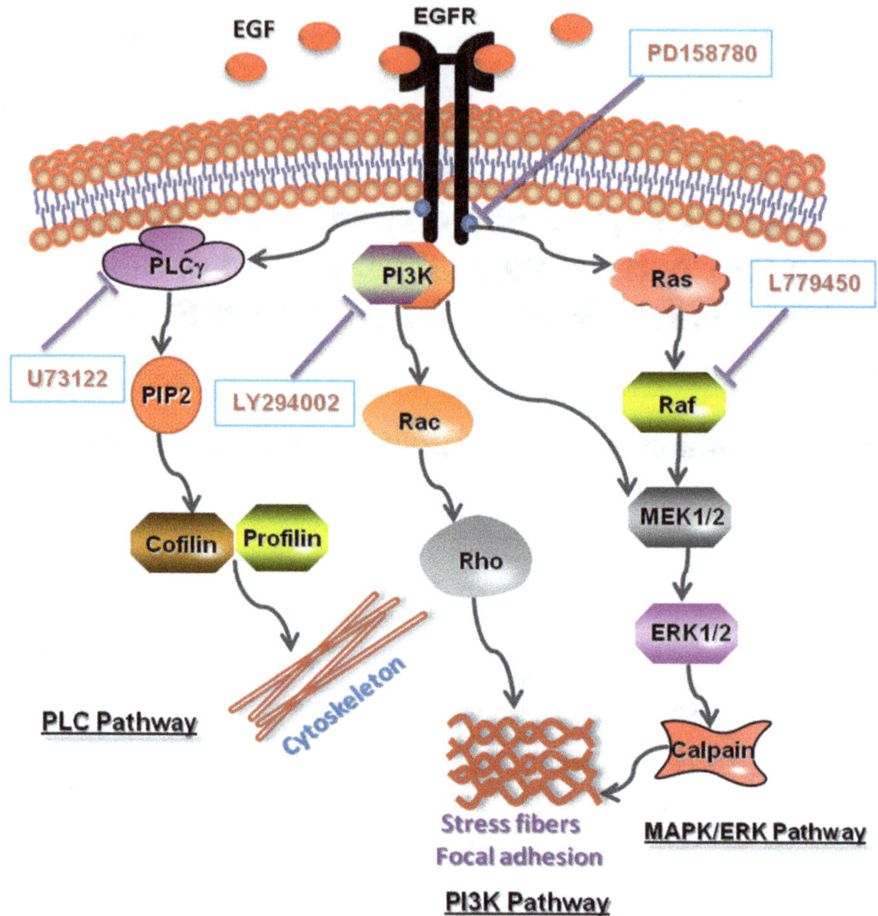

Fig. 1 The three main downstream pathways of EGFR-mediated cell signaling. Adapted from Chen et al. 2012 Copyright 2012 Elsevier B.V

of focal adhesions [9, 10] is mediated by the downstream signaling pathways of EGFR and is thought to be a critical step in tumor cell metastasis [11]. Mutant MCF-10A cells possess a high level of EGFR [12], a situation that mimics the abnormal levels of EGFR in many types of solid tumors [13]. Suppression of the EGFR-mediated de-adhesion process in mutant MCF-10A cells with pathway-specific inhibitors will potentially provide a useful lead for finding effective cancer treatment.

1.2 Conventional Approaches

The conventional approach to examining inhibition of cell signaling pathways is based on quantitation of proteins and/or small molecules involved in the specific signaling process using biochemical methods (e.g., western blot) [14]. The major drawback of this type of approach is that it is usually limited to end-point detection and therefore cannot provide information concerning the kinetics of inhibition. Tagging signaling proteins with fluorescent labels allows real-time tracking of inhibitory effects on cell signaling activities. However, the introduction of fluorescent labels can potentially create a nonnative cellular environment that can lead to ambiguous results [15, 16]. These problems can be overcome with the use of a real-time and label-free approach.

1.3 Quartz Crystal Microbalance with Dissipation Monitoring

The quartz crystal microbalance with dissipation monitoring (QCM-D) is a mechanical sensing device capable of simultaneously measuring changes in frequency and energy dissipation factor of the sensing element and any material that is coupled to it. The sensing element of the QCM-D is a thin AT-cut quartz crystal of disc-like geometry sandwiched between two metal electrodes. Because it is piezoelectric, the quartz crystal can oscillate when a current is applied through the electrodes [17]. The resonant frequency of the oscillating crystal is sensitive to nanogram-scale changes in mass coupled to the surface. The relationship between changes in frequency and mass is governed by the Sauerbrey equation, $\Delta m = -\dfrac{C}{n}\Delta f_n$. In this equation, Δm is the mass deposited per unit area of crystal, Δf_n is the change in resonant frequency of the vibrational mode n, and C is the mass sensitivity constant of the instrument [18]. When the mass coupled to the sensor is rigid, elastic, and evenly distributed on the surface of the crystal [19], the Sauerbrey equation is valid. However, it is often invalid for soft materials such as cells and hydrogels, which dissipate a large portion of any energy input. The ability of the QCM-D to measure changes in energy while simultaneously measuring changes in resonant frequency is extremely useful. The change in energy dissipation is related to changes in mechanical properties (e.g., viscoelasticity) of the material attached to the surface of the sensor. Energy dissipation is expressed as dissipation factor, D, and the change in this factor is defined as $\Delta D = \dfrac{E_{dissipated}}{2\pi E_{stored}}$, where $E_{dissipated}$ is the energy dissipated and E_{stored} is the energy stored in the oscillating system during one cycle of oscillation, or vibration [20].

The QCM-D has been widely used in chemical [21], physical [22], biological [23, 24], and biomedical [25] fields. This sensing device provides highly sensitive and label-free measurement of real-time changes in mass and mechanical properties of the material coupled to the sensor surface. This unique capability has enabled the QCM-D to evolve into a powerful bioanalytical tool capable of assessing properties of biomaterials such as proteins [26, 27], lipid layers [28], DNA [29], and whole cells [24, 30–33]. Special applications in the areas of kinetics of protein adsorption and desorption [34, 35], binding of surface-bound receptors and ligands [36], and characterization of lipid films [28] have been developed. In recent years, the use of the QCM-D has been focused primarily on evaluation of attachment and spreading of cells on the surface of the sensor crystal [37–39], on evaluation of cellular mechanics [40–42], on monitoring of the pathway-mediated cell-substrate de-adhesion [31], and on evaluation of cellular biomarkers [32].

1.4 QCM-D Method

To assess inhibitors of EGFR-mediated pathways, a QCM-D-based method has been developed to examine the inhibition of the EGF-induced cell de-adhesion process. Previously, it was shown that the ΔD-response profile is an indicator of time-dependent changes in cell adhesion induced by EGF in MCF-10A cells, whereas the Δf-response is neither sensitive to nor consistent with such events [31]. This EGF-induced change in cell adhesion is known to be mediated by downstream signaling pathways of EGFR. By tracking real-time changes in the ΔD-response of MCF-10A cells in the presence of pathway-specific inhibitors (PD158780 for the EGFR activation pathway, LY294002 for the PI3K pathway, U73122 for the PLC pathway, and L-779450 for the MAPK/ERK pathway), the effects of these inhibitors can be evaluated and IC_{50}-values of these inhibitors can be determined from the dose-inhibition responses.

2 Materials

2.1 Instrumentation

1. Quartz crystal microbalance with dissipation monitoring (QCM-D E4) (Biolin Scientific Q-Sense, Stockholm, Sweden) (Fig. 2).

2. Q-Sense open module (QOM 401) (Biolin Scientific).

3. AT-cut quartz crystals in the form of 14 mm-discs with a top surface coating of a 50-nm-thick film of deposited gold (QSX 301) (Biolin Scientific).

2.2 Reagents and Materials

1. MCF-10A cell line (American Type Cell Culture, ATCC; Manassas, Virginia, USA).

2. Mutant MCF-10A cell line overexpressing EGFR (provided by Dr. Mauricio Reginato, Drexel University College of Medicine, Philadelphia, PA, USA) [12].

3. Dulbecco's modified Eagle's medium: nutrient mix F12 (DMEM/F12) cell culture media, horse serum, penicillin/streptomycin antibiotics solution, 0.25 % trypsin–EDTA, HEPES buffer, phosphate buffered saline (PBS) buffer, and Hank's balanced salt solution (HBSS) (Invitrogen, Carlsbad, CA, USA).

4. Growth medium: DMEM/F12 medium contains 5 % horse serum, 20 ng/mL EGF, 0.5 µg/mL hydrocortisone, 50 ng/mL cholera toxin, 10 µg/mL insulin, 100 IU/mL penicillin, and 100 µg/mL streptomycin.

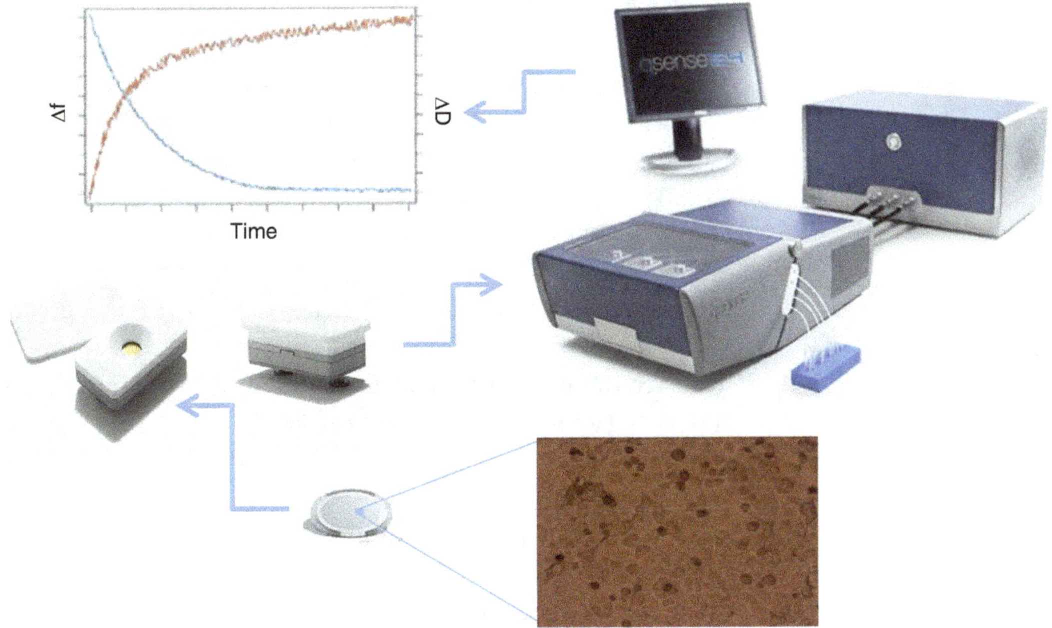

Fig. 2 Illustration of setup of QCM-D experiments. The Q-Sense E4 images were adapted from the Biolin Scientific Q-Sense web site (http://www.biolinscientific.com/q-sense/products)

5. Assay buffer: 1× HBSS, 20 mM HEPES, pH 7.2.

6. Hydrocortisone, cholera toxin, and insulin (Sigma-Aldrich, St. Louis, MO, USA).

7. Epidermal growth factor (human EGF) (Peprotech, Rocky Hill, NJ, USA).

8. PD158780 and L779450 (Raf kinase inhibitor IV) (EMD Biosciences, La Jolla, CA, USA).

9. U73122 and LY294002 (Cayman Chemical, Ann Arbor, MI, USA).

2.3 Data Analysis Software

1. Qsoft 401 2.0.0.275 software (Biolin Scientific).

2. Qtools software (Qsoft 3.0.1.178) (Biolin Scientific).

3. Origin software (Origin, Northampton, MA, USA).

3 Methods

3.1 Cell Culture

MCF-10A cells and mutant MCF-10A cells are cultured in T75 Corning culture flasks in the growth medium. The cells are maintained in a humidified atmosphere at 37 °C and 5 % CO_2.

The cells are usually harvested for experiments at 90–95 % confluency by means of trypsin–EDTA treatment.

1. Remove the growth medium in flask containing a monolayer of cell culture (90–95 % confluency) and rinse the cells with PBS buffer twice to remove residual medium.

2. Add 0.25 % trypsin–EDTA to the monolayer of cells; allow the cells to detach from the flask in the 37 °C/5 % CO_2 incubator for 10 min.

3. Stop the cell detachment with the addition of the growth medium.

4. Transfer the cell suspension to a 15-mL centrifuge tube and spin it at 1,200 rpm ($290 \times g$) for 4 min.

5. Remove the supernatant by aspiration and replace it with fresh growth medium.

6. Gently force the growth medium up and down in a pipette to break up the pellet of cells.

7. Count the number of cells.

8. Seed cells onto freshly prepared sensor crystals by depositing 1 mL of cell suspension.

3.2 Sensor Preparation

The following protocol provides an optimized method for coating the QCM-D sensors with a monolayer of live epithelial cells with a normal and healthy morphology. This is critical to the success of the QCM-D-based cell studies. If sensors are carefully cleaned and sterilized (*see* **Note 1**), the sensors can be reused many times without substantial reduction of the quality of the data.

1. Wash the sensors with ethanol.

2. Expose the sensors to UV/ozone for 20 min.

3. Expose the sensors to UV light in a tissue culture hood for 30 min.

4. Place each sensor with gold surface facing upward into an individual well in a 12-well tissue culture plate (*see* **Note 2**).

5. Seed the cells detached from a T75 culture flask at a specific cell density.

6. Place the 12-well plate with sensors in a humidified atmosphere at 37 °C and 5 % CO_2 to allow the cells to adhere to the sensors and grow.

7. After 90–95 % confluency has been reached, wash the cells with PBS and starve the cells in serum-free DMEM/F12 medium for 18 h prior to QCM-D measurements.

3.3 QCM-D Assays

3.3.1 Baseline Equilibrium

The following procedure allows cells to reestablish a stable physiological state in the QCM-D after being transferred from the CO_2 incubator. A stable physiological state of the cells, indicated by a stable baseline response, is essential for obtaining reliable and reproducible results in the QCM-D-based cell studies.

1. On the day of the QCM-D measurement, carefully rinse the sensor crystals bearing adhered cells with the assay buffer.

2. Wipe the underside of each sensor crystal with a Kimwipe to remove any buffer solution that could interfere with electrical circuitry.

3. Mount each sensor crystal in an open module (Q-sense) and cover each with 400 µL of the assay buffer.

4. Place the modules in the QCM-D platform.

5. Set the module temperature at 37 °C and allow the frequency ($\Delta f_n/n$) and dissipation factor (ΔD_n) to achieve stable baselines (*see* **Note 3**).

3.3.2 EGF Dose-Dependency Study

The following procedure describes how to obtain QCM-D profiles for the EGF-induced, dose-dependent cellular response. This study provides the necessary data for deriving the dose–response curve and for determining the corresponding EC_{50}-value of EGF (*see* Section 3.4).

1. Start a new measurement by zeroing the QCM-D and acquiring a baseline with assay buffer for 8 min.

2. Once the 8-min baselines are obtained, carefully remove the solution surmounting the cell layer in the module and add 400 µL of the assay buffer (pre-warmed to 37 °C) containing a specific concentration of EGF (*see* **Note 4**).

3. Repeat **step 2** for the remaining three modules with varying doses of EGF.

4. Record both frequency ($\Delta f_n/n$) and dissipation factor (ΔD_n) simultaneously at 37 °C for 3 h.

3.3.3 Inhibition Study

The following procedure is optimized for obtaining the QCM-D response profile of cells that are inhibited by an inhibitor of EGFR-mediated signaling pathways. This study provides the necessary data for deriving the dose-inhibition curve and for determining the corresponding IC_{50}-value of the inhibitor (*see* Section 3.4). This study may also provide mechanistic insight into the potential impact of each pathway on the cellular response.

1. Start a new measurement by zeroing the QCM-D and acquiring a baseline with assay buffer for 8 min.

2. Carefully remove the solution surmounting the cell layer in the module and add 400 µL of the assay buffer (pre-warmed to 37 °C) containing a specific dose of an inhibitor.

3. Repeat **step 2** for the remaining three modules with various doses of the inhibitor.

4. Record the frequency ($\Delta f_n/n$) and dissipation factor (ΔD_n) at 37 °C for a minimum of 30 min to complete the pretreatment step.

5. After the pretreatment, zero the QCM-D instrument measurement and acquire baselines for 8 min.

6. Replace the solution in each module with a pre-warmed 10-nM solution of EGF containing the same dose of the inhibitor in the assay buffer.

7. Record both frequency ($\Delta f_n/n$) and dissipation factor (ΔD_n) simultaneously at 37 °C for 3 h.

3.4 Data Analysis

3.4.1 Raw Data Treatment

The following procedure describes how the raw data is exported from the QCM-D and converted into a readable file in the format of various data analysis softwares.

1. Once experiments are complete, save the data as a qSoft data file (.qsd).

2. Using the Qsoft software, condense the data to a data point every 120 s and save again as a qTool data file (.qtd).

3. Open the condensed qTool data file with Qtools software and export the data as an Excel file.

4. Import the data from Excel into Origin software for data analysis.

3.4.2 Dose–Response Curve

The following procedure describes how to derive an EC_{50}-value based on the QCM-D response profiles. The resulting EC_{50}-values can be used to quantitatively assess the EGF-induced response of various cell lines under desired conditions.

1. Generate dose–response curves by plotting the average amplitudes (± 1 std. dev.) of ΔD-responses at a selected time point (e.g., 60 min) as a function of EGF concentration. Typically ΔD-responses at the vibrational mode $n=3$ are used (*see* **Note 3**). The amplitude is defined as the difference between the experimental value (with EGF) and the control value (no EGF), where the values of ΔD are taken at 60 min.

2. Use $\Delta D = \dfrac{ax}{EC_{50} + x}$ to fit the data, where x is the concentration of the EGF and a is the maximum ΔD-response.

3. Determine EC_{50}-values from curve-fitting of the equation above with the aid of Origin software. The use of either log functional plot or sigmoid plot for this analysis gives rise to essentially the same EC_{50}-values.

3.4.3 Dose-Inhibition Curve

The following procedure describes how to derive an IC_{50}-value based on the QCM-D response profiles of inhibited cells. The resulting IC_{50}-values can be used to quantitatively assess the potency of individual pathway inhibitors.

1. Generate dose-inhibition curves by plotting the average amplitudes (±1 std. dev.) of ΔD at a specific time point (e.g., 40 min) as a function of inhibitor concentration. The amplitude is defined as the difference between the experimental value (with an inhibitor) and the control value (no inhibitor), where the values of ΔD are taken at 40 min. ΔD-responses at the vibrational mode $n = 3$ are used (*see* **Note 3**).

2. Use $\Delta D = \dfrac{ax}{IC_{50} + x}$ to fit the data, where x is the concentration of the EGF inhibitor and a is the maximum ΔD-response.

3. Determine the IC_{50}-values from curve-fitting of the equation above with the aid of Origin software. The use of either log functional plot or sigmoid plot for this analysis gives rise to essentially the same IC_{50}-values.

3.5 Interpretation of Data

3.5.1 EC_{50}-Values

The EC_{50}-value of the EGF-induced response in MCF-10A cells was determined from the ΔD-responses induced at various concentrations of EGF, shown in Fig. 3a. The results show that as the concentration of EGF increases, the amplitude of the ΔD-response increases. Figure 3b shows the amplitude of the ΔD-response at 60 min as a function of the EGF concentration. An EC_{50}-value of 1.2 nM was computed from the curve-fitting of the dose–response. This EC_{50}-value is comparable to the k_d-values of EGFR obtained by others [43].

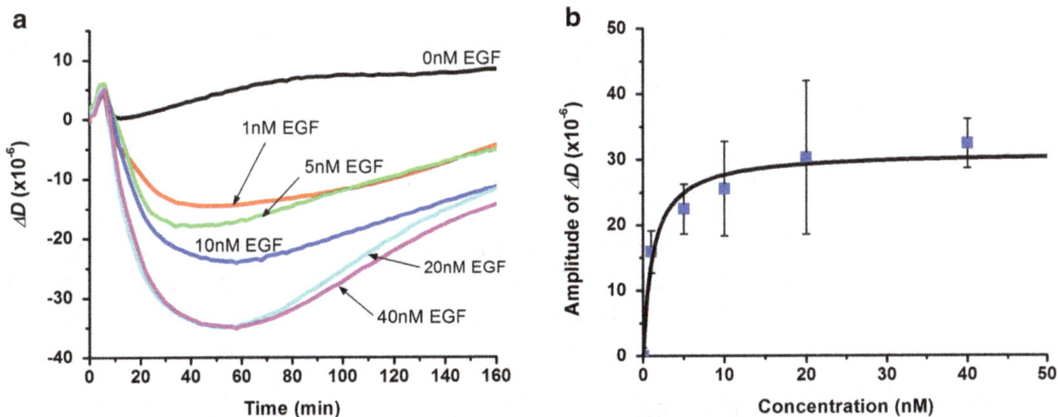

Fig. 3 Real-time QCM-D measurements (at the order of vibrational mode $n = 3$) of the responses of MCF-10A cells to EGF at 37 °C. (**a**) The ΔD-responses at the following concentrations: 0, 1, 5, 10, 20, and 40 nM of EGF. (**b**) The amplitudes of ΔD-responses at 60 min as a function of EGF concentrations. The EC_{50}-value for EGFR was 1.2 nM, determined from a curve fit of the dose–response curve. Adapted from Chen et al. 2012 Copyright 2012 Elsevier B.V

3.5.2 Profiling EGFR-Mediated Pathway Inhibition

Each of the three main EGFR-mediated pathways in MCF-10A cells was inhibited with a pathway-specific inhibitor. To determine if the ΔD-response was due to the EGFR-mediated pathway, cells were treated with 20- and 100-nM solutions of PD158780 [44], a potent inhibitor of EGFR tyrosine kinase (Fig. 1), for 40 min prior to stimulation with EGF. Figure 4a shows that the ΔD-response was significantly reduced, which indicates that the ΔD-response is a specific measure of the EGFR-mediated signaling after stimulation with EGF. For examination of the MAPK/ERK pathway (Fig. 1), cells were treated with 1- and 10-μM solutions of L779450 [45], a potent cell-permeable inhibitor of Raf kinase, for 30 min prior to stimulation with EGF. To examine the PI3K pathway, cells were treated with LY294002 (Fig. 1), a potent inhibitor of PI3K [46]. For examination of the PLC pathway, cells were treated with U73122 (Fig. 1), a potent inhibitor of PLCγ [47]. All three pathways were found to be responsible for regulation of cell de-adhesion in MCF-10A cells, as indicated by the dose-dependent suppression of the ΔD-responses. Interestingly, cells exhibited a distinct ΔD-response depending on which pathway that was selectively inhibited. When the MAPK/ERK pathway was inhibited, the initial portions of the phase I (de-adhesion) responses at all three inhibitor concentrations appeared superimposed on one another (Fig. 4b). By contrast, when the PI3K pathway was inhibited, the initial portions of the phase I responses were clearly separated from one another (Fig. 4c). While the ΔD-response in phase III was rising when either the MAPK/ERK or PI3K pathway was inhibited (Fig. 4b, c), the rise was absent when the PLC pathway was inhibited (Fig. 4d). The differences in the inhibitory profiles clearly indicate that each of these pathways has a distinct role at different stages of EGFR-mediated cell signaling. Obviously, continuous monitoring of the effects of pathway-specific inhibitors has the potential to advance our understanding of how these and other pathways regulate EGFR-mediated cell signaling.

3.5.3 IC$_{50}$-Values

The IC$_{50}$-value of each inhibitor of the EGFR-mediated pathways in mutant MCF-10A cells was determined from the ΔD-responses prior to stimulation with 10 nM EGF at various concentrations of inhibitor. Figure 5 shows the dose-inhibition curves used to obtain IC$_{50}$-values for the inhibitors [30]. In Table 1, the IC$_{50}$-values obtained from the QCM-D method were compared to literature values obtained from biochemical and biomechanical methods. The values obtained from the QCM-D method agree well with the reported values, strongly supporting the notion that the QCM-D method has the sensitivity and reliability to be used for drug screening.

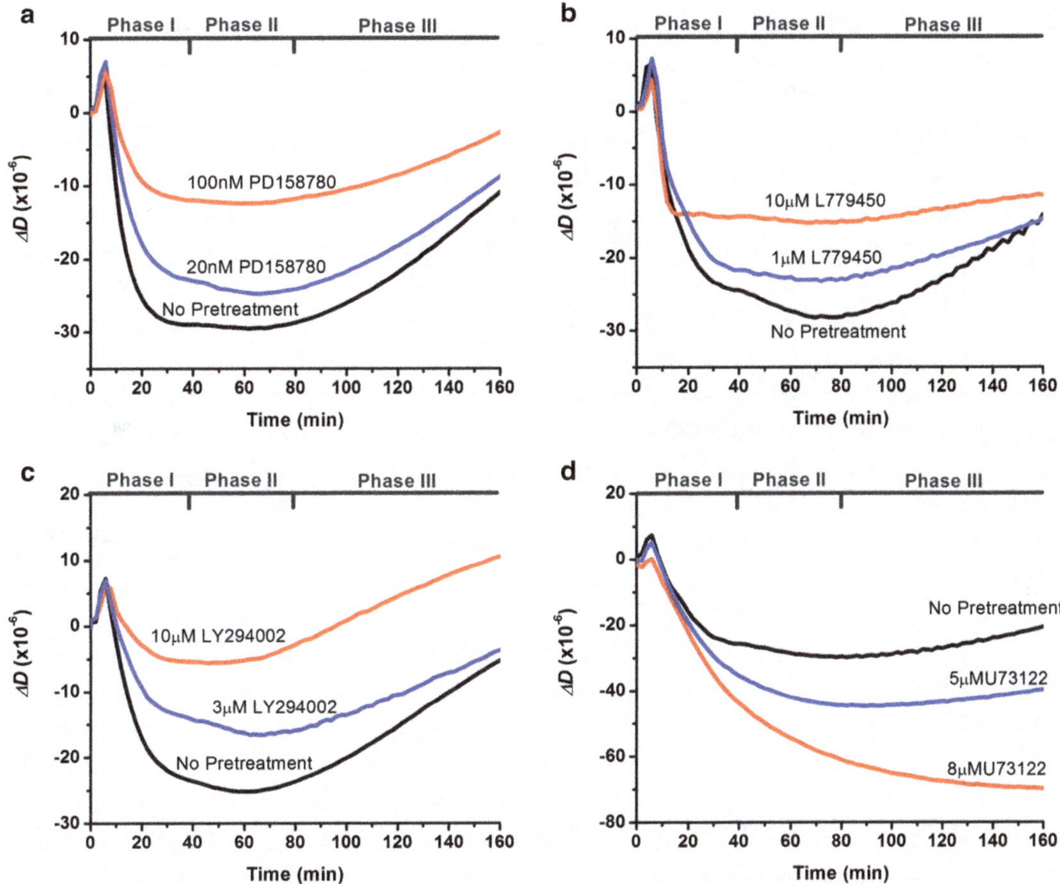

Fig. 4 Assessment of EGFR signaling in the presence of pathway inhibitors in MCF-10A cells at 37 °C. (**a**) The ΔD-response of the cells induced by 10 nM EGF was suppressed by PD158780, a known inhibitor of Raf kinase kinase of the mitogen-activated protein kinase/extracellular signal-regulated kinase (MAPK/ERK) pathway. (**b**) The ΔD-response of the cells induced by 10 nM EGF was suppressed by L779450, a known inhibitor of Raf kinase of the mitogen-activated protein kinase/extracellular signal-regulated kinase (MAPK/ERK) pathway. (**c**) The ΔD-response of the cells induced by 10 nM EGF was suppressed by LY294002, a known PI3K inhibitor of the PI3K pathway. (**d**) The ΔD-response of the cells induced by 10 nM EGF was enhanced by U73122, a known PLC inhibitor of the PLC pathway. Adapted from Chen et al. 2012 Copyright 2012 Elsevier B.V

4   Notes

1. The gold-surfaced crystals can be cleaned and sterilized after each use. For removal of cells, each sensor crystal is first soaked in 0.5 mL of trypsin–EDTA for 30 min at room temperature, and then rinsed three times with 2 mL of water. The resulting cell-free crystals are submerged in 0.5 mL of 1 % SDS solution at room temperature for 20 min to remove any cell and protein residues and then rinsed with a large amount of water.

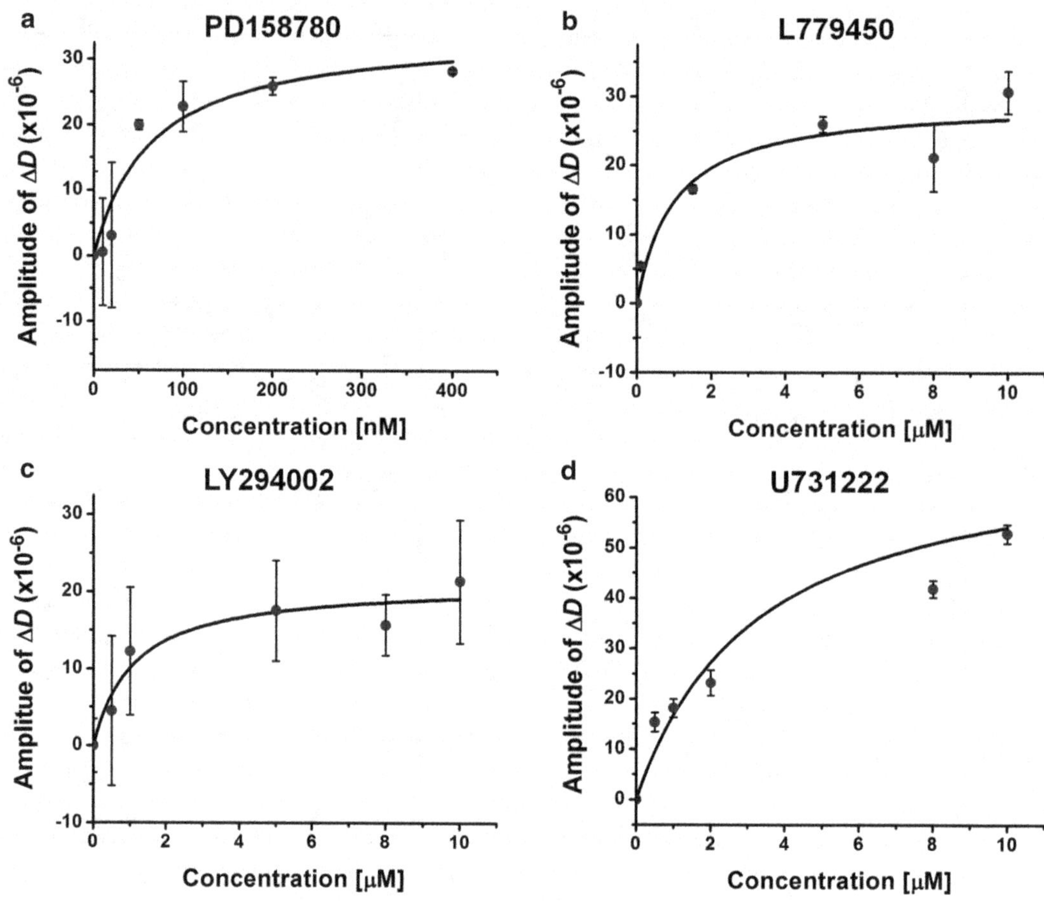

Fig. 5 The amplitudes of EGF-induced ΔD-responses as a function of inhibitor concentrations in mutant MCF-10A at 37 °C. The IC_{50}-values were determined for each inhibitor. (**a**) The dose-inhibition curve of PD158780 gave $IC_{50} = 64 \pm 30$ nM. (**b**) The dose-inhibition curve of L779450 gave $IC_{50} = 1.0 \pm 0.6$ µM. (**c**) The dose-inhibition curve of LY294002 gave $IC_{50} = 1.1 \pm 0.5$ µM. (**d**) The dose-inhibition curve of U73122 gave $IC_{50} = 2.5 \pm 0.9$ µM. Adapted from ref. 30 with the Creative Commons Attribution License

Next the sensors are soaked in 100 % ethanol for 30 min at room temperature. Lastly, the sensors are dried with flowing nitrogen gas and are placed in UV/ozone for 30 min for final sterilization. We found this protocol permits reuse of these sensor chips without comprising data quality.

2. The gold surface of the QCM-D sensors is more durable than silica-surfaced sensors, and permits repeated usage while still giving rise to stable and consistent results. MCF-10A cells grow well on this type of surface, yielding results comparable in every way to the results obtained on silica-surfaced sensors [31, 48].

3. The data at vibrational mode $n = 3$ is usually used in the cell studies. The QCM-D at this vibrational mode has a penetration depth into the coupled material of approximately 100–150 nm

Table 1
Comparison of IC$_{50}$-values of EGF inhibitors to literature values [30]

Inhibitor	IC$_{50}$ (QCM-D)	IC$_{50}$ (literature)
PD158780	64±30 nM	52 nM [44]
L779450	1.0±0.6 µM	1 µM [50]
LY294002	1.1±0.5 µM	1.4 µM [46]
U73122	2.5±0.9 µM	1–2.1 µM [5]

from the surface of a 5-MHz sensor [49]. This sensing depth corresponds with the basal region of the cell monolayer, allowing the QCM-D to interrogate the interaction between the basal region of the cells and the surface of the sensor.

4. Adding and removing solution from the cells in the open modules before and after the QCM-D measurement can cause a minor mechanical perturbation to the cells. This perturbation can produce an artifact in the form of a small, sharp peak within the first 5 min of the ΔD-response. To minimize such artifacts, the original solution in the module needs to be carefully removed with a P1000 pipet that does not make contact with the sensor surface. Addition of the next solution (400 µL) must also be done carefully; this is best done by allowing it to slowly trickle down the side wall of the module onto the cells. The entire transfer, both removal and addition of solutions, for all four modules should be completed within 30 s.

References

1. Carpenter G (1987) Receptors for epidermal growth factor and other polypeptide mitogens. Annu Rev Biochem 56(1):881–914. doi:10.1146/annurev.bi.56.070187.004313

2. Lemmon MA, Schlessinger J (2010) Cell signaling by receptor tyrosine kinases. Cell 141(7): 1117–1134. doi:10.1016/j.cell.2010.06.011

3. Scaltriti M, Baselga J (2006) The epidermal growth factor receptor pathway: a model for targeted therapy. Clin Cancer Res 12(18):5268–5272. doi:10.1158/1078-0432.ccr-05-1554

4. Osaki M, Oshimura M, Ito H (2004) PI3K-Akt pathway: its functions and alterations in human cancer. Apoptosis 9(6):667–676. doi:10.1023/B:APPT.0000045801.15585.dd

5. Xie W, Peng H, Zalkow LH, Li Y-H, Zhu C, Powis G, Kunkel M (2000) 3β-Hydroxy-6-aza-cholestane and related analogues as phosphatidylinositol specific phospholipase C (PI-PLC) inhibitors with antitumor activity. Bioorg Med Chem 8(4):699–706. doi:10.1016/S0968-0896(00)00014-6

6. Zandi R, Larsen AB, Andersen P, Stockhausen M-T, Poulsen HS (2007) Mechanisms for oncogenic activation of the epidermal growth factor receptor. Cell Signal 19(10):2013–2023. doi:10.1016/j.cellsig.2007.06.023

7. Sebastian S, Settleman J, Reshkin SJ, Azzariti A, Bellizzi A, Paradiso A (2006) The complexity of targeting EGFR signalling in cancer: from expression to turnover. Biochim Biophys Acta 1766(1):120–139. doi:10.1016/j.bbcan.2006.06.001

8. Murphy-Ullrich JE (2001) The de-adhesive activity of matricellular proteins: is intermediate cell adhesion an adaptive state. J Clin Invest 107(7):785–790

9. Welsh JB, Gill GN, Rosenfeld MG, Wells A (1991) A negative feedback loop attenuates EGF-induced morphological changes. J Cell

Biol 114(3):533–543. doi:10.1083/jcb.114.3.533

10. Xie H, Pallero MA, Gupta K, Chang P, Ware MF, Witke W, Kwiatkowski DJ, Lauffenburger DA, Murphy-Ullrich JE, Wells A (1998) EGF receptor regulation of cell motility: EGF induces disassembly of focal adhesions independently of the motility-associated PLCgamma signaling pathway. J Cell Sci 111(5):615–624

11. Lauffenburger DA, Horwitz AF (1996) Cell migration: a physically integrated molecular process. Cell 84(3):359–369. doi:10.1016/S0092-8674(00)81280-5

12. Reginato MJ, Mills KR, Paulus JK, Lynch DK, Sgroi DC, Debnath J, Muthuswamy SK, Brugge JS (2003) Integrins and EGFR coordinately regulate the pro-apoptotic protein Bim to prevent anoikis. Nat Cell Biol 5(8):733–740. doi:10.1038/ncb1026

13. Dei Tos AP, Ellis I (2005) Assessing epidermal growth factor receptor expression in tumours: what is the value of current test methods. Eur J Cancer 41(10):1383–1392. doi:10.1016/j.ejca.2005.03.018

14. Oda K, Matsuoka Y, Funahashi A, Kitano H (2005) A comprehensive pathway map of epidermal growth factor receptor signaling. Mol Syst Biol 1:2005.0010. doi:10.1038/msb4100014

15. Abbitt KB, Rainger GE, Nash GB (2000) Effects of fluorescent dyes on selectin and integrin-mediated stages of adhesion and migration of flowing leukocytes. J Immunol Methods 239(1–2):109–119. doi:10.1016/S0022-1759(00)00189-7

16. Xi B, Yu N, Wang X, Xu X, Abassi Y (2008) The application of cell-based label-free technology in drug discovery. Biotechnol J 3(4):484–495. doi:10.1002/biot.200800020

17. Rodahl M, Kasemo B (1996) Frequency and dissipation-factor responses to localized liquid deposits on a QCM electrode. Sens Actuator B: Chem 37(1–2):111–116. doi:10.1016/S0925-4005(97)80077-9

18. Sauerbrey G (1959) Verwendung von Schwingquarzen zur Wägung dünner Schichten und zur Mikrowägung. Zeitschrift für Physik 155(2):206–222. doi:10.1007/bf01337937

19. Reviakine I, Johannsmann D, Richter RP (2011) Hearing what you cannot see and visualizing what you hear: interpreting quartz crystal microbalance data from solvated interfaces. Anal Chem 83(23):8838–8848. doi:10.1021/ac201778h

20. Zhang Y, Du B, Chen X, Ma H (2008) Convergence of dissipation and impedance analysis of quartz crystal microbalance studies.

Anal Chem 81(2):642–648. doi:10.1021/ac8019762

21. Cheng CI, Chang Y-P, Chu Y-H (2012) Biomolecular interactions and tools for their recognition: focus on the quartz crystal microbalance and its diverse surface chemistries and applications. Chem Soc Rev 41(5):1947–1971. doi:10.1039/c1cs15168a

22. Urbakh M, Tsionsky V, Gileadi E, Daikhin L (2007) Probing the solid/liquid interface with the quartz crystal microbalance. In: Janshoff A, Steinem C (eds) Piezoelectric sensors. Vol. 5. Springer series on chemical sensors and biosensors. Springer, Berlin, pp 111–149. doi:10.1007/978-3-540-36568-6_3

23. Höök F, Kasemo B (2007) The QCM-D technique for probing biomacromolecular recognition reactions. In: Janshoff A, Steinem C (eds) Piezoelectric sensors. Vol. 5. Springer series on chemical sensors and biosensors. Springer, Berlin, pp 425–447. doi:10.1007/978-3-540-36568-6_12

24. Marx K (2007) The quartz crystal microbalance and the electrochemical qcm: applications to studies of thin polymer films, electron transfer systems, biological macromolecules, biosensors, and cells. In: Steinem C, Janshoff A (eds) Piezoelectric sensors. Vol. 5. Springer series on chemical sensors and biosensors. Springer, Berlin, pp 371–424. doi:10.1007/5346_033

25. Hunter AC (2009) Application of the quartz crystal microbalance to nanomedicine. J Biomed Nanotechnol 5(6):669–675. doi:10.1166/jbn.2009.1083

26. Cabré EJ, Malmström J, Sutherland D, Pérez-Gil J, Otzen DE (2009) Surfactant protein sp-b strongly modifies surface collapse of phospholipid vesicles: insights from a quartz crystal microbalance with dissipation. Biophys J 97(3):768–776. doi:10.1016/j.bpj.2009.04.057

27. Lee H-S, Contarino M, Umashankara M, Schön A, Freire E, Smith A III, Chaiken I, Penn L (2010) Use of the quartz crystal microbalance to monitor ligand-induced conformational rearrangements in HIV-1 envelope protein gp120. Anal Bioanal Chem 396(3):1143–1152. doi:10.1007/s00216-009-3313-8

28. Keller CA, Kasemo B (1998) Surface specific kinetics of lipid vesicle adsorption measured with a quartz crystal microbalance. Biophys J 75(3):1397–1402. doi:10.1016/S0006-3495(98)74057-3

29. Marques BF, Schneider JW (2005) Sequence-specific binding of DNA to liposomes containing di-alkyl peptide nucleic acid (PNA) amphiphiles. Langmuir 21(6):2488–2494. doi:10.1021/la047962u

30. Garcia M, Shahid A, Chen J, Xi J (2012) Evaluating inhibition of the epidermal growth factor (EGF)-induced response of mutant MCF-10A cells with an acoustic sensor. Biosensors 2(4):448–464. doi:10.3390/bios2040448

31. Chen JY, Shahid A, Garcia MP, Penn LS, Xi J (2012) Dissipation monitoring for assessing EGF-induced changes of cell adhesion. Biosens Bioelectron 38(1):375–381

32. Chen JY, Li M, Penn LS, Xi J (2011) Real-time and label-free detection of cellular response to signaling mediated by distinct subclasses of epidermal growth factor receptors. Anal Chem 83(8):3141–3146. doi:10.1021/ac200160u

33. Xi J, Chen JY, Garcia MP, Penn LS (2013) Quartz crystal microbalance in cell biology studies. J Biochip Tissue Chip S5, 10.4172/2153-0777.S5-001

34. Höök F, Kasemo B, Nylander T, Fant C, Sott K, Elwing H (2001) Variations in coupled water, viscoelastic properties, and film thickness of a Mefp-1 protein film during adsorption and cross-linking: a quartz crystal microbalance with dissipation monitoring, ellipsometry, and surface plasmon resonance study. Anal Chem 73(24):5796–5804. doi:10.1021/ac0106501

35. Yin Y, Bilek MMM, McKenzie DR, Nosworthy NJ, Kondyurin A, Youssef H, Byrom MJ, Yang W (2009) Acetylene plasma polymerized surfaces for covalent immobilization of dense bioactive protein monolayers. Surf Coatings Technol 203(10–11):1310–1316. doi:10.1016/j.surfcoat.2008.10.035

36. Hovgaard MB, Dong M, Otzen DE, Besenbacher F (2007) Quartz crystal microbalance studies of multilayer glucagon fibrillation at the solid-liquid interface. Biophys J 93(6):2162–2169. doi:10.1529/biophysj.107.109686

37. Fredriksson C, Kihlman S, Rodahl M, Kasemo B (1998) The piezoelectric quartz crystal mass and dissipation sensor: a means of studying cell adhesion. Langmuir 14(2):248–251. doi:10.1021/la971005l

38. Nimeri G, Fredriksson C, Elwing H, Liu L, Rodahl M, Kasemo B (1998) Neutrophil interaction with protein-coated surfaces studied by an extended quartz crystal microbalance technique. Colloids Surf B Biointerfaces 11(5):255–264. doi:10.1016/S0927-7765(98)00038-1

39. Saitakis M, Gizeli E (2012) Acoustic sensors as a biophysical tool for probing cell attachment and cell/surface interactions. Cell Mol Life Sci 69(3):357–371. doi:10.1007/s00018-011-0854-8

40. Yang R, Chen JY, Xi N, Lai KWC, Qu C, Fung CKM, Penn LS, Xi J (2012) Characterization of mechanical behavior of an epithelial monolayer in response to epidermal growth factor stimulation. Exp Cell Res 318(5):521–526. doi:10.1016/j.yexcr.2011.12.003

41. Xi J, Penn LS, Chen JY, Xi N, Yang R (2012) Dynamic mechanical response of epithelial cells to epidermal growth factor. In: de Vicente J (ed) Viscoelasticity - From theory to biological applications. InTechOpen, pp 171–185. doi:10.5772/49977

42. Xi N, Yang R, Song B, Lai KWC, Chen H, Chen JY, Penn LS, Xi J (2013) Developing a dynamics model for epidermal growth factor (EGF)-Induced cellular signaling events. In: Xi N, Zhang M, Li G (eds) Modeling and Control for Micro/Nano devices and systems. Automation and control engineering. CRC Press, pp 69–86. doi:10.1201/b16071-6

43. Martin-Fernandez M, Clarke DT, Tobin MJ, Jones SV, Jones GR (2002) Preformed oligomeric epidermal growth factor receptors undergo an ectodomain structure change during signaling. Biophys J 82(5):2415–2427. doi:10.1016/S0006-3495(02)75585-9

44. Fry DW, Nelson JM, Slintak V, Keller PR, Rewcastle GW, Denny WA, Zhou H, Bridges AJ (1997) Biochemical and antiproliferative properties of 4-[Ar(alk)ylamino]pyridopyrimidines, a new chemical class of potent and specific epidermal growth factor receptor tyrosine kinase inhibitor. Biochem Pharmacol 54(8):877–887. doi:10.1016/S0006-2952(97)00242-6

45. Gollob JA, Wilhelm S, Carter C, Kelley SL (2006) Role of Raf Kinase in Cancer: therapeutic potential of targeting the Raf/MEK/ERK signal transduction pathway. Semin Oncol 33(4):392–406. doi:10.1053/j.seminoncol.2006.04.002

46. Vlahos CJ, Matter WF, Hui KY, Brown RF (1994) A specific inhibitor of phosphatidylinositol 3-kinase, 2-(4-morpholinyl)-8-phenyl-4H-1-benzopyran-4-one (LY294002). J Biol Chem 269(7):5241–5248

47. Smith RJ, Sam LM, Justen JM, Bundy GL, Bala GA, Bleasdale JE (1990) Receptor-coupled signal transduction in human polymorphonuclear neutrophils: effects of a novel inhibitor of phospholipase C-dependent processes on cell responsiveness. J Pharmacol Exp Ther 253(2):688–697

48. Garcia M, Shahid A, Chen J, Xi J (2013) Effects of the expression level of epidermal growth factor receptor on the ligand-induced restructuring of focal adhesions: a QCM-D study. Anal Bioanal Chem 405(4):1153–1158. doi:10.1007/s00216-012-6558-6

49. Le Guillou-Buffello D, Gindre M, Johnson P, Laugier P, Migonney V (2011) An alternative quantitative acoustical and electrical method for detection of cell adhesion process in real-time. Biotechnol Bioeng 108(4):947–962. doi:10.1002/bit.23005

50. Shelton JG, Moye PW, Steelman LS, Blalock WL, Lee JT, Franklin RA, McMahon M, McCubrey JA (2003) Differential effects of kinase cascade inhibitors on neoplastic and cytokine-mediated cell proliferation. Leukemia 17(9): 1765–1782. doi:10.1038/sj.leu.2403052

Chapter 15

Profiling Sodium-Dependent Phosphate Transporter NaPi-IIb with Resonant Waveguide Grating Biosensor

Soo-Hang Wong, Alice Gao, and Paul H. Lee

Abstract

The development of label-free resonant waveguide grating (RWG) technology in microplate format in the last decade has stimulated interests from academic and industrial scientists, leading to evaluation of the technology in a broad range of biochemical and cell-based assays. In cellular assays the plasma membrane and immediate cellular volume are within the sensing region from the surface of the RWG biosensor. Any rearrangement of intracellular proteins or molecules in this region of the cells, termed dynamic mass redistribution (DMR), can be detected by the RWG biosensor. The biosensor monitors a global cellular output that can amplify the activity of a few active receptors into a measurable response; therefore, it is a useful tool for measuring physiological responses of live cells.

Most membrane transporter studies still rely on measurement of the accumulation of radiolabeled substrates or on using electrophysiology techniques. Thus, there is an unmet need for a homogeneous and high-throughput assay for transporter research. The biological process of transporting substrates across the plasma membrane of cells and their subsequent interactions with intracellular proteins or molecules presents an ideal case study for the RWG biosensor. In this report, we describe a detailed protocol using an RWG biosensor to monitor DMR signals in cells following the activation of the type IIb sodium-dependent phosphate transporter (NaPi-IIb) in a homogeneous, 384-well assay format. Results suggest that the DMR signals could serve as novel and quantifiable physiological responses of activated NaPi-IIb transporters and the technology can be used to query transporter pharmacology.

Key words Cellular assay, Dynamic mass redistribution (DMR), High-throughput, Label-free, NaPi-IIb, Resonant waveguide grating (RWG), Transporter

---

1 Introduction

In the last decade, new cellular assay methods in microplate format have expanded exponentially because of significant advancements in both fluorescent and label-free technologies. Despite this improvement, few cellular assays are available for studying the functional activity of membrane surface transporters. To date, the most widely used transporter assay measures the accumulation of radiolabeled substrates in tissues or cells that express the target transporters. Recent use of the scintillation proximity assay (SPA)

Ye Fang (ed.), *Label-Free Biosensor Methods in Drug Discovery*, Methods in Pharmacology and Toxicology, DOI 10.1007/978-1-4939-2617-6_15, © Springer Science+Business Media New York 2015

method eliminates the wash procedure, which is required for the separation of excess free radiolabeled substrates from those transported and accumulated in cells, allowing a homogeneous assay in 384-well format [1]. The SPA method, however, retains a number of drawbacks, including the use of radioisotopes, storage and disposal of radioactive waste, and limitation to low concentrations of radiolabeled substrates because high concentration would result in background issue without the wash procedure.

Another popular method for studying electrogenic transporters is to express the target transporters in *Xenopus* oocytes and record the substrate transport by electrophysiology techniques. This assay measures the amount of current necessary to clamp the cell membrane of an oocyte at a given applied voltage in the presence or absence of expressed transporters, substrates, or inhibitors. Electrophysiology measurements offer the advantage of a functional, nonradioactive readout with exquisite time resolution. This method, however, has a low throughput and requires highly skilled technical staff to perform assays. In addition, this technique depends on the electrogenicity of the transporter and measures the net charge being transported. Therefore, it is not suitable for all transporters, resulting in an unmet need for a label-free, homogeneous, and high-throughput assay for studying membrane transporters.

Label-free resonant waveguide grating (RWG) biosensor in microplate format was developed a decade ago and since then has gained applications in biological research. Its universal principle of detection and amenability to high-throughput screening stimulated interest in its applicability as a generic methodology to facilitate a broad range of assays in drug discovery [2, 3]. The RWG biosensor utilizes the resonant coupling of light into a waveguide by means of a diffraction grating. The microplate has a waveguide grating bottom surface onto which proteins are attached or cells are plated. When live cells are in contact with the surface of a biosensor at the bottom of the well, their plasma membranes and immediate cellular volume, meaning the bottom portion of the cells, are within the sensing region (150 nm from the surface of the biosensor) [2]. An induced change in intracellular contents, especially those in close proximity to the plasma membrane, will lead to an alteration in local refractive index near the sensor surface, resulting in a dynamic mass redistribution (DMR) signal. DMR is an integrated response that involves cellular events, including cytoskeleton or microfilament rearrangement, and movement of signaling cascade proteins.

Unlike other conventional assay platforms which are generally limited to measurement of a single signaling event, this technology uses the integrated signature of DMR to study cell signaling and network interactions. The biosensor monitors a global cellular output that can amplify the activity of a few active receptors, even though which might not be detected by a binding or second messenger assay, into a measureable response. Owing to the noninvasive nature of the biosensor, multiple relevant cell lines can be measured simultaneously to determine the pharmacological profile of a drug in development. Furthermore, primary cells, or theoretically any cell type, can be studied to determine drug efficacy in a more physiological or tissue relevant manner. This would permit comparison of drug effects on primary cells obtained from patients and normal subjects without further manipulation.

The cytoskeleton of eukaryotic cells is implicated in many cellular activities, from maintaining cell shape to providing docking sites for signaling and trafficking [4–6]. The translocation of intracellular proteins and molecules is fundamental to control the amplitude and/or kinetics of cell responses, including signal transmission, morphological changes, and cell migration. An example is illustrated in G protein-coupled receptor (GPCR) signaling. GPCRs are membrane-bound proteins. Their activation by agonists can lead to a series of spatial and temporal events that are precisely controlled by intracellular signaling machinery. Many of these events occur in close proximity to the plasma membrane, which is within the sensing region of the RWG biosensors. Many GPCRs have been studied using the RWG biosensor and the measured pharmacological profiles are in accord with those reported in second messenger studies [7, 8].

A type IIb sodium-dependent phosphate transporter, NaPi-IIb, is responsible for absorbing more than half of dietary phosphorous in the small intestine. It is electrogenic and exhibits a $Na^+:HPO4^{2-}$ stoichiometry of 3:1 [9]. However, potassium phosphate does not elicit detectable currents using the manual patch-clamp method in CHO cells expressing NaPi-IIb [10]. This lack of detectable current suggests that a high expression level of the transporters or using an overexpression system, such as *Xenopus* oocytes, is necessary for studying transporter proteins with electrophysiological methods. In this report, we describe a detailed protocol for a label-free assay using an RWG biosensor to monitor DMR signals in cells following the activation of the NaPi-IIb transporter in a homogeneous, 384-well assay format. DMR allows kinetic measurements at physiological concentrations of the substrate without labeling either the substrate or the transporter. Results suggest that the DMR signals could serve as novel and quantifiable physiological responses of activated NaPi-IIb transporters and the technology can be used to query NaPi-IIb pharmacology.

2 Materials

2.1 Cell Culture

1. Chinese hamster ovary (CHO) cell line stably expressing the human NaPi-IIb transporter gene SLC34A2 (NaPi-IIb-CHO) (Amgen).

2. Dulbecco's Modified Eagle Medium with Glutamax (DMEM) (Life Technologies cat. 10566-016).

3. Dulbecco's Modified Eagle Medium without phenol red (Life Technologies cat. 31053-028).

4. Fetal bovine serum (FBS) (Life Technologies cat. 16000-044).

5. Geneticin selective antibiotic solution (Life Technologies cat. 10131-035).

6. Non-essential amino acids solution (Life Technologies cat. 11140-050).

7. HT supplement solution (Life Technologies cat. 11067-030).

8. Penicillin-streptomycin solution (Life Technologies cat. 15140-122).

9. Penicillin-streptomycin-glutamine solution (Life Technologies cat. 10378-016).

10. Growth media for NaPi-IIb-CHO cells: DMEM with Glutamax, 10 % FBS, 1 mg/mL geneticin selective antibiotic, 1× nonessential amino acids, 1× HT supplement, 100 U/mL penicillin-100 µg/mL streptomycin.

11. Plating media for NaPi-IIb-CHO cells: DMEM without phenol red, 10 % FBS, 1 mg/mL geneticin selective antibiotic, 1× nonessential amino acids, 1× HT supplement, 100 U/mL penicillin-100 µg/mL streptomycin-1 mM glutamine.

12. Dulbecco's Phosphate Buffer Saline (DPBS) (Life Technologies cat. 14190-136).

13. 0.05 % Trypsin with EDTA solution (Life Technologies cat. 25300-054).

14. Cell viability analyzer (Vi-Cell XR, Beckman Coulter).

2.2 Dynamic Mass Redistribution Assay

1. Potassium phosphate (K-Pi) 1 M solution: Mix 1 volume of 1 M KH_2PO_4 to 2 volumes of 1 M K_2HPO_4 (prepare fresh on the day of assay).

2. Assay buffer: 10 mM Hepes pH 7.2, 137 mM NaCl, 5.4 mM KCl, 2.8 mM $CaCl_2$, 1.2 mM $MgCl_2$, 10 mM D-glucose, 5 mM $NaHCO_3$ (prepare fresh on the day of assay from stock solutions).

3. Test compounds: Solubilized in 100 % dimethyl sulfoxide (DMSO) at 20 mM concentration (for long-term storage of 20 mM stock, store at −20 °C; intermediate concentration of test compounds prepared fresh on the day of the assay).

4. 384-Well Epic microplate, fibronectin coated (Corning cat. 5042).

5. 384-Well microplate (Greiner Bio-one cat. 781280).

6. Microplate washer dispenser (EL406 Biotek Instruments).

7. Epic instrument equipped with Liquid Handling Accessory (LHA) (Corning).

8. Low volume liquid handler (Echo 555 instrument, Labcyte).

9. 384-Well low dead volume Echo qualified microplate (Labcyte cat. LP-0200).

10. Liquid handler for 384-well microplates (e.g., Multimek-384, Beckman Coulter).

2.3 Data Analysis Software

1. Epic Offline Viewer software (Corning).

2. GraphPad Prism software (GraphPad Software Inc., La Jolla, CA, USA).

---

3 Methods

3.1 NaPi-IIb-CHO Cell Culture

3.1.1 Cell Maintenance

NaPi-IIb-CHO cells were split when they reached 75–90 % confluence in the T-75 tissue culture flasks. The growth media was warmed to 37 °C before use.

1. Remove growth media from flask and wash cells with 10 mL of DPBS.

2. Add 2 mL of 0.05 % trypsin/EDTA and place flask in a 37 °C incubator in an atmosphere of 5 % CO_2 for 3 min.

3. Add 2 mL of growth media to the cells to quench the trypsin and transfer the detached cells to a 50 mL conical centrifuge tube.

4. Centrifuge cells at $800\,g$ in a Beckman GS-6KR centrifuge (or equivalent) for 5 min.

5. Discard the supernatant and resuspend the cells with 10 mL of growth media. Dilute the cellular suspension to the desired concentration in a new T-75 flask. For example, for a 1:10 dilution of the initial flask, transfer 1 mL of the cellular suspension to a new T-75 flask and add 14 mL of fresh growth media.

6. Place the flask in the 37 °C cell culture incubator for continued growth.

3.1.2 Plating Cells for the Assay

1. Follow steps 1–4 of Section 3.1.1.

2. After centrifugation of the cells, discard the supernatant and resuspend the cells with 10 mL of plating media.

3. Count a 1 mL aliquot of the cellular suspension on a Vi-Cell XR cell viability analyzer (or equivalent).

4. Plate cells at a density such that they will become confluent on the day of the assay. Specifically, suspend NaPi-IIb-CHO cells to a concentration of 2.25×10^5 cells/mL for plating. Using an electronic multichannel pipettor, dispense 40 µL of the cellular suspension per well into an Epic 384-well fibronectin-coated microplate, resulting in 9,000 cells per well.

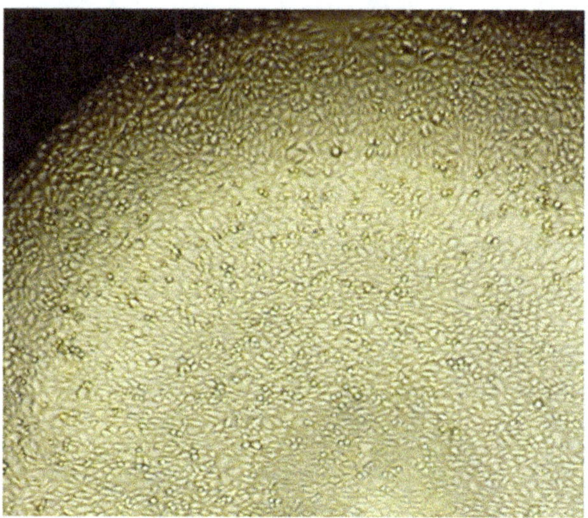

Fig. 1 Light microscopic image of NaPi-IIb-CHO cells in the Epic fibronectin-coated microplate on the day of the dynamic mass redistribution (DMR) measurement. 4× magnification

5. Incubate the cell plate in the laminar flow hood for 25 min (*see* **Note 1**).

6. Place the plate in a 37 °C cell culture incubator for 24-h growth, resulting in the NaPi-IIb-CHO cell plate for assays. The appearance of the cells in the microplate should be confluent as shown in Fig. 1.

3.2 Measurement of NaPi-IIb-CHO Cell DMR Responses Elicited by K-Pi

The protocol below was optimized specifically for DMR measurements of NaPi-IIb transporter using NaPi-IIb-CHO cell line and LHA-equipped Epic system (Fig. 2). Assays that use other cell lines with different NaPi-IIb expression levels or different biosensor systems may require further optimization of the assay protocol. Figure 3a is a representative DMR kinetic profile stimulated by K-Pi at various concentrations (0.1, 0.3, 0.6, 1.0, 1.8, 3.0, 10, 30, 100 μM) on NaPi-IIb-CHO cells. K-Pi elicited a DMR response in a concentration-dependent manner in the presence of 137 mM NaCl with a maximum signal equivalent to a wavelength shift of 50 pm (Fig. 3b). The calculated K_m value for Pi is 1.4 ± 0.3 μM ($n = 4$).

1. Prepare a 1 M solution of K-Pi, pH 7.3 (*see* Section 2.2). Prepare intermediate K-Pi solutions (3× final concentration) in assay buffer at concentrations between 0.03 and 300 μM for a concentration-response study. The final K-Pi concentrations after addition to the cell plate will be 0.01–100 μM. Dispense 35 μL of each concentration to a standard microplate using an electric multichannel pipette. Also dispense 35 μL of assay buffer to the buffer control wells which does not contain K-Pi.

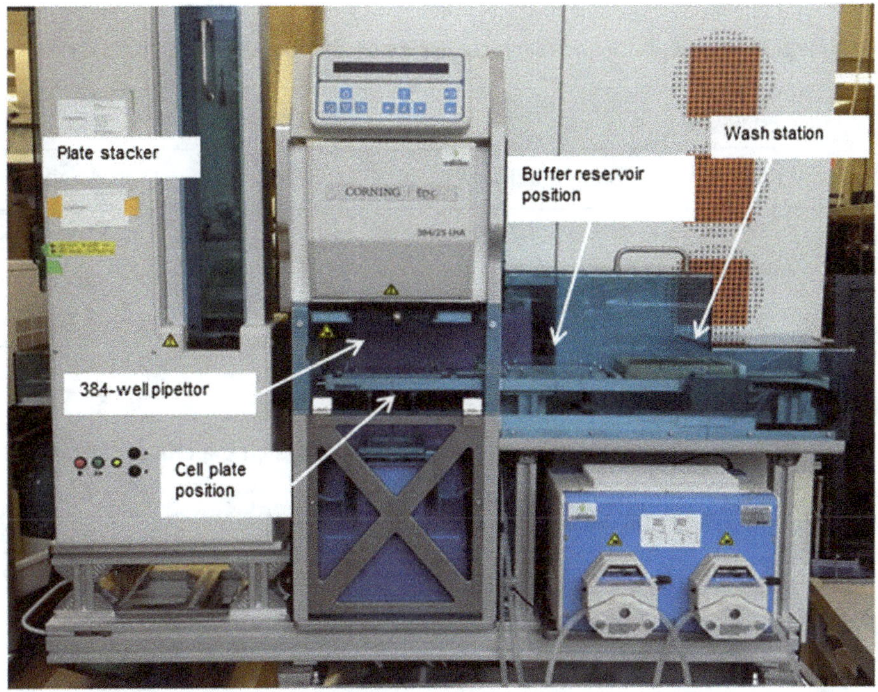

Fig. 2 Photo of the liquid-handling accessory (LHA) on the Epic instrument. The LHA is equipped with a plate stacker. The cell plate position is pictured below the 384-well pipettor. Adjacent are the position for a buffer reservoir and tip wash station

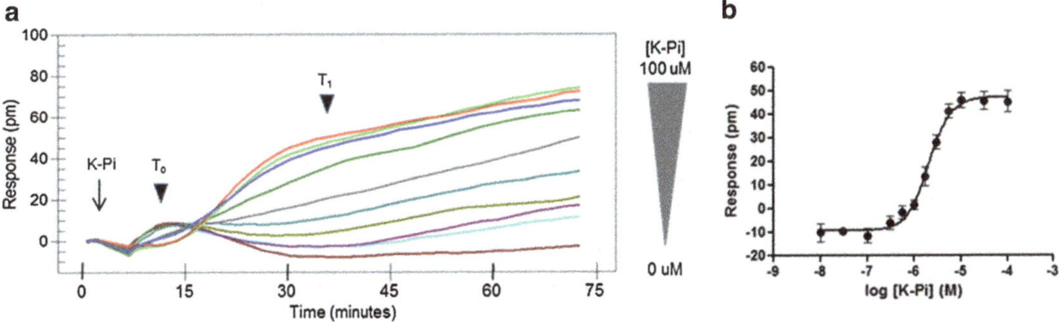

Fig. 3 Potassium phosphate (K-Pi)-elicited dynamic mass redistribution (DMR) kinetic profile in NaPi-IIb–CHO cells. (**a**) A 5-min baseline measurement was taken prior to the addition of K-Pi at various concentrations (0.01–100 μM) into different wells. The plate was then measured for an additional 65 min. *Arrow* indicates the addition of K-Pi. *Closed black arrows* indicate typical baseline time point (T_0) and test time point (T_1) at which DMR responses were used to generate concentration-response curves. (**b**) The DMR response as a function of Pi concentration. Data are mean ± S.D. values of four separate wells from a representative experiment. Reproduced from ref. 10 with permission from SAGE Publications

2. Aspirate the growth media from the NaPi-IIb-CHO cell plate 24 h after cell plating and perform two wash cycles of 50 μL of assay buffer using a plate washer. Leave a residual amount of assay buffer in the well since the aspirator height is offset from

Table 1
Parameter settings for the aspirate and dispense cycles on the Biotek EL406 plate washer

Parameter	Aspirate		Dispense	
	Steps	Step detail	Steps	Step detail
Z offset	58	7.37 mm above carrier	355	16.23 mm above carrier
X offset	−6	0.27 mm left of center	22	1.01 mm left of center
Y offset	0	Center of well	0	Center of well

Table 2
Parameter settings for the wash cycles on the LHA of the Epic instrument

Parameter	Aspirate	Dispense
Tip height	1.5 mm	2 mm
Flow rate	2.5 µL/s	5 µL/s

the bottom of the well to prevent disturbance of the cell monolayer. Table 1 lists the parameters of the plate washer.

3. Perform two aspirations of 25 µL of the residual assay buffer left by the plate washer and then one wash cycle of 25 µL using the LHA of the Epic instrument (*see* **Note 2**).

4. Replace the disposable tips on the LHA and use new assay buffer in the reservoir. Flush the wash station on the LHA with water for a minimum of 1 min. Continue with four wash cycles of 25 µL of assay buffer on the LHA. Steps 3 and 4 comprise the two-step wash method on the LHA. Refer to Table 2 for LHA parameters (*see* **Notes 2** and **3**).

5. Dispense 30 µL (two cycles of 15 µL) of assay buffer into the wells of the cell plate using the LHA.

6. Equilibrate the intermediate K-Pi concentration-response plate and cell plate in the Epic instrument at 26 °C for 1 h (*see* **Note 4**).

7. Measure the baseline DMR of the cells for 5 min, for example, seven reads every 0.7 min.

8. Pre-wet pipette tips with K-Pi solution and transfer 20 µL to the cell plate using the LHA. Perform two mix cycles of 20 µL in the cell plate. Continue to monitor DMR response for 65 min, for example, 30 reads every 0.5 min for 15 min and then an additional 25 reads every 2 min for 50 min.

9. Select the baseline time point (T_0) and test time point (T_1) from the DMR kinetic profile using Epic Offline Viewer

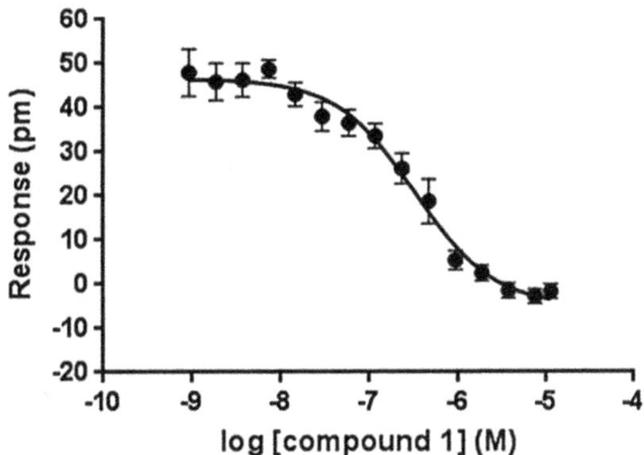

Fig. 4 Concentration-response curve of compound 1, a benchmark NaPi-IIb inhibitor, in the inhibition of potassium phosphate (K-Pi)-elicited dynamic mass redistribution responses in NaPi-IIb-CHO cells. The cells were pretreated with various concentrations of compound 1 for 1 h during plate equilibration in the Epic reader. A 5-min baseline measurement was taken before the addition of 100 µM K-Pi. Data are mean ± S.D. values of four separate wells from a representative experiment

software. Select 35 min post-stimulation for T_1 since it is the time point at which the buffer effect remained at the baseline prior to the gradual increase for the NaPi-IIb-CHO cells tested. Plot the resulting DMR response values ($T_1 - T_0$) as a function of the K-Pi concentrations. Determine the K_m value for K-Pi by nonlinear regression analysis of the concentration-response curve using GraphPad Prism software.

3.3 Assay Procedure for Compound Testing

This protocol is to examine the effect of compounds on the transport activity of NaPi-IIb. Here, the cells are pretreated with the test compounds, followed by stimulation with K-Pi. The DMR elicited by K-Pi is recorded and used to determine the compound inhibitory potency. Compound 1 (JTP-59557) is a noncompetitive inhibitor of the NaPi-IIb transporter [11]. As expected, compound 1 inhibited the K-Pi-induced DMR response in a concentration-dependent manner with an IC_{50} of 0.44 µM (Fig. 4), which is similar to the IC_{50} of 0.12 µM reported by Matsuo et al. using a radiolabel accumulation assay. Table 3 summarizes DMR IC_{50} values for six additional NaPi-IIb inhibitors as compared to a [^{33}P]-uptake assay using this NaPi-IIb-CHO cell line. The IC_{50} values between the two assays are within a threefold difference, suggesting that DMR measurement can be an alternative assay platform to study NaPi-IIb inhibitors.

1. Prepare K-Pi in assay buffer at a concentration of 300 µM and dispense 35 µL to wells of a standard 384-well microplate using an electric multichannel pipette. The final concentration of K-Pi in the cell plate will be 100 µM (*see* **Note 3**).

Table 3
Comparison of DMR measurement to [³³P]-uptake assay in NaPi-IIb-CHO cells

Compound	[³³P]-uptake assay IC$_{50}$ (μM)	DMR measurement IC$_{50}$ (μM)
1	0.82 ± 0.28	0.44 ± 0.27
2	1.58 ± 0.25	0.81 ± 0.28
3	6.28 ± 0.86	2.05 ± 0.87
4	9.06 ± 3.24	4.61 ± 0.74
5	3.72 ± 1.39	3.50 ± 1.73
6	1.84 ± 0.54	2.58 ± 1.47
7	4.95 ± 1.47	6.31 ± 1.37

The seven compounds were tested in the [³³P]-uptake assay and Epic DMR measurement using the NaPi-IIb-CHO cells. Data are mean $\pm$ S.D. values of 3–5 separate determinations (reproduced from Ref. 10 with permission from SAGE Publications)

2. Prepare a 384-well compound plate containing 0.1 μL of various concentrations of the test compounds in DMSO for concentration-response determination (*see* **Notes 5** and **6**). Add 67 μL of assay buffer to the compound plate using an electric multichannel pipette. Using the LHA, perform eight mix cycles of 25 μL volume in the diluted compound plate to ensure complete mixing.

3. Aspirate the growth media from the NaPi-IIb-CHO cell plate 24 h after cell plating and perform two wash cycles of 50 μL of assay buffer using a plate washer. Leave a residual amount of assay buffer in the well since the aspirator height is offset from the bottom of the well to prevent disturbance of the cell monolayer.

4. Perform the two-step wash method on the LHA (*see* Section 3.2, steps 3 and 4).

5. Transfer 30 μL (two cycles of 15 μL) of test compounds from the diluted compound plate to the cell plate using the LHA and perform one mix cycle of 20 μL in the cell plate.

6. Equilibrate both the K-Pi plate and the cell plate containing test compounds in the Epic instrument at 26 °C for 1 h.

7. Measure the DMR baseline for 5 min and using the LHA, add 20 μL of K-Pi from the K-Pi plate. Perform two mix cycles of 20 μL in the cell plate. Continue to monitor DMR response for 65 min.

8. Plot the DMR response of K-Pi as a function of compound concentrations to determine the compound IC$_{50}$ value.

4   Notes

1. After NaPi-IIb-CHO cells were seeded in an Epic 384-well fibronectin-coated plate, the plate was incubated at room temperature in the laminar flow hood for 25 min before transfer to a 37 °C cell culture incubator. This practice minimizes plate edge effects and variations between inner and outer wells, thus improving the uniformity of cell confluence in all wells of the microplate and ensuring consistent DMR responses among different wells.

2. The wash procedure for the cells prior to equilibration in the Epic instrument was important for obtaining the largest DMR assay window for the NaPi-IIb-CHO cells described here. Performing the wash steps on a Biotek EL406 microplate washer dispenser in combination with the LHA of the Epic instrument allows the complete removal of residual Pi, which is present at high concentration in the growth media. This residual Pi can cause a higher background signal and hence a smaller assay window.

   The EL406 plate washer was used to remove the cell growth media. It was critical to add a large volume of assay buffer to dilute residual growth media remaining in the wells. In addition, the plate washer was used for this initial wash to avoid multiple pipetting steps with the LHA, which would have been necessary due to the limitation on the disposal pipette tip volume of 25 μL for the 384-channel manifold head. Employing a plate washer alone was insufficient because the aspirate cycle could not remove the cell growth media completely from the well. The dispense cycle simply adds buffer on top due to the small volume of the wells on the Epic microplate. A subsequent two-step wash method on the LHA ensured removal of residual growth media to minimize any carryover of the media from the first wash step on the LHA. Thus, employing both the plate washer and LHA achieved the largest assay window for NaPi-IIb-CHO DMR measurements.

   A comparison of the K-Pi-elicited DMR responses when the cells were washed with either the plate washer or the LHA alone is summarized in Fig. 5. Figure 5a shows results when only the plate washer was employed with six wash cycles of 40 μL each. A small DMR response was obtained, which could have been misinterpreted as a lack of response. Data generated from washing cells with only the LHA and the two-step wash method described in Section 3.2, steps 3 and 4, are represented in Fig. 5b. A relatively larger DMR response was generated in comparison to using the plate washer alone. A significantly larger assay window was generated for the NaPi-IIb-CHO cells when the plate washer was used in combination with the LHA as depicted in Fig. 3b and as reported earlier [10].

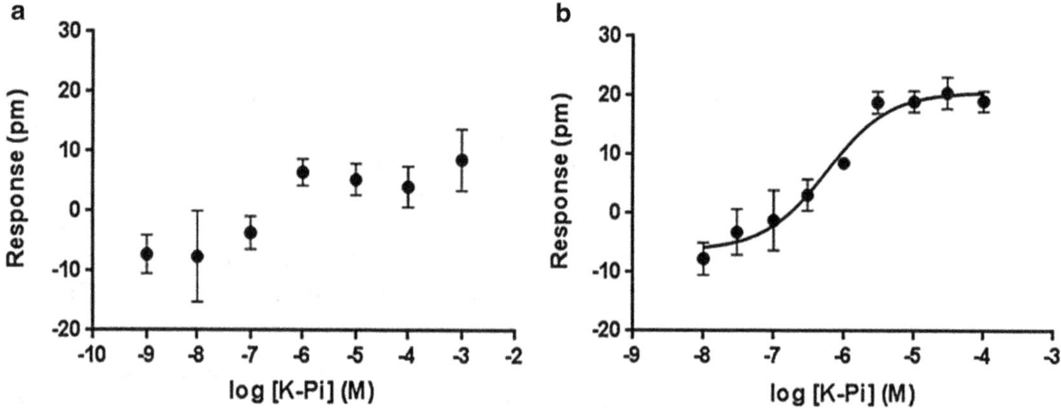

Fig. 5 Influence of wash procedure on potassium phosphate (K-Pi) (100 μM)-elicited dynamic mass redistribution response in NaPi-IIb-CHO cells. (**a**) Data generated when a plate washer alone was used for the wash procedure: six wash cycles of 40 μL assay buffer. (**b**) Data generated when only the LHA of the Epic instrument was employed with a two-step wash method. The two-step wash method consisted of the first step with one wash cycle of 25 μL using the LHA and then a change of the assay buffer in the reservoir and LHA tips. The second step had four additional wash cycles of 25 μL on the LHA. Data are mean ± S.D. values of four separate wells from a representative experiment

3. After aspiration of the assay buffer in the last wash cycle on the LHA, 10 μL of residual volume was left in the well at a tip aspiration height of 1.5 mm on the LHA (*see* Table 2). The final concentration of K-Pi in the cell plate takes into account of this 10 μL of residual buffer remaining in the well.

4. When the microplate containing intermediate concentrations of K-Pi was equilibrated at 26 °C for 1 h in the Epic instrument simultaneously with the cell plate, the variability in the DMR response was noticeably reduced for replicate wells. In addition, the reproducibility of the NaPi-IIb-CHO cell response was improved. Allowing the intermediate K-Pi plate to equilibrate to 26 °C may be particularly important when there is a large difference between the laboratory temperature and the interior chamber (26 °C) of the Epic instrument [2].

5. An intermediate 384-well microplate containing 30 μL of 1,333× concentrated test compounds at a range of concentrations in 100 % DMSO could be stored for a long term at −20 °C. This plate also includes wells which contain only DMSO as negative controls. If the intermediate plate has been stored at −20 °C, a sufficient amount of time must be allowed for the plate to reach room temperature and a brief low-speed centrifugation must be performed. The intermediate compound plate was then used to prepare the 384-well Echo qualified source plate by transferring 12 μL of compound to the Echo source plate using an automated liquid handler such as the Multimek-384. The Echo liquid handler is then used to

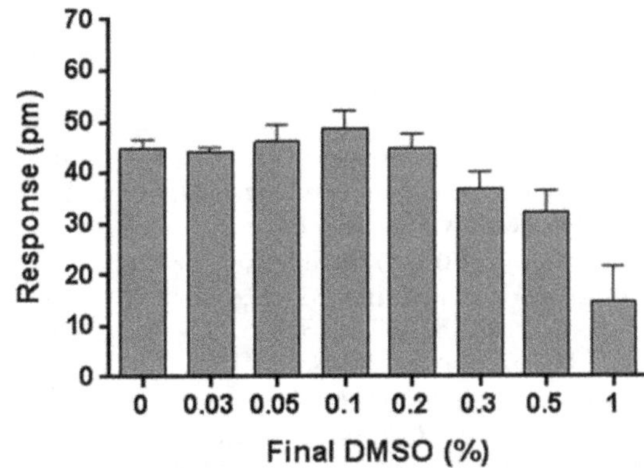

Fig. 6 Effects of DMSO on potassium phosphate (K-Pi)-elicited dynamic mass redistribution (DMR) responses in NaPi-IIb-CHO cells. Cells in different wells were equilibrated with various concentrations of DMSO for 1 h in the Epic instrument prior to baseline readings and then followed by the addition of K-Pi (100 μM). The final DMSO concentration in the well was 0–1 % as shown in the figure. Data are mean ± S.D. values of three separate wells from a representative experiment

transfer 0.1 μL of test compound from the Echo source plate to a standard daughter 384-well microplate. Due to the ultralow volume of the compounds and sensitivity of the DMR assay, the reproducibility of compound data on NaPi-IIb-CHO cells was significantly improved when these microplates containing 0.1 μL of compound were prepared fresh on the day of the assay. In addition, at least four replicate wells of each compound concentration were run on the same microplate.

6. The DMSO tolerance level of each individual cell line can vary considerably. The optimal final DMSO concentration needs to be determined for each cell line to achieve the largest DMR response without compromising the solubility of the test compounds. The DMSO tolerance of this NaPi-IIb-CHO cell line is summarized in Fig. 6. A final DMSO concentration of 0.1 % was used for the NaPi-IIb-CHO cells.

References

1. Williams JB, Mallorga PJ, Lemaire W, Williams DL, Na S, Patel S, Conn PJ, Pettibone DJ, Austin C, Sur C (2003) Development of a scintillation proximity assay for analysis of Na+/Cl–dependent neurotransmitter transporter activity. Anal Biochem 321:31–37. doi:10.1016/S0003-2697(03)00431-7

2. Fang Y (2006) Label-free cell-based assays with optical biosensors in drug discovery. Assay Drug Dev Technol 4:583–595. doi:10.1089/adt.2006.4.583

3. Fang Y, Ferrie AM, Li G (2006) Cellular functions of cholesterol probed with optical biosensors. Biochim Biophys Acta 1763:254–261. doi:10.1016/j.bbamcr.2006.01.006

4. Schafer DA (2002) Coupling actin dynamics and membrane dynamics during endocytosis. Curr Opin Cell Biol 14:76–81. doi:10.1016/S0955-0674(01)00297-6

5. Stamnes M (2002) Regulating the actin cytoskeleton during vesicular transport. Curr Opin Cell Biol 14:428–433. doi:10.1016/S0955-0674(02)00349-6

6. Janmey PA (1998) The cytoskeleton and cell signaling: component localization and mechanical coupling. Physiol Rev 78:763–781

7. Fang Y, Li G, Peng J (2005) Optical biosensor provides insights for bradykinin B2 receptor signaling in A431 cells. FEBS Lett 579:6365–6374. doi:10.1016/j.febslet.2005.10.019

8. Lee PH, Gao A, van Staden C, Ly J, Salon J, Xu A, Fang Y, Verkleeren R (2008) Evaluation of dynamic mass redistribution technology for pharmacological studies of recombinant and endogenously expressed G protein-coupled receptors. Assay Drug Dev Technol 6:83–94. doi:10.1089/adt.2007.126

9. Virkki LV, Biber J, Murer H, Forster IC (2007) Phosphate transporters: a tale of two solute carrier families. Am J Physiol Renal Physiol 293:F643–F654. doi:10.1152/ajprenal.00228.2007

10. Wong S-H, Gao A, Ward S, Henley C, Lee PH (2012) Development of a label-free assay for sodium-dependent phosphate transporter NaPi-IIb. J Biomol Screen 17:829–834. doi:10.1177/1087057112442961

11. Matsuo A, Negoro T, Seo T, Kitao Y, Shindo M, Segawa H, Miyamoto K (2005) Inhibitory effect of JTP-59557, a new triazole derivative, on intestinal phosphate transport *in vitro* and *in vivo*. Eur J Pharmacol 517:111–119. doi:10.1016/j.ejphar.2005.05.003

Chapter 16

Label-Free Impedance Measurements for Profiling Drug-Induced Cardiotoxicity

Filomain Nguemo, Judith Semmler, and Jürgen Hescheler

Abstract

Cardiotoxicity is an important cause for concern in drug development. In recent years a number of noncardiac drugs have been withdrawn from markets because of cardiotoxicity concerns, while some other drugs have either been withdrawn prior to marketing or required labeling changes that significantly restrict their use. The prediction of arrhythmic risk based on preclinical trials during drug development remains limited despite intensive and costly investigation. Moreover, drug testing using stem cell-derived cardiomyocytes requires a sophisticated platform of sensitive and cell compatible bioanalytical tools with sufficient and accurate recording capacity for key physiological and biochemical changes in the cells. The label-free impedance technology has emerged as a leading platform for detecting spontaneous beating activities of cardiomyocyte. Impedance based assays provide an exceptionally diverse pattern of functional end points, each with the robustness characteristics required to support drug development process and screening. This chapter reviews the techniques for measuring the impact of pharmacologic compounds on the beating rate of pluripotent stem cell-derived cardiomyocytes with cellular impedance systems.

Key words Cardiomyocytes, Cardiotoxicity, Drugs, Electrophysiology, Label-free impedance, Stem cells

---

1 Introduction

Despite considerable progress in the last decade, safety assessment remains a crucial step in drug development. A significant number of drugs have been withdrawn from the market due to their adverse effects (e.g., cardiotoxicity), while for many other drugs safety labels have been revised to state adequate warning about their potential cardiac side effects. It has been mandated by regulatory authorities that all lead drug candidates should be subjected to a series of stringent screens to identify and rectify potential adverse cardiac side effects before drugs enter into clinical trials and are ultimately placed on the market [1–4]. In cardiac treatment a special liability lies in the occurrence of cardiotoxicity, arrhythmia, or dysfunction. Many drugs can induce heart dysfunction by a variety of mechanisms from direct cardiomyocytes injury to the alteration

Ye Fang (ed.), *Label-Free Biosensor Methods in Drug Discovery*, Methods in Pharmacology and Toxicology,
DOI 10.1007/978-1-4939-2617-6_16, © Springer Science+Business Media New York 2015

of biochemical and biophysical processes (e.g., disturbances in the well-coordinated electrical pathways that control the heart's rhythmic contractions) [5, 6].

Ion channels are present in the cell membrane of all cells and regulate ionic passage across the membrane. The flux of ions such as Ca^{2+}, K^+, and Na^+ into and out of the cell generates electrical charges which, in turn, stimulate and coordinate cardiomyocyte (CM) contractions. Alteration of these ion pathways may lead to heart dysfunction. For example, in most of the cases cardiotoxicity arises when the compound interacts with ion channels or transporters to increase the risk for developing arrhythmias such as life-threatening Torsade de pointes (TdP) [7]. The molecular mechanisms resulting in TdP are still not fully understood; but, the concerning delayed ventricular repolarization and prolongation of the QT interval that gives rise to early afterdepolarizations (EADs) triggering TdP is well accepted [8–10]. An assessment of drug-induced QT interval prolongation risk is one of the main aspects of preclinical drug evaluation [11]. In humans, the ion channel playing the most important responsibility in the repolarization phase of an action potential (AP) is the ether-á-go-go-related gene (hERG) channel, transporting the rapidly activated delayed rectifier potassium current IKr. In case of QT prolongation, this ion current is inhibited [4, 12]. However, the hERG channel interaction alone is not predictive of ventricular arrhythmia, given that there are some drugs that block the hERG channels but do not cause arrhythmia, and there are some other drugs that cause arrhythmia but do not block the hERG channel, like verapamil [4, 13]. Besides hERG, other ion channels are also known to play critical roles in physiology and diseases. Indeed, ion channels represent the second largest class of drug targets after G-protein coupled receptors [14].

In the last decades, several systems have been implemented to assess the effect of compounds on the cardiac system. Some have been adapted for high-throughput screening (HTS), whereas others are further in implementation phase into HTS. Microelectronics-based monitoring of cells using impedance has been intensively described [15, 16]. The key features of this approach are the non-invasive readout and the possibility to sample cellular responses to drug treatments continually for a long time [17]. Recently ACEA Biosciences (San Diego, USA) developed a system called "xCELLigence RTCA Cardio System" which allows for continuous monitoring the activity of CMs based on impedance measurement. The assay is performed using specially designed microtiter plates that are integrated with gold microelectrodes [1]. The concept of investigating cardiac contractility based on impedance measurement as an in vitro real-time system realizes a provision of important information about compound action. During such investigations the respective chemical compound influences the expression and development of a protein of interest in different manners.

Numerous factors play important roles in such an experimental setup, like the expression level of the protein, the effective concentration, as well as the dwell time of the drug. A morphologic and kinetic profiling approach for the long-term monitoring of cell response allows for a multidimensional investigation of drug action. The xCELLigence RTCA system has been validated using both pluripotent stem cell-derived CMs and primary CMs and is able to sensitively and quantitatively detect the effect of drugs on cardiac function in real time [2]. These capabilities are extended with a more specialized system which allows for functional monitoring of the manufacturing process and label-free assessment of the physiological status of beating CMs as well as the detection of both short- and long-term responses to compound exposure.

The creation of induced pluripotent stem (iPS) cells from adult somatic cells opened an important new approach not only for basic research but also for regenerative medicine, disease modeling, and toxicology. Several recent studies have reported the generation and differentiation of iPS cell-derived cardiomyocytes (iPS-CMs) from different sources and species [18–21]. Studying the beating activity of spontaneously active iPS-CMs can provide considerable information on the effects of compounds on the cardiovascular system. The use of iPS-CMs has a potential to improve the confidence in the predictive value of tests and considerably reduces the number of animal experiments for toxicological testing [22, 23]. However, drug testing using iPS-CMs requires a sophisticated platform of sensitive and cell compatible bioanalytical tools such as xCELLigence RTCA cardio with sufficient and accurate recording capacity for key physiological and biochemical changes in the cells.

In this chapter, taking into consideration the sensitivity, predictivity, real-time data acquisition, measurement of periodicity of beating over both short and prolonged time windows in 96-well format of the xCELLigence RTCA system, we describe the utility of this system for early cardiotoxicity assessment of compounds using pluripotent stem cells and neonatal-derived CMs.

2   Materials

1. *xCELLigence Real-Time Cell Analysis (RTCA) Cardio Instrument (ACEA Biosciences, San Diego, USA)*. This system is developed by ACEA Biosciences and Roche Diagnostics (Penzberg, Germany) [1, 2] and used to measure cell viability as well as the electrical activities of any spontaneous beating cells such as stem cell-derived CMs from mouse and human origin (Fig. 1). This system can be utilized to record the short- and long-term effect of various compounds on CMs. It consists of four key components (Fig. 1a): (1) RTCA Cardio Station that holds one E-plate, is placed inside a humidified CO_2

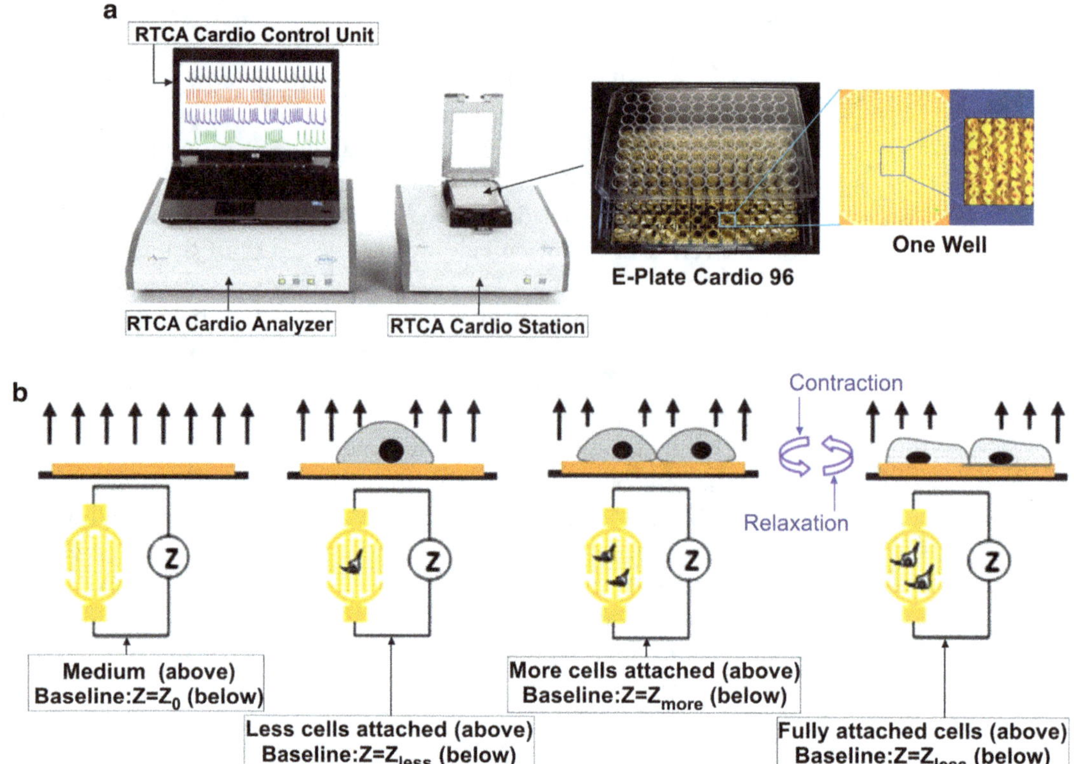

Fig. 1 Components and detection principle of the xCELLigence system. (**a**) The impedance signal Z is generated by application of the AC signal, which creates an ion current between the electrodes. The interaction of cells with the electrodes blocks the current and generates the impedance signal Z, which is proportional to the number of cells covering the electrode and the morphologic and adhesive characteristics of cells. In the form of the cell index, the impedance signal represents the ratio of a change in impedance to the background impedance. (**b**) The beating signal is based on the rhythmic changes of cardiomyocyte attachment and morphology due to contraction and relaxation of the cells, which induces the fluctuation of the impedance signal. Adapted with permission from website of ACEA Bioscience Inc

incubator and connected to the Cardio Analyzer via ribbon cable; (2) RTCA Control Unit that performs the software and collects and displays the data; (3) RTCA Analyzer that is an interface outside the incubator used to receive and send the electronic signals between the control unit and the station; and (4) E-Plate Cardio 96-well. This system uses impedance readout to noninvasively quantify cardiomyocyte status in real time (Fig. 1b). The presence of the cells on top of the electrodes will affect the local ionic environment at the electrode/solution interface, leading to an increase in the electrode impedance. Impedance measurements use weak alternating current (AC) between the electrodes with tissue culture medium as the electrolyte. The electronic hardware monitors the voltage across the electrodes, and the impedance is calculated using the AC version of Ohm's law where impedance (Z) rather than simple resistance (R) is calculated as $Z = V/I$ [26]. Thus, this system measures impedance signals, processes and calculates the data by converting the impedance into a cell index (CI) value, an arbitrary unit which is the ratio of the well impedance change $Z_X - Z_0$ to the well background impedance Z_0: $(Z_X - Z_0)/Z_0$. The CI value is affected by multiple factors such as cell growth, proliferation, cell–cell contact, and cell–substrate adhesion. Therefore, it can be used to reflect cell viability, number, morphology, and adhesion degree in the cell-based impedance assay and allows high temporal resolution for recording spontaneous beating activities of cells such as cardiomyocytes [25, 26]. As impedance measurement is noninvasive, the millisecond data acquisition rate can be combined with longer-term monitoring to study both the short-term and long-term effects of compounds on cardiomyocytes [26].

2. *E-plate Cardio 96 wells (ACEA Biosciences)*. This plate is a specially designed 96-well microtiter plate with integrated gold microelectrode arrays in the bottom of each well. The bottom diameter of each well is 5.0 mm ± 0.05 mm, with a total volume of 243 µl ± 5 µl. The plate is designed to be used in an environment of +15 °C to +40 °C, relative humidity 98 % maximum without condensation.

3. *Cardiomyocytes (Center for Physiology and Pathophysiology, University of Cologne)*. Cardiac differentiation of transgenic iPS cells was performed in spinner flasks as previously and prepared as described [2].

4. *Chemicals and media*. Basic culture media were purchased from Gibco/Invitrogen (GIBGO, Invitrogen GmbH, Karlsruhe, Germany); supplements and chemicals were from Sigma (Sigma-Aldrich Chemie GmbH, Steinheim, Germany), unless otherwise specified.

5. Fibronectin used was from Sigma (Sigma-Aldrich, St. Louis, MO, USA).

---

3 Methods

3.1 Preparation of Cell Model Systems

One of the main challenges in preclinical cardio-safety assessment has been the lack of a predictive and biologically relevant model system available in sufficient quantity and purity for cardiotoxicity testing in a high-throughput platform [1]. Although primary cardiomyocytes from mouse, rat, chick, rabbit, and human systems can be used, technical difficulties in obtaining high numbers of pure cardiomyocytes has been an obstacle to wider adoption. Functional cardiomyocytes can now be derived routinely from human origin using embryonic and induced pluripotent stem cells.

This technology presents a new opportunity to develop physiologically and pharmacologically relevant in vitro screens for the detection of cardiotoxicity, with a view to improve patient safety while reducing the economic burden to industry arising from high drug attrition rates.

Significant efforts have been invested in both academic institutions and companies concerning embryonic and induced pluripotent stem cells of human origin. The intention is to devise optimal maintenance and differentiation protocols that deliver large quantities of well-characterized, stable, and reproducible cell lineages, which express the important phenotypic properties and functions found in vivo. Different cardiomyocytes of high purity have been used for the assessment of drug-induced cardiotoxicity using xCELLigence RTCA system (Table 1). The most common cardiomyocytes used in RTCA system are: primary CMs that are freshly harvested following the standard protocols as described previously [26, 30, 31]; differentiated and purified CMs from murine ES/iPS cells [2, 28, 29]; and high purity cryopreserved CMs such as Cor.At™ (Axiogenesis, Cologne Germany) and iCells™ (Cellular Dynamics Int., Madison, WI, USA) that are commercially available [37].

Cardiomyocytes obtained should be handled according to the User's Guide of the respective supplier. Figure 2 illustrates the general workflow of a typical xCELLigence RTCA cardio measurement (*see* **Note 1**).

3.1.1 Preparation of the E-Plate Cardio-96 and Background Measurement

Many proteins of the extracellular matrix (ECM) interact with cells via cell surface receptors. The resulting focal contacts are important for the maintenance of tissue architecture and for supporting a variety of cellular processes. ECM protein binding initiates a complex network of signal transduction cascades that, depending on the context, plays an important role in cell spreading, migration,

Table 1
Cardiomyocytes used in xCELLigence RTCA system

Cell type (species)	Origin	Purity	Cells/well	References
iPSC CMs (mouse)	University of Cologne, Germany	~99 %	$15\text{–}20 \times 10^3$ cells/well	[2, 27]
ESC CMs (mouse)	Cor.At™; Axiogenesis, Cologne, Germany	100 %	$30\text{–}70 \times 10^3$ cells/well	[1, 28, 29]
neonatal primary CMs (rat)	Molecular Toxicology/Safety Pharmacology, Waltham, Massachusetts	~100 %	$15 \times 10^3\text{–}3 \times 10^4$ cells/well	[26, 31, 40]
iPSC CMs (human)	iCells™; Cellular Dynamics Int. (CDI), Madison, WI, USA	Highly purity	$40 \times 10^3\text{–}2 \times 10^6$ cells/well	[1, 28, 29, 32–36]

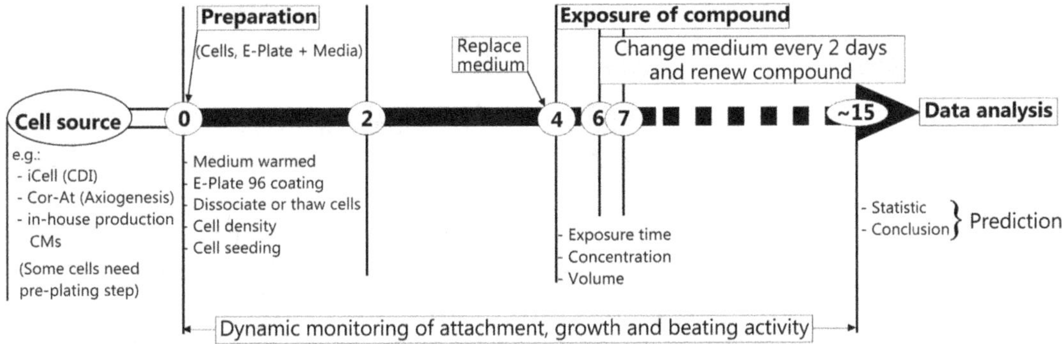

Fig. 2 Work flow for preparing, culturing, growing, and recording beating of cardiomyocytes using the xCEL-Ligence RTCA Cardio System. On day 0 cardiomyocytes are dissociated from clusters or thawed and plated onto an E-Plate 96-well previously coated with fibronectin. On days 2, 4, and 6 post-plating, medium is changed. Depending to the cell types, after day 4, 5, 6, or 7 post-plating, a clear and regular/stable rhythmic beating pattern can be recorded, allowing compound treatment

proliferation, and functional activity. Thus, it is important to choose the right substrates for appropriate cell culture on biosensor plates.

The E-Plate is generally prepared at the same day of cardiomyocytes plating.

1. Dilute 1 mg/ml fibronectin solution in sterile phosphate buffered saline (PBS) without Ca^{2+} and Mg^{2+} to a final concentration of 10 μg/ml (*see* **Note 2**).

2. Transfer 50 μL of the diluted fibronectin solution into each well of the E-Plate Cardio 96 (*see* **Note 3**).

3. Place the freshly coated E-Plate Cardio 96 into the 37 °C incubator for 3 h or overnight at 2–4 °C.

4. Carefully aspirate the fibronectin coating solution and fill up with 150 μl of culture medium.

5. Incubate the prepared E-Plate for 10–20 min at 37 °C (*see* **Note 4**).

6. Place the E-Plate Cardio 96 containing only 180 μl culture medium on the RTCA Cardio Station inside the CO_2 incubator.

7. Record the background impedance according to the RTCA Cardio Instrument Operator's Guide.

3.1.2 Plating Procedure of Cardiomyocytes onto the E-Plate

The thawing and plating procedures are stressful to frozen cells, therefore using a good technique and working quickly ensures that a high proportion of the cells survive the procedure. For any cell culture procedures, one needs to closely follow the instructions provided with the cells and other reagents for best results.

1. Prepare/dissociate the cells or remove the frozen vial containing the cardiomyocytes from storage place (generally –80 °C or liquid N_2).

2. Thaw the cells or resuspend the cells in the new tube according to the User's Guide or protocol and count the cells using hemocytometer (*see* **Note 5**).

3. Dilute the cell suspension in Plating Medium at a final concentration as indicated in the User's Guide to obtain the correct cell plating density.

4. Transfer the E-plate Cardio 96 from the incubator into the laminar hood and aspirate the culture medium from each well (*see* **Note 6**).

5. Add immediately 150–180 μL of medium containing appropriate number of cells to each labeled well of the E-plate Cardio 96 using a multichannel pipette (*see* **Note 7**).

6. Leave the E-Plate undisturbed in the laminar hood at room temperature to allow the cardiomyocytes to settle and ensure an equal distribution.

7. After at least 30 min, transfer and place the E-Plate 96 into the RTCA Cardio Station inside the CO_2 incubator.

8. Start directly the measurement (*see* **Note 8**).

3.1.3 Medium Change and Compound Addition

The culture medium provides the necessary nutrients, growth factors, and hormones for cell growth, the pH and regulates and the osmotic pressure of the culture. During culture, nutrients become depleted and metabolic products increase in concentration. The latter may be toxic to the cells. How frequently the medium need to be changed depends on the cell line and the type of medium. Therefore, for optimal experimental reproducibility, the cells should be grown for a standard number of days after being plated on E-Plate 96. Medium changes and compound treatment should be performed as indicated below.

1. Perform the medium change every 2 days. From each well of the E-Plate, carefully exchange 75–90 μL of culture medium with fresh pre-warmed culture medium by applying a multichannel pipette to the side of the well to avoid disturbing the cardiomyocyte monolayer behavior.

2. Monitor the activity of the cardiomyocytes on the E-Plate to ensure regular beating rate, beating amplitude, similar and regular beating rhythm pattern.

3. Prepare test compounds by dissolving the compound stock solutions in culture medium at 2× the final concentration in a regular 96-well cell culture plate (*see* **Note 9**).

4. Design the experimental layout and program the steps for compound measurement as described in RTCA software manual (*see* **Note 10**)

5. Immediately before the addition of the compounds, perform the baseline measurement of the E-plate. This baseline value will be used to normalize the effects of compound in each well.

6. Pause the RTCA Cardio Instrument, disengage the E-Plate Cardio 96 from the RTCA Cardio Station, and transfer it to the laminar flow hood.

7. To add the compound, remove 75–90 μL of the culture medium from the top of each well and, following the layout labeled, replace it with 75–90 μL of the respective double-concentrated stock solution.

8. Take the E-Plate 96 back into the RTCA Cardio Station inside the CO_2 incubator immediately and go on with the measurement by clicking the Start/Continue button.

9. Change medium and renew compound as described above every 2 days (*see* **Note 11**).

10. At the end of compound exposure time, perform a washout step (*see* **Note 12**). This step consists of: (1) warm indicated culture medium without compounds to 37 °C; (2) pause the RTCA Cardio Instrument and disengage the E-Plate Cardio 96 from the RTCA Cardio Station; (3) after transferring the E-Plate 96 to the laminar flow hood, gently remove 75–90 μL of the compound solution from every well using a multichannel pipette; (4) immediately add 75–90 μL of fresh medium to each well using a multichannel pipette ; (5) return the E-Plate Cardio 96 back into the Cardio Station as quickly as possible and resume the measurement for additional 24–48 h.

3.2 Impedance Data Acquisition and Analysis

The xCELLigence RTCA Cardio Instrument Software offers a wide variety of options for data acquisition and analysis. The instructions provided here are collected from different publications and meant to serve as a general guideline. For specific instructions, see the RTCA Cardio Instrument Operator's Guide. Data analysis can be conducted during every sweep and generally deals with the following parameters: contraction amplitude, beating rate, and beating rhythm as described in RTCA Cardio Instrument Software Guide, Version Sept 2010 and by Xi et al. [1]. Brief changes in the beating rate of CMs are quantified based on beating cycle and appearance of the abnormal or irregular beat (IB) rhythm [16, 34, 37]. The RTCA software allows for real-time recording and display of beating activity across the entire 96 wells of the Cardio Plate. In theory, each beating signal corresponds to one excitation–contraction coupling of the CMs. The beating profiles contain information about transmembrane currents and action potential (AP) properties and are composed of multiple parameters [1]. The contribution of individual transmembrane currents to the AP and their change could be distinguished in the single beating signal waveform, from which parameters can be used to characterize functional differences in different conditions [36]. All parameters are calculated for every beating within one recording period and the average and standard deviation are derived correspondingly.

To determine the effect of any compounds, data of parameters such as beating rate and amplitude after treatment are normalized to the same time point in control condition (that is, no treatment). To evaluate the degree of arrhythmia, the beating rhythm irregularity index is derived based on the coefficient of variation (that is, standard deviation divided by average) of the beating period during a record period. It is also possible to evaluate beat-to-beat variability under between control conditions and under treatment [1].

4   Results

4.1   Cell Index (CI)

The RTCA Cardio System records relative changes in impedance signals, resulting from the application of a low voltage signal that induces a current between the interdigitated electrodes of the E-plate. A change in the electrical impedance results from alterations in the current, which is impeded by the cells spreading out on the bottom of the wells [16]. This system processes and displays the data by converting the impedance value into an arbitrary unit, the Cell Index (CI) value [1, 28]. It is influenced by a complex mixture of factors like the cell growth, the proliferation, cell–cell interactions, and adhesion. Thereby, it enables the reflection of the cell number, morphology, viability, adhesion, and beating activity [17, 24, 26]. The CMs grow in the well under fresh medium condition during the whole experiment. Thereby, the CI of an initially low mouse iPS-CMs density (5,000 cells/well) increases continuously, whereas the CI of a high density (15,000 and 20,000 cells/well) increases and reaches its maximum approximately 24 h after plating, thereafter remains unchanged during 200 h (Fig. 3a), suggesting the early optimal saturation period with high cell density culture [2].

The duration till reaching a steady-state level that is indicative of rhythmic beating varies dependent on the cell type. While the human iCell™-derived CMs spread out slowly and require about 6 days, the mouse Cor.At™-CMs spread out faster reaching a steady-state level for the overall CI after 36–48 h. Spontaneous rhythmic changes of the CI become detectable at ≥24 h after plating in both cell types [24].

Medium exchange 12 and 24 h after cell seeding significantly influences the CI negatively (Fig. 3b), suggesting a medium

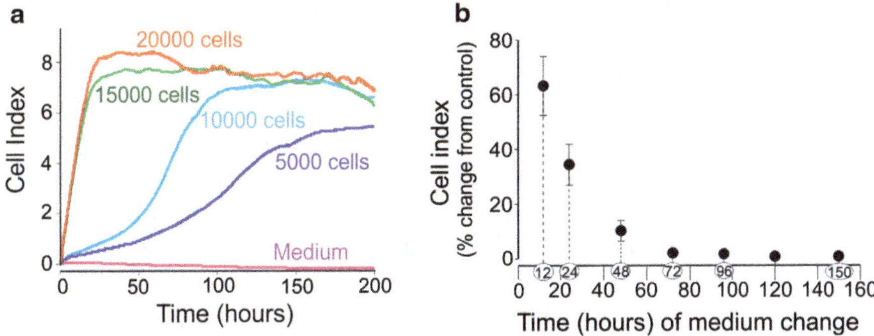

Fig. 3 Dynamic monitoring of the correlation between cardiomyocyte density and cell index (CI) using the xCELLigence RTCA Cardio system. (**a**) Cardiomyocytes at a density of 0 (cell culture medium), 5,000, 10,000, 15,000, and 20,000 cells/well were observed during 200 h. (**b**) Effect of medium change on Cell Index (CI) of CMs at the density of 15,000 cell/well. In control condition, medium was not changed. Values are presented as mean ± SEM of at least 8 wells from three independent experiments

change after 48 h to maintain iPS-CMs in optimal condition for attachment [2]. Impedance measurements can be performed at selected time points. Guo et al. [34] identified the origin of arrhythmic beats by comparing the waveforms and pattern, the CI values, and onset time associated with beating rate changes between cardiac ion channel modulators and compounds that cause structural cardiotoxicity or general cytotoxicity. They determined the arrhythmic beats to occur concurrently with substantial CI reduction and often to be followed by transient tachycardia/fibrillation-like pattern and an irreversible arrest of beating [35]. Thus, it was reasonable to define a threshold for the CI value. A loss of ≥10 % was identified as the threshold capable of delineating "false" cytotoxicity-induced arrhythmic beats from arrhythmia caused primarily by cardiac ion channel modulation [35].

4.2 Beating Rate

One of the main features of the RTCA Cardio System is the fast data acquisition rate, 12.9 ms for entire 96-well Cardio Plate, which allows for monitoring CM beating cycles with high temporal resolution [16]. By measurement of the impedance signal which is precisely and rhythmically interrupted by contraction and relaxation processes of spontaneously beating CMs, this system does not provide detailed electrophysiological readouts and mechanistic insight on the single cell level or on cell clusters. Instead, it offers a relevant physiological readout of CM contraction on interconnected CMs in a thin layer. Moreover, this system can measure in vitro synchronized CM beating for an extended period of time at a remarkable steady performance, thus representing a viable model for the study of chronotropy and ultimately arrhythmia, once optimized. The system is able to detect even small changes in beating frequency in the presence of any activating or inhibiting agents of the cell contraction. Irregular beating or complete disappearance of beating as a result of compound addition indicates arrhythmias and cardiotoxicity [29].

For identification of the optimal cell density for analysis of the beating frequency and amplitude of confluent cultures at different time points, different cell concentrations have been tested. Within the first 120 h after plating miPS-CMs at low concentrations (5,000 cells/well), a regular and stable beating signal could not be detected, but the signal appeared later and consistently increased over time. However, with high miPS-CMs seeding density (20,000 cells/well) consistent and synchronized beating signal was observed already 60 h post-plating and remained stable thereafter. After seeding miPS-CMs at 15,000 and 20,000 cells/well the maximum beating rate and amplitude were observed approximately 72 h later as compared to cells seeded at low density (5,000 and 10,000 cells/well), which exhibited irregular and unsynchronized beating signals. Thus, the appearance of reproducible contraction signals mainly depends on the cell density (Fig. 4) [2].

4.3 Compound Effects

Several recent presentations of electrophysiological and pharmacological results on cardiomyocytes have been conducted for a large amount of different classes of cardioactive or references compounds using the xCELLigence RTCA Cardio System as screening model by different groups (Table 2), with the aim to:

1. Test varying doses and durations (short- and long-term) of compound exposure.

2. Investigate the compound effects on the cardiomyocytes beating frequency (inhibition or stimulation).

3. Determine different compound effects (e.g., initiation of arrhythmia, loss of ionic homeostasis).

4. Find a model that is capable of incrementally improving the ability to assess in vitro drug's arrhythmogenic potential.

Individual contraction curves and the overall CI measured by the xCELLigence unit provide important information regarding the effect of a given compound on the beating signal of the CMs with respect to the concentration and time of exposure. For example treatment of miPS cell-derived CMs with isoproterenol, a β-adrenergic receptor agonist, increased the beating frequency in a dose- and time-dependent manner (Fig. 5).

The nondestructive impedance measurements thereby offer a proper tool to uncover previously unappreciated safety aspects for a given molecule. For confirmation of the synchronous oscillations of impedance over time being attributed to the physical movement of the CMs during contraction, the addition of blebbistatin (a widely used inhibitor of myosin heavy chain ATPase activity) completely abolished the contractility of CM monolayers.

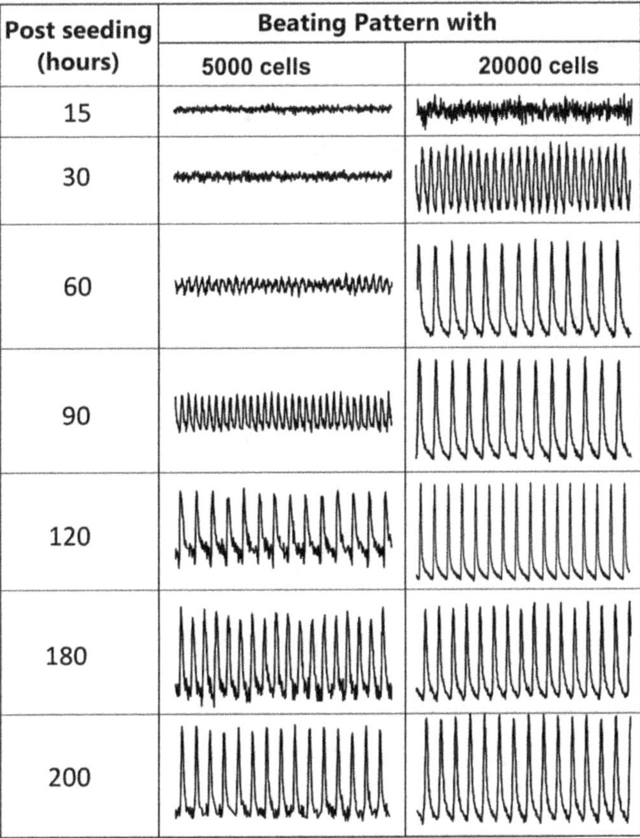

Fig. 4 Beating activity profile of mouse iPS cell-derived CMs at a density of 5,000 and 20,000 cells/well recorded by the RTCA Cardio Instrument at the indicated time points after cell seeding. Duration of 5 s of recording time is shown (Adapted from [2])

This could be detected by measurement of the impedance, and was restored by washing out the compound. Under the same conditions, no effects on field potential morphology recorded with MEAs (Fig. 6) or on AP signals of single iPS-derived CMs recorded via the conventional current-clamp technique were observed [2]. Thus, impedance measurements reflect the physical movement of the confluent monolayer of iPS-CMs and impedance is a property that is distinct from electrical field potential.

Exposure of the CMs to different classes of cardioactive compounds can have different effects, dependent on the modulator type. Modulators of ion channels and receptors often generate rapid changes in the beating rate and amplitude causing arrhythmic beats shortly after compound application. Pure structural cardiotoxicants, on the other hand, induce a delayed onset of beating rate and/or amplitude changes whereas the structural toxicants which exhibit acute effects on ion channels and receptors induce a rapid effect on beating rate and amplitude [37, 38].

Table 2
Reference compounds tested in xCELLigence RTCA Cardio System for their activities on cardiomyocytes

Compound	Mode of action	Cell line	Concentration	Effect on CMs	References
Amlodipine	L-type Ca^{2+} channel blocker	Cor.At™, iCells™	0.09–0.36 µM	Increase in BR	[29]
As_2O_3	hERG channel inhibitor	Cor.At™	1–30 µM	Dose-dependent decrease in CA and BR	[28]
ATX-II	Delays inactivation of Na^+ channels	Cor.At™, iCells™	1–100 nM	Dose-dependent decrease in BR (human), decrease in CA (mouse)	[28]
Bay K8644	Ca^{2+} channel agonist	Neonatal primary CMs (rat)	0.01–10 µM	Increase in BR, decrease in CA	[31]
Blebbistatin	Excitation–contraction uncoupler	miPSCs (TiB7.4)	10 µM	Inhibits BR	[2, 34]
Carbachol (Cch)	Cholinergic agonist	miPSCs (TiB7.4), Cor.At™, iCells™, neonatal primary CMs (rat)	0.01–10.84 µM	Decrease in BR	[2, 31, 35]
Crizotinib	Tyrosine kinase inhibitor	iCells™	10 nM–10 µM	Induces beating irregularities, decreases BR	[32]
Dimethyl sulfoxide (DMSO)	Solvent, vehicle	Cor.At™, iCells™	0.03–3 %	Dose-dependent increase in BR and decrease CA (human), unchanged BR and decreased CA (mouse)	[28, 29]
Dobutamine	β-adrenergic agonist	Neonatal primary CMs (rat)	0.01–10 µM	Increase in BR, decrease in CA	[31]
Dofetilide	hERG channel inhibitor	Cor.At™, iCells™	3–300 nM	Dose-dependent increase of BR, decrease of CA	[28]

(continued)

Table 2
(continued)

Compound	Mode of action	Cell line	Concentration	Effect on CMs	References
Doxorubicin (Doxo)	intercalates DNA	miPSCs (TiB7.4), iCells™	0.1–10 μM	Dose-dependent decrease of BR and CA 24 h pretreatment with NRG (100 ng/ml) attenuated effect of 1 μM Doxo 24 h pretreatment with 1 μM trastuzumab potentiated effect of Doxo	[2, 33]
E4031	hERG channel inhibitor	Cor.At™, iCells™	3–360 nM	Dose-dependent decrease of BR and CA	[1, 28, 29, 34, 35]
Flecainide	Lass Ic antiarrhythmic agent	Neonatal primary CMs (rat)	1.56–50 μM	Dose-dependent decrease of BR	[26]
Heptanol	Reversible inhibitor of cell-to-cell coupling	miPSCs (TiB7.4)	0.5 μM	Inhibits impedance signals, no influence on AP frequency	[2]
HMR1556	KvLQT1 K$^+$ channel blocker	Cor.At™, iCells™	0.01–1 μM	No effect on contraction parameters	[28]
Isoproterenol (Iso)	β-Adrenergic agonist	miPSCs (TiB7.4), neonatal primary CMs (rat)	0.01–10 μM	Increase in BR, decrease in CA	[2, 29, 31]
Isradapine	Voltage-gated calcium-channel inhibitor	Cor.At™	40 nM	Decrease in BR and CA	[1]
Jaspamide	Blocks several ion channels (e.g., Kv1.5, Cav1.2, Cav3.2, HCN2)	iCells™	30 nM–30 μM	Increase in BR at ≥0.3 μM (1 h) Increase in BR at 1–3 μM (6 h) Decrease in BR at 10–30 μM (6 h) Dose-dependent Decrease in BR, no BR at ≥3 μM (>6 h)	[36]

(continued)

Table 2
(continued)

Compound	Mode of action	Cell line	Concentration	Effect on CMs	References
Mibefradil	T-type Ca^{2+} channel blocker	Cor.At™, iCells™	0.09–0.36 μM	No effect on contraction parameters (human), decrease in BR (mouse)	[29]
Mitoxantrone	Structural cardiotoxicant	iCells™	0.03–30 μM	Decrease in BR at 30 μM (1 h) Decrease in BR at 10–30 μM (6 h) Increase in BR at 0.1–0.3 μM (≥24 h) Decrease in BR, no BR at ≥3 μM (≥24 h)	[36]
Nifedipine	L-type Ca^{2+} channel blocker	Cor.At™	0.03–3 μM	Dose-dependent inhibition of BR and CA	[28]
Nilotinib	Tyrosine kinase inhibitor	iCells™	10nM–10 μM	Induces beating irregularities, decreases BR	[32]
Ouabain	Blocks the Na$^+$/K$^+$-ATPase and elevates intracellular Na$^+$ and Ca^{2+}	Cor.At™, iCells™	0.03–3 μM	Increases BR and CA (human), no effect on contraction parameters (mouse)	[28]
Pentamidine	hERG channel inhibitor	Cor.At™, iCells™	0.3–30 μM	Dose-dependent increase/variations in BR and decrease CA (human), decreased BR and increased CA (mouse)	[28]
Ranolazine	hERG channel inhibitor				
Sotalol	Class III antiarrhythmic agent	miPSCs (TiB7.4)	0.01–10 μM	Induces beating irregularities	[2]
Sunitinib	Tyrosine kinase inhibitor, hERG channel inhibitor	iCells™	10 nM–10 μM	Induces beating irregularities, decreases BR	[32]

(continued)

Table 2
(continued)

Compound	Mode of action	Cell line	Concentration	Effect on CMs	References
Terfenadine	Nonsedating antihistamine drug, blocks multiple cardiac ion channels (hERG, Na$^+$, and Ca^{2+})	miPSCs (TiB7.4)	0.01–10 μM	Dose-dependent reversible inhibition of BR	[2, 34]
Tetrodotoxin (TTX)	Selective Na$^+$ channel blocker	Cor.At™, iCells™, neonatal primary CMs (rat)	0.01–30 μM	Complete reduction of BR and CA (human), no effect on contraction parameters (mouse), decrease in BR (rat)	[1, 28, 31]
Verapamil	L-type Ca^{2+} channel blocker, hERG channel inhibitor	Neonatal primary CMs (rat), Cor.At™, iCells™	0.065–10 μM	Dose-dependent inhibition of BR and CA	[26, 28]
Zatebradine	Pacemaker channel blocker	Cor.At™, iCells™	1.11–4.34 μM	Decrease in BR, induces beating irregularities	[29]

AP action potential, *BR* beating rate, *CA* contraction amplitude, *CI* Cell index

In addition, numerous compounds inhibit the hERG K+ channel assembly or prolong the QT interval, but do not clinically induce TdP. Arrhythmogenic drugs such as ranolazine, alfuzosin, verapamil, moxifloxacin, pentamidine, As$_2$O$_3$, or geldanamycin decrease the hERG channel function and consequently display delayed onset of beating rate reduction and lengthened repolarization-mediated arrhythmic beats. However, acute effects on cardiac ion channels do not arise [35, 39]. The inhibition of other ion channels (e.g., the plasma membrane Na$^+$/K$^+$-ATPase) with compounds like ouabain, digoxin, and digitoxin induced arrhythmia by producing an acute effect on CMs followed by a delayed effect due to blocking hERG protein trafficking [23, 40].

The response of mouse and human stem cell-derived CMs to cardioactive drugs have been shown to differ from each other and these responses also vary in comparison to already established in vitro and in vivo models. For example, applying the selective hERG channel blockers E-4031 and dofetilide on mouse and human iPSC-derived CMs, a decrease in the contraction amplitude and an

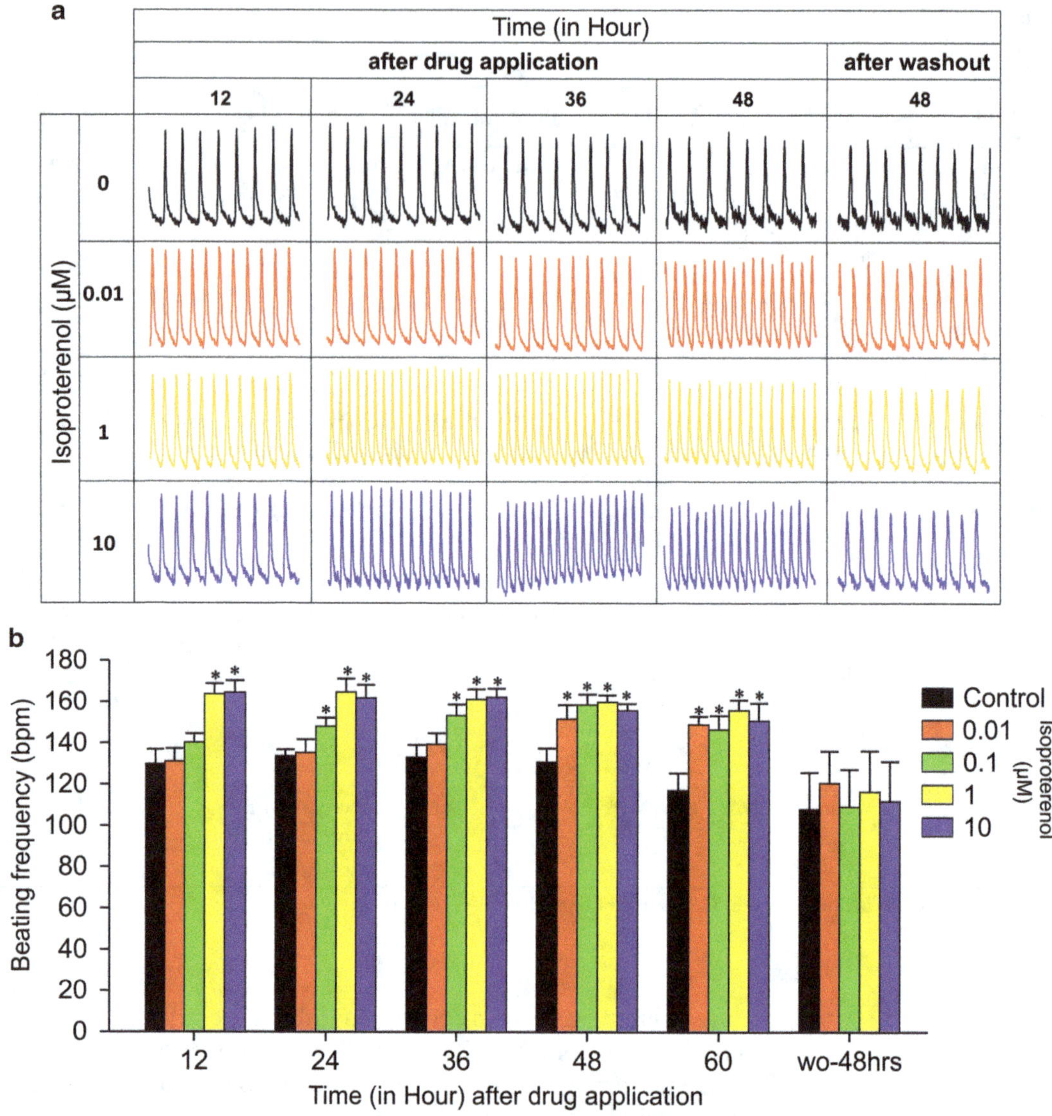

Fig. 5 Concentration and time dependent effect of Isoproterenol on beating frequency (bpm, beats per minute) of mouse iPS cell-derived cardiomyocytes. Values are presented as mean ± SEM of at least 6 wells from three independent experiments

increase in the beating rate were detected, with more pronounced effect on mouse cells [28]. On the other hand, E-4031 caused arrhythmia in both cell types with a more pronounced effect in human iPS-CMs [29]. In primary CMs and in tissue preparations, both drugs showed an increase in cell shortening and contractile force and a decrease in the beating rate. In contrast, the effect of verapamil was almost identical in mouse and human iPSC-derived CMs, namely a concentration-dependent reduction of the contraction amplitude with rhythmic changes of the CI [26]. The T-type calcium channel blocker amlodipine strongly decreased the beating

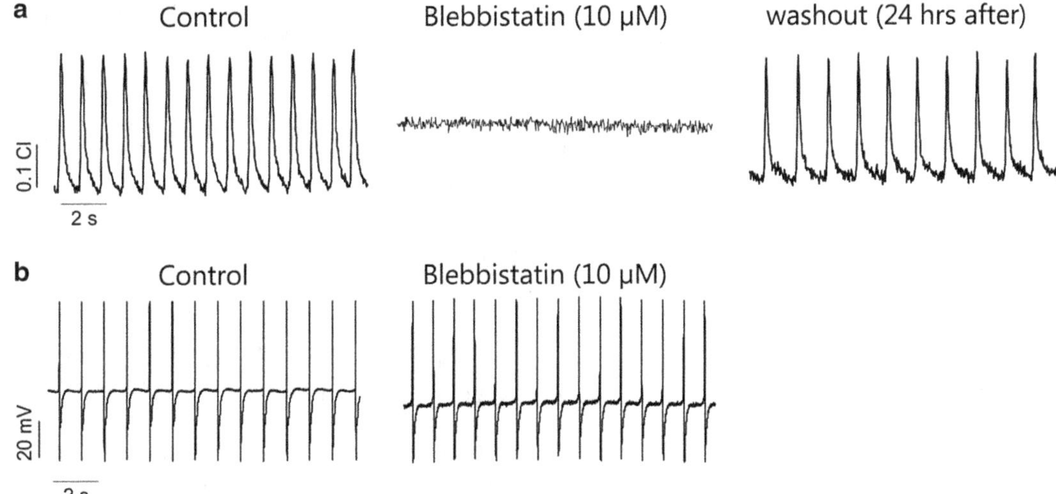

Fig. 6 Effect of blebbistatin on mouse iPS cell-derived CMs. (**a**) Impedance recordings show inhibition of CM contractions after blebbistatin (myosin II inhibitor, at 1 μM) application. (**b**) Blebbistatin has no effect on field potential of CMs recorded with MEA system

rate with a smaller effect on hiPS CMs [29]. Also the application of the antitumor activity exhibiting cyclodepsipeptide jaspamide has been shown to be strongly concentration-dependent, but also species-dependent, as a narrow margin of safety was observed between the doses required for efficacy in mouse tumor models and the doses that caused severe acute toxicity, include cardiotoxicity, in rats and dogs [36].

With the RTCA Cardio System it has also been shown that adequate tests can be performed to test the cytotoxicity of medicinal plants to accommodate wider acceptance, recognition and utilization of traditional medicine [27]. The xCELLigence RTCA cardio system can be used to access the biological and pharmacological activities of natural products or plant extracts in concentration-dependent manner as well (*see* Fig. 7 for example of compound derived from plant extract). In a recent study by Nembo et al. the effect of *Brillantaisia nitens* Lindau (Acanthaceae), a plant commonly used in traditional medicine in Africa for the treatment of many disorders including heart diseases and malaria, was tested for its activity on miPS-CMs. The addition of *Brillantaisia nitens* extract on undifferentiated pluripotent cells and on synchronous beating layer of iPS cell-derived CMs inhibits the proliferative capacity of pluripotent stem cells and induced significant changes in the beating pattern in a concentration- and time-dependent manner, respectively, approving its depressant action on the heart [27].

In summary, despite the important advances in science and technology concerning drug toxicity in the last two decades,

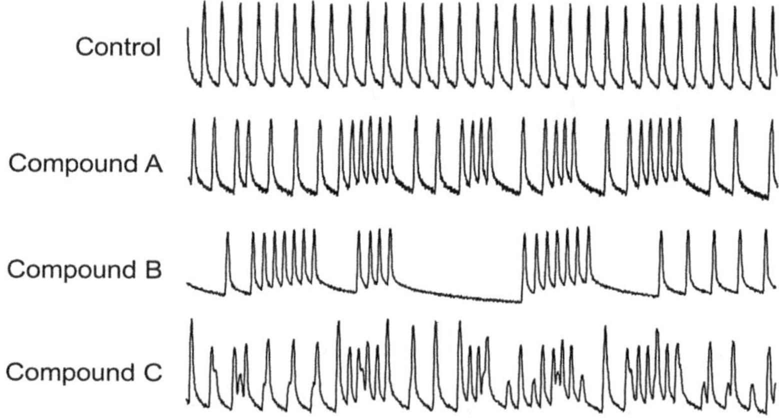

Fig. 7 Typical example of spontaneously beating signal of cardiomyocytes recorded after 2 days in the absence (control) and presence of indicated compound. Each trace represents 10 s of recording time. This data show that the xCELLigence system is a reliable and efficient tool for real-time screening of cardiotoxic effect of compounds in cell-based in vitro assays

progress in pharmaceutical industry is still restricted by a high rate of attrition of compounds during the drug development process. Cardiotoxicity issues are still amongst the most frequent reasons for retaining drugs from the market. Thus, the implementation of a new tool for in vitro cardiotoxicity screening tests is still crucial to prevent this. In this chapter, we describe the physiologically relevant and predictive assay of xCELLigence System RTCA Cardio Instrument, especially in combination with pluripotent stem cell-derived CMs, for preclinical cardiac safety assessment of new compounds. The features of this assay system, including time resolution and dynamic monitoring of mechanical beating activity of cardiomyocytes, as well as the 96-well throughput, which provide important mechanistic and cardiotoxicity information of drug molecules. Additionally, it also possesses some useful properties such as noninvasive, continuous monitoring of changes in beating activities during compound exposure, which are unique to its design. Therefore, this system can be easily applied to screen for potential problems with promising drug candidates at an early stage of their development.

5   Notes

1. Before starting any experiment read carefully the RTCA Cardio xCELLigence manual and documentation.

2. This should be done immediately before use and the reconstituted fibronectin should be diluted with sterile water to a

concentration of 1 mg/ml according to the manufacturer's instructions. Aliquot and store at –20 °C.

3. It is important to ensure no damage of the sensors by avoiding touching the bottom of the plate.

4. During the time of E-Plate incubation, start the RTCA Cardio program and enter requested information (labeled) regarding the cells, cell number, compounds and concentrations, this for each well as indicated on the RTCA Cardio Instrument Operator's Guide.

5. Make sure the cell suspension to be counted is well mixed by either gentle agitation of the tube. For some cells a pre-plating step is recommended before starting the experiment.

6. Be careful not to damage the bottom of the plate when pipetting with the pipette tips.

7. It is important to include control wells, which contain the same volume of culture medium without cells.

8. It is recommended to minimize opening the incubator's door during the first 2 days of experiment to reduce the interference in measurements.

9. If stock solution was dissolved in dimethyl sulfoxide (DMSO), its final concentration should not exceed 0.1 %.

10. Generally, the impedance signals reach stable status between day 4 and day 6 after cell seeding. However, cardiomyocytes from different sources may behave differently.

11. It is important to ensure temperature stability during experimental procedures, which can be achieved, for example, by keeping the E-Plate 96 on RTCA Cardio Temperature Tool while compounds are added.

12. Repeat washout step at least three times to perform an almost complete removal of the compound.

Acknowledgements

We thank Susan Rohani and Annette Köster for their technical assistance as well as Suzanne Wood and Elke Lieske for the secretarial assistance. We also thank Matthias Matzkies, Erastus Nembo, Julie Albrecht, Nermeen El Dabah, and Christoph Schäfer for fruitful discussion. We owe many thanks to Dr. Yama Abassi and ACEA biosciences for the fruitful collaboration.

This work was funded by DETECTIVE (Grant Agreement No. 266838) projects through the EU Seventh Framework Programme HEALTH-2010-4.2.9 Alternative Testing Strategies (Health-F5-2010-267042) and Cosmetics Europe.

References

1. Xi B, Wang T, Li N, Ouyang W, Zhang W, Wu J, Xu X, Wang X, Abassi YA (2011) Functional cardiotoxicity profiling and screening using the xCELLigence RTCA cardio system. J Lab Autom 16(6):415–421. doi:10.1016/j.jala. 2011.09.002

2. Nguemo F, Saric T, Pfannkuche K, Watzele M, Reppel M, Hescheler J (2012) In vitro model for assessing arrhythmogenic properties of drugs based on high-resolution impedance measurements. Cell Physiol Biochem 29(5–6):819–832. doi:10.1159/000188069

3. Fermini B, Fossa AA (2003) The impact of drug-induced QT interval prolongation on drug discovery and development. Nat Rev Drug Discov 2(6):439–447. doi:10.1038/nrd1108

4. Braam SR, Tertoolen L, van de Stolpe A, Meyer T, Passier R, Mummery CL (2010) Prediction of drug-induced cardiotoxicity using human embryonic stem cell-derived cardiomyocytes. Stem Cell Res 4(2):107–116. doi:10.1016/j. scr.2009.11.004

5. Natarajan A, Stancescu M, Dhir V, Armstrong C, Sommerhage F, Hickman JJ, Molnar P (2011) Patterned cardiomyocytes on micro-electrode arrays as a functional, high information content drug screening platform. Biomaterials 32(18):4267–4274. doi:10.1016/j.biomaterials.2010.12.022

6. Kannankeril PJ, Roden DM (2007) Drug-induced long QT and torsade de pointes: recent advances. Curr Opin Cardiol 22(1): 39–43

7. Anson BD, Kolaja KL, Kamp TJ (2011) Opportunities for use of human iPS cells in predictive toxicology. Clin Pharmacol Ther 89(5):754–758. doi:10.1038/clpt.2011.9

8. Brown AM (2005) HERG block, QT liability and sudden cardiac death. Novartis Found Symp 266:118–131. doi:10.1002/047002142X.ch10, discussion 131-115, 155-118

9. Valentin JP (2010) Reducing QT liability and proarrhythmic risk in drug discovery and development. Br J Pharmacol 159(1):5–11. doi:10.1111/j.1476-5381.2009.00547.x

10. Wallis RM (2010) Integrated risk assessment and predictive value to humans of non-clinical repolarization assays. Br J Pharmacol 159(1):115–121. doi:10.1111/j.1476-5381.2009.00395.x

11. Chain AS, Krudys KM, Danhof M, Della Pasqua O (2011) Assessing the probability of drug-induced QTc-interval prolongation during clinical drug development. Clin Pharmacol Ther 90(6):867–875. doi:10.1038/clpt.2011.202

12. Moss AJ, Kass RS (2005) Long QT syndrome: from channels to cardiac arrhythmias. J Clin Invest 115(8):2018–2024. doi:10.1172/JCI25537

13. Moller C (2010) Keeping the rhythm: hERG and beyond in cardiovascular safety pharmacology. Expert Rev Clin Pharmacol 3(3):321–329. doi:10.1586/ecp.10.24

14. Overington JP, Al-Lazikani B, Hopkins AL (2006) How many drug targets are there? Nat Rev Drug Discov 5(12):993–996. doi:10.1038/nrd2199

15. Atienza JM, Yu N, Wang X, Xu X, Abassi Y (2006) Label-free and real-time cell-based kinase assay for screening selective and potent receptor tyrosine kinase inhibitors using microelectronic sensor array. J Biomol Screen 11(6):634–643. doi:10.1177/1087057106289334

16. Abassi YA, Xi B, Zhang W, Ye P, Kirstein SL, Gaylord MR, Feinstein SC, Wang X, Xu X (2009) Kinetic cell-based morphological screening: prediction of mechanism of compound action and off-target effects. Chem Biol 16(7):712–723. doi:10.1016/j.chembiol.2009.05.011

17. Giaever I, Keese CR (1993) A morphological biosensor for mammalian cells. Nature 366(6455):591–592. doi:10.1038/366591a0

18. Takahashi K, Yamanaka S (2006) Induction of pluripotent stem cells from mouse embryonic and adult fibroblast cultures by defined factors. Cell 126(4):663–676. doi:10.1016/j.cell.2006.07.024

19. Takahashi K, Tanabe K, Ohnuki M, Narita M, Ichisaka T, Tomoda K, Yamanaka S (2007) Induction of pluripotent stem cells from adult human fibroblasts by defined factors. Cell 131(5):861–872. doi:10.1016/j.cell.2007.11.019

20. Mauritz C, Schwanke K, Reppel M, Neef S, Katsirntaki K, Maier LS, Nguemo F, Menke S, Haustein M, Hescheler J, Hasenfuss G, Martin U (2008) Generation of functional murine cardiac myocytes from induced pluripotent stem cells. Circulation 118(5):507–517. doi:10.1161/CIRCULATIONAHA.108.778795

21. Yu J, Vodyanik MA, Smuga-Otto K, Antosiewicz-Bourget J, Frane JL, Tian S, Nie J, Jonsdottir GA, Ruotti V, Stewart R, Slukvin II, Thomson JA (2007) Induced pluripotent stem cell lines derived from human somatic cells. Science 318(5858):1917–1920. doi:10.1126/science.1151526

22. Pistollato F, Bremer-Hoffmann S, Healy L, Young L, Stacey G (2012) Standardization of pluripotent stem cell cultures for toxicity testing. Expert Opin Drug Metab Toxicol 8(2):239–257. doi:10.1517/17425255.2012.639763

23. Savla JJ, Nelson BC, Perry CN, Adler ED (2014) Induced pluripotent stem cells for the study of cardiovascular disease. J Am Coll Cardiol 64(5):512–519. doi:10.1016/j.jacc.2014.05.038

24. Peters MF, Lamore SD, Guo L, Scott CW, Kolaja KL (2014) Human stem cell-derived cardiomyocytes in cellular impedance assays: bringing cardiotoxicity screening to the front line. Cardiovasc Toxicol. doi:10.1007/s12012-014-9268-9

25. Urcan E, Haertel U, Styllou M, Hickel R, Scherthan H, Reichl FX (2010) Real-time xCELLigence impedance analysis of the cytotoxicity of dental composite components on human gingival fibroblasts. Dent Mater 26(1): 51–58. doi:10.1016/j.dental.2009.08.007

26. Wang T, Hu N, Cao J, Wu J, Su K, Wang P (2013) A cardiomyocyte-based biosensor for antiarrhythmic drug evaluation by simultaneously monitoring cell growth and beating. Biosens Bioelectron 2013(49):9–13. doi:10.1016/j.bios.2013.04.039

27. Nembo EN, Dimo T, Bopda MO, Hescheler J, Nguemo F (2014) The proliferative and chronotropic effects of Brillantaisia nitens Lindau (Acanthaceae) extracts on pluripotent stem cells and their cardiomyocytes derivatives. J Ethnopharmacol 156:73–81. doi:10.1016/j.jep.2014.07.046

28. Himmel HM (2013) Drug-induced functional cardiotoxicity screening in stem cell-derived human and mouse cardiomyocytes: effects of reference compounds. J Pharmacol Toxicol Methods 68(1):97–111. doi:10.1016/j.vascn.2013.05.005

29. Jonsson MK, Wang QD, Becker B (2011) Impedance-based detection of beating rhythm and proarrhythmic effects of compounds on stem cell-derived cardiomyocytes. Assay Drug Dev Technol 9(6):589–599. doi:10.1089/adt.2011.0396

30. Lamore SD, Kamendi HW, Scott CW, Dragan YP, Peters MF (2013) Cellular impedance assays for predictive preclinical drug screening of kinase inhibitor cardiovascular toxicity. Toxicol Sci 135(2):402–413. doi:10.1093/toxsci/kft167

31. Peters MF, Scott CW, Ochalski R, Dragan YP (2012) Evaluation of cellular impedance measures of cardiomyocyte cultures for drug screening applications. Assay Drug Dev Technol 10(6):525–532. doi:10.1089/adt.2011.442

32. Doherty KR, Wappel RL, Talbert DR, Trusk PB, Moran DM, Kramer JW, Brown AM, Shell SA, Bacus S (2013) Multi-parameter in vitro toxicity testing of crizotinib, sunitinib, erlotinib, and nilotinib in human cardiomyocytes. Toxicol Appl Pharmacol 272(1):245–255. doi:10.1016/j.taap.2013.04.027

33. Eldridge S, Guo L, Mussio J, Furniss M, Hamre J 3rd, Davis M (2014) Examining the protective role of ErbB2 modulation in human-induced pluripotent stem cell-derived cardiomyocytes. Toxicol Sci 141(2):547–559. doi:10.1093/toxsci/kfu150

34. Guo L, Abrams RM, Babiarz JE, Cohen JD, Kameoka S, Sanders MJ, Chiao E, Kolaja KL (2011) Estimating the risk of drug-induced proarrhythmia using human induced pluripotent stem cell-derived cardiomyocytes. Toxicol Sci 123(1):281–289. doi:10.1093/toxsci/kfr158

35. Guo L, Coyle L, Abrams RM, Kemper R, Chiao ET, Kolaja KL (2013) Refining the human iPSC-cardiomyocyte arrhythmic risk assessment model. Toxicol Sci 136(2):581–594. doi:10.1093/toxsci/kft205

36. Schweikart K, Guo L, Shuler Z, Abrams R, Chiao ET, Kolaja KL, Davis M (2013) The effects of jaspamide on human cardiomyocyte function and cardiac ion channel activity. Toxicol In Vitro 27(2):745–751. doi:10.1016/j.tiv.2012.12.005

37. Abassi YA, Xi B, Li N, Ouyang W, Seiler A, Watzele M, Kettenhofen R, Bohlen H, Ehlich A, Kolossov E, Wang X, Xu X (2012) Dynamic monitoring of beating periodicity of stem cell-derived cardiomyocytes as a predictive tool for preclinical safety assessment. Br J Pharmacol 165(5):1424–1441. doi:10.1111/j.1476-5381.2011.01623.x

38. Scott CW, Zhang X, Abi-Gerges N, Lamore SD, Abassi YA, Peters MF (2014) An impedance-based cellular assay using human iPSC-derived cardiomyocytes to quantify modulators of cardiac contractility. Toxicol Sci 142(2):331–338. doi:10.1093/toxsci/kfu186

39. Drew BJ, Ackerman MJ, Funk M, Gibler WB, Kligfield P, Menon V, Philippides GJ, Roden DM, Zareba W (2010) Prevention of torsade de pointes in hospital settings: a scientific statement from the American Heart Association and the American College of Cardiology Foundation. Circulation 121(8):1047–1060. doi:10.1161/CIRCULATIONAHA.109.192704

40. Wang L, Wible BA, Wan X, Ficker E (2007) Cardiac glycosides as novel inhibitors of human ether-a-go-go-related gene channel trafficking. J Pharmacol Exp Ther 320(2):525–534. doi:10.1124/jpet.106.113043

Digital Holographic Imaging for Label-Free Phenotypic Profiling, Cytotoxicity, and Chloride Channels Target Screening

Benjamin Rappaz, Fabien Kuttler, Billy Breton, and Gerardo Turcatti

Abstract

Cellular assays using label-free Digital Holographic Microscopy (DHM) have been previously validated for cell viability assays in a drug screening context. Our automated DHM system allows performing fast and cost-effective screening assays for a wide range of applications for monitoring cell morphological changes and cell movements upon interaction with interfering compounds. In addition to these classic phenotypic assays, it has been demonstrated that target-based cellular assays can also be addressed by DHM for therapeutically relevant chloride channel receptors. Our DH-imaging (DHI) technology, potentially scalable for screening by imaging approaches in a high-throughput manner can also deliver highly informative data through long term experiments. Three examples of phenotypic screens are detailed in the present chapter: a label-free profiling approach, a cell proliferation assay, and methods for monitoring the activity of the $GABA_A$ chloride channel receptor.

Key words Cell migration, Cell proliferation, CFTR, Chloride channels, Cytotoxicity profiling, Digital holographic microscopy, $GABA_A$, High-content screening, Label-free quantitative microscopy, Phenotypic drug discovery

1 Introduction

The use of high-content cell-based assays has increased over the past years and is presently widely applied for chemical biology, systems biology research, and drug discovery [1, 2]. This fast evolution triggered hardware and software developments from instruments manufacturers, resulting in commercialization of automated fluorescence microscopes with improved performance in terms of autofocusing speed and precision, and capabilities for processing very large sets of images. In addition, current trends in screening suggest to move back from target-based assays to phenotypic screening and to critically redefine the global screening strategy [3].

Ye Fang (ed.), *Label-Free Biosensor Methods in Drug Discovery*, Methods in Pharmacology and Toxicology, DOI 10.1007/978-1-4939-2617-6_17, © Springer Science+Business Media New York 2015

As a general and widely applied approach for fluorescence imaging, cells are individually identified through the use of nuclear staining procedures with standard dyes such as Hoechst and DAPI. Often an additional dye, such as DRAQ5, CellMask, or Calcein AM, is also used for staining the cytoplasm and precisely defining the contours of the cell object. The use of these exogenous labels to determine the spatial location of cells and their morphological parameters has several disadvantages. First, these labelling steps contribute to the increased heterogeneity of the cell-based assay due to the extra pipetting and fluidic dispensing steps required that might play against the throughput and global quality of the cell-based assay. Second, this invasive method may alter the intactness of cells, in particular due to phototoxic effects resulting from long term light exposure of DNA stains, thus preventing continuous cell monitoring over periods of several hours [4–6]. Finally, the use of one or two labels for defining the cell objects reduces the global multiplexing capacity in terms of fluorescent probes that can be used for detecting specific cellular markers describing the events or the phenotype investigated.

Noninvasive label-free imaging techniques have recently emerged for fulfilling the requirements of minimal cell manipulation for cell-based assays in a high-content screening (HCS) context. Moreover, instruments manufacturers have also included solutions to implement label-free approaches in HCS-based image acquisition protocols, with, for example, imaging of transmitted light capabilities for detecting and counting cells in the new generation of automated microscopes for high-content analysis (for instance in the software-based "phase contrast" or "DIC" imaging modes of the IN Cell Analyzer 2200 from GE Healthcare) [7].

Among these label-free techniques, Digital Holographic Microscopy (DHM) is the only image-based technology providing quantitative information that is automated for end-point and time-lapse HCS using 96 and 384 well plates [8, 9].

DHM is a label-free interferometric microscopy technique that provides a quantitative measurement of the optical path length (OPL, related to the optical density of the cell) [8, 10, 11]. In short, a hologram consisting of a 2D interference pattern is first recorded on a digital camera and the contrast (phase) images are reconstructed numerically using a specific algorithm [10]. The DHM setup is illustrated in Fig. 1. The DHM phase image is quantitatively related to the optical path difference (OPD), expressed in terms of physical properties as:

$$\mathrm{OPD}(x, y) = d(x, y)\left[\bar{n}_c(x, y) - n_m\right], \tag{1}$$

where $d(x,y)$ is the cell thickness, $\bar{n}_c(x, y)$ is the mean z-integrated intracellular refractive index at the (x,y) position, and nm is the refractive index of the surrounding culture medium.

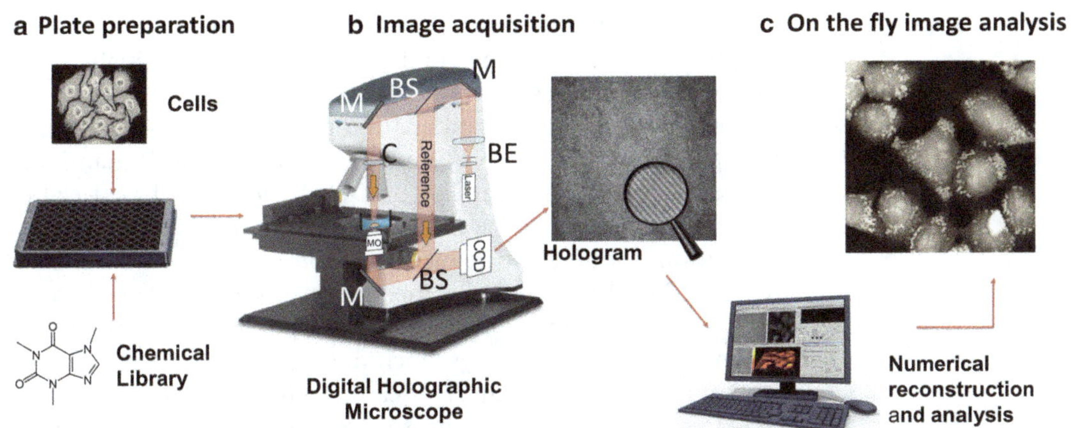

Fig. 1 Digital Holographic Imaging, acquisition workflow. (**a**) Plate preparation procedure: compounds to be tested are added to a well plate before or after cell seeding. (**b**) Image acquisition: diagram of a Digital holographic Microscope (DHM). Holograms are recorded out of focus by a digital camera on a DHM system equipped with a motorized stage for automated multi-well plate experiments. Legend: M, mirror, BS, beam splitter, BE, beam expander, MO, microscope objective, C, condenser. (**c**) The hologram is reconstructed by a computer to form an in-focus quantitative phase image

Simply put, Eq. (1) means that the OPD signal is proportional to both the cell thickness and the intracellular refractive index. DHM systems generally use a low intensity laser as light source for specimen illumination and a digital camera to record the hologram. Here, the 684 nm laser source delivers roughly 200 $\mu W/cm^2$ at the specimen plane for an exposure time of only 400 μs. The light intensity is six orders of magnitude lower than intensities typically associated with confocal fluorescence microscopy and well below phototoxicity levels. An extensive quality control protocol for DHM can be found in ref. [12].

DH imaging (DHI) relies on a signal that is proportional to both the cell thickness and the intracellular refractive index—a parameter linked to the protein content of the cell [10, 13]. In addition, the sensitivity of the technique to ion and water fluxes through the membrane makes DHM applicable for optically monitoring the activity of pharmacologically relevant targets such as the chloride channel $GABA_A$ [14] and the Cystic fibrosis transmembrane conductance regulator (CFTR) [15]. Furthermore, DHM provides extended depth-of-focus images, allowing to refocus the images, a strong advantage for high-throughput applications [16, 17]. Practically, DHM was applied to live cell imaging [10], determination of transmembrane ion fluxes in neurosciences [18], early cell death diagnosis [19], time-lapse studies of cancerous cell mitosis and duct cells water permeability analysis, to name only a few of the validated DHM applications. Each of these cellular assays has the potential to be implemented in a DH Imaging instrument for their further validation as screening applications.

In order to validate the use of DHM for monitoring morphological cell changes in a HCS context, we initially developed cell viability assays and compared the experimental outputs of this technique with standard fluorescence microscopy methods [8]. After this first reported demonstration and quantitative assessment of the applicability of DHM for image-based cellular screening in 96 and 384 well plate format, we validated a range of applications for their future incorporation as informative cell-based assays during the screening campaigns performed at our platform.

The focus of this chapter is on the practical aspects of three screening-compatible assays, including cytotoxic assays and cell profiling methods for cancer research, cell proliferation assay, and DHM as an optical electrode for monitoring the activity of the $GABA_A$ chloride channel.

2 General Methodological Workflow

The methodological workflow is graphically described in Fig. 1. Unless described for each particular application, the following generic methods and materials have been applied for DHM cell based screening assays.

2.1 Sample Preparation

HeLa (ATCC®, CCL-2™) cells were maintained in Dulbecco's modified Eagle's GlutaMAX medium (Life Technologies Ltd., ref. 32430) supplemented with 10 % gamma irradiated and heat inactivated fetal bovine serum (Life Technologies Ltd., ref. 10101-145), and were grown at 37 °C in 5 % CO_2 with ~95 % relative humidity. Before drug treatment, cells were trypsinized, seeded in 96-well BD-falcon imaging plate (ref. 353219) at a density of 4,000 to 6,000 cells per well and grown for 24–48 h. Cells were at 25–60 % confluency at the time of measurement.

For end-point measurements, compounds were diluted in media from a 10 mM stock solution to a final concentration of 10 μM and 0.1 % DMSO. Control wells mimic this final DMSO concentration. Alternatively, for primary screens, compounds were pre-plated in wells using an ECHO acoustic dispenser (Labcyte Echo 555, Dublin, Ireland), prior to the addition of cells. In this case, 0.1 μl of compounds was dispensed in wells, and cells were then added in a final volume of 100 μl. For the dose–response curves, dilution series were prepared in culture medium for each of the tested compounds in the concentration range of 0.1–30 μM.

2.2 Image Acquisition

DHM time-lapse measurements on live cells were achieved in a Chamlide WP incubator system for 96-well plate (LCI, South Korea) set at 37°/5 % CO_2 with high humidity. Time-lapse images were acquired each 10 or 15 min for 24–48 h (*see* **Note 1**).

For each experiment, in general four images per well were acquired with appropriate objective magnification (*see* **Note 2**) and the corresponding measurements were averaged to yield a mean value per well. DHM images were acquired on a commercially available DHM T-1001 from LynceeTec SA (Lausanne, Switzerland) equipped with a motorized xy stage (Märzhäuser Wetzlar GmbH & Co. KG, Wetzlar, Germany, ref. S429).

2.3 Image Segmentation and Data Analysis

With DHM images, phenotypic changes were quantified using two distinct analysis workflows: direct raw OPD measurement for a global population analysis and single-cell image analysis performed with CellProfiler (Broad Institute, MA, http://www.cellprofiler.org, r11710) [20] and CellProfiler Analyst [21] software.

Average OPD measurement is performed automatically during the reconstruction of the images and thus offers a fast way to directly quantify the experiments on-the-fly.

1. Determine the confluency mask by thresholding the images using a fixed value (Fig. 2). We generally use 512 Å which allows removing all the pixels from background.

2. Obtain the total OPD value by adding the OPD value recorded in each of the (x,y) masked pixel of the image (obtained to measure the confluency, see above).

3. Obtain the average OPD by dividing the total OPD by the surface of the mask. Average OPD is a measure of the optical density of the cells normalized by the confluency. This value is dependent on the cell shape (it increases with rounded cells) and is independent of cell confluency. Average OPD is an unbiased parameter that can be used to categorize phenotypes, as it is calculated without human intervention [8].

Cell profiler analysis is performed when single cells quantification of subcellular structure or complex subpopulations are investigated. It can be performed in parallel to the *Average OPD measurement* presented above. DHM phase signal has a similar signal as a fluorescent cytoplasmic dye, so analysis developed for such modality can be used with few modifications for DHM. For this, CellProfiler is able to successfully detect, segment, and analyze individual cells in DHM images [8].

1. Segment single images using CellProfiler pipeline slightly modified for DHM phase images.

2. Perform training (with CellProfiler Analyst and machine-guided learning) to separate different object classes (*see* **Note 3**).

3. Classify cells based on a selection of parameters (including intensity, texture, granularity, area, and shape) measured by CellProfiler. Results are presented as number of cells expressing the round phenotype divided by the total number of cells minus the number of segmentation errors objects.

1. Population average

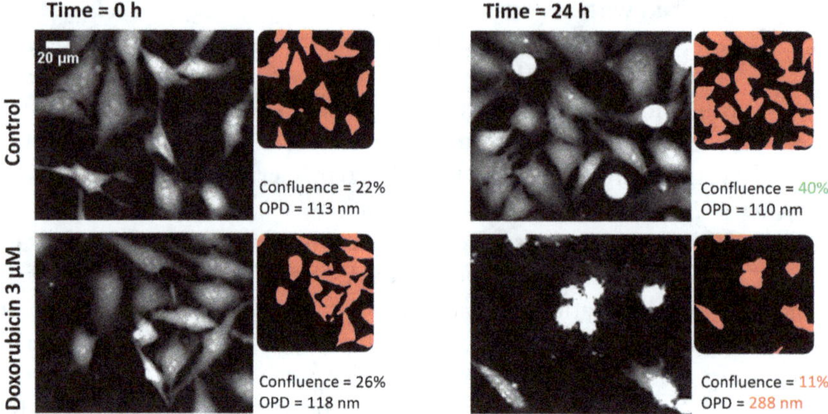

2. Individual cell

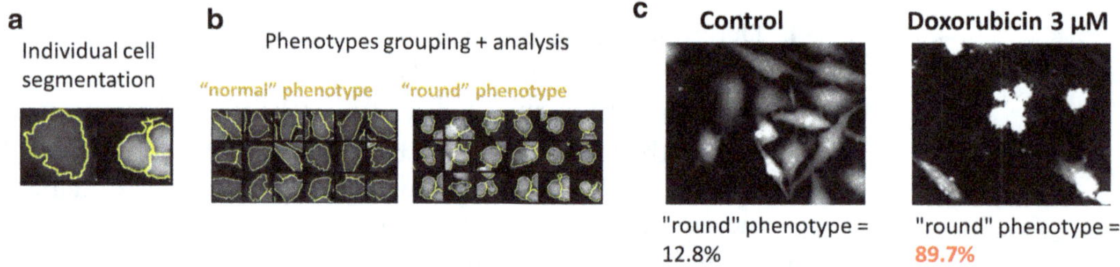

Fig. 2 Digital Holographic Imaging, analysis workflow. (1) Population average analysis. Images are thresholded using a fixed-value; this provides information on the confluence of cells (pink mask, yielding information about proliferation). The mean OPD signal (providing information about cytotoxicity) is obtained by measuring the OPD value of each pixel in the pink mask. We observed that HeLa cells treated with 3 µM doxorubicin for 24 h have a smaller confluence and a higher OPD than the control condition, thus indicating a proliferation inhibition and a cytotoxic effect. (2) Individual cell analysis. Single cells are segmented with CellProfiler software and then grouped into two phenotypes (normal and round) using CellProfiler Analyst. Each image is then automatically scored to provide the percentage of each phenotype. We observed that doxorubicin treatment induces an increase in the round phenotype, compared to the control. The same data set was analyzed using both approaches

2.4 Assay Validation

For statistical analyses, the mean value and the standard deviation for each parameter (avg. OPD, confluence, or phenotype as determined by CellProfiler Analyst classification) were measured from 12 to 16 different wells (mean of 4 fields of view) for each condition. These values were then used to calculate the Z'-factor [22] for each condition (cell type and phenotype). It can be argued that this statistical parameter is not the best criteria for the assessment of the quality of a screen concerning image-based assays [23]. However, the Z'-factor is appropriate for comparisons of different readouts technologies using different microscopic techniques tested under the same experimental conditions and evaluated using similar or identical analysis methods [9].

3 Selected Drug Discovery Applications of DHM

3.1 Cytotoxic Assays and Cell Profiling Methods for Cancer Research

DHM technology can be used for an important range of early drug discovery applications, in particular cell death assays which are of great importance for toxicological profiling of bioactive compounds, or for the search of cytotoxic agents in cancer research or cytoprotective compounds in the context of various therapeutic applications. We have shown that DHM easily delivers basic cell viability data with results comparable to fluorescence-based methods in a faster and more effective way [8].

In the present approach we show the usefulness of clustering the screened compounds in OPD vs. confluence plots for a fast classification of potential interesting drug candidates and a preliminary estimation of their mode of action based on the phenotype generated through both end-point and time-lapse experiments.

1. Assemble a library of 80 compounds as the "cancer set" (Table 1). A series of cancer-specific toxic compounds are selected from the Prestwick Chemical Collection (PCL, Prestwick) composed of 1,200 FDA approved drugs. Other drugs from external sources and non-cancer related control compounds are also selected as part of this library.

2. Test the effect of each compound on HeLa cells using DHM.

3. Plot DHM data at different time-points as a scatter plot of OPD signal versus confluency, both normalized by the results of control sample (0.1 % DMSO-treated cells). This allows the visualization of clusters of compounds according to their phenotype, reflecting differences in activity, potency, speed or mode of action.

A Z'-factor between 0.6 and 0.9 was obtained for the different assays using HeLa cells in 96 or 384 well plates, validating the robustness of DHM assay for phenotypic screening. Furthermore, EC_{50} curves generated for selected compounds and analyzed by DHM either using cell populations (OPD) or individual cells (CellProfiler analysis) are in excellent agreement with standard fluorescence-based methods [8, 9]. Having a fast informative method of analysis though the OPD signal and the possibility to further investigate cellular phenotypes at the single cell level with a single acquisition represents a major advantage of DHM as a high-throughput/high-content approach. The advantage of the OPD analysis and its excellent correlation with image analysis data obtained by CellProfiler is illustrated in Fig. 3. Dose–response plots for doxorubicin generated with the two methods gave rise to comparable EC_{50} values.

Clustering of compounds using OPD vs. confluence plots (indicating cytotoxicity or proliferation, respectively) was initially performed for the whole screen of 1,200 drugs (PCL), in order to

Table 1
List of 80 "cancer set" compounds selected from the Prestwick Chemical Collection and other external sources

Mode of action	Compounds			
Microtubule poisons	Colchicine	Nocodazole	Docetaxel	Paclitaxel
Aromatase inhibitors	Anastrozole	Formestane	Fadrozole hydrochloride	Glutethimide, para-amino
Topoisomerase inhibitors	Topotecan	Irinotecan hydrochloride	Mitoxantrone dihydrochloride	Camptothecine (S,+)
	Etoposide			
Antiandrogen/antiestrogen	Bicalutamide	Fulvestrant	Epitiostanol	Nilutamide
	Tamoxifen citrate	Hexestrol	Cyproterone acetate	Chlormadinone acetate
	Flutamide	Toremifene		
Antimetabolites	5-fluorouracil	Fludarabine	Azaguanine-8	Methotrexate
	Amethopterin (R,S)	Gemcitabine	Azathioprine	Thioguanosine
	Azacytidine-5	Mercaptopurine	Capecitabine	N6-methyladenosine
	Floxuridine			
Kinase inhibitors	Erlotinib	Regorafenib	Imatinib	Vatalanib
Alkylating/DNA targeting agents	Altretamine	Etanidazole	Cytarabine	Streptozotocin
	Busulfan	Ifosfamide	Dacarbazine	Temozolomide
	Chlorambucil	Oxaliplatin	Cyclophosphamide	TH-302
	Doxorubicin hydrochloride	Daunorubicin hydrochloride	Procarbazine hydrochloride	Tirapazamine (TPZ)

Other specific inhibitors	Auranofin	Everolimus	Bortezomib	Iobenguane sulfate
	Atractyloside potassium salt	Hesperidin	Cladribine	Mitotane
Controls: non-cancer specific or related molecules	Aripiprazole	Enoxacin	Cilnidipine	Perhexiline maleate
	Atorvastatin	Lovastatin	Digoxin	Pravastatin
	Caffeine	Imiquimod	Diclazuril	Simvastatin
	Carvedilol	Fluvastatin sodium salt	Clomiphene citrate (Z, E)	Triclosan

Molecules are classified according to their known or putative mode of action

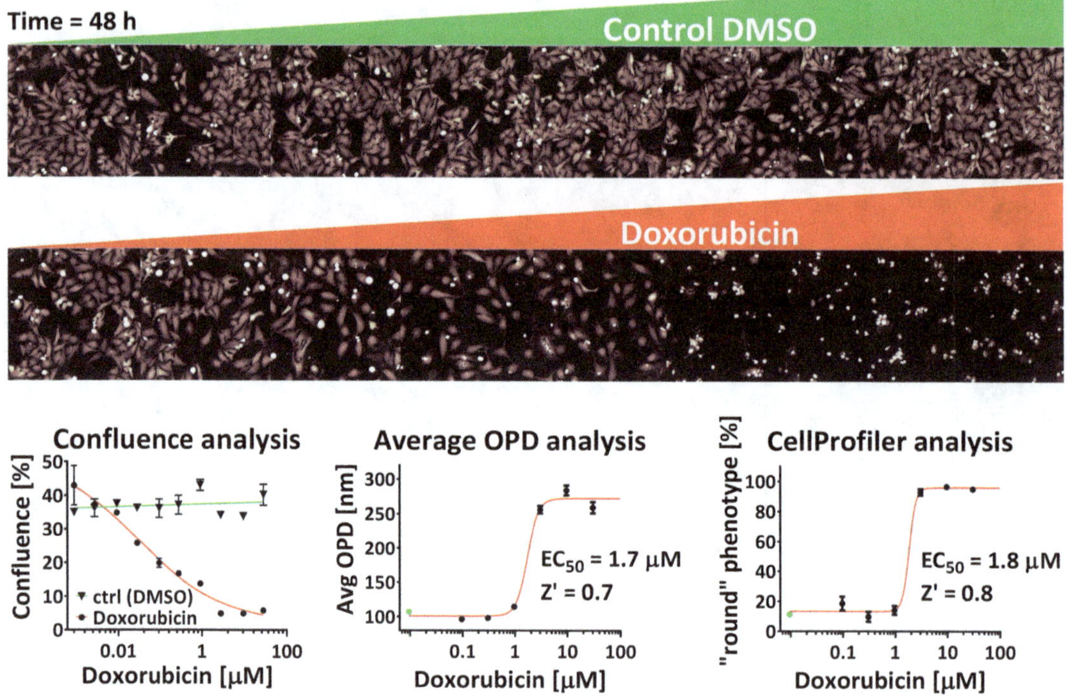

Fig. 3 Dose–response curves for an end-point DHI cytotoxycity assay. HeLa cells were treated with serial dilutions of doxorubicin or DMSO as control, and DHI was performed after 48 h of culture. Both population (avg. OPD) and individual cell (CellProfiler) analyses allow measuring EC$_{50}$ values in a cell density independent manner. Data are mean ± SEM

facilitate a preliminary classification of compounds according to the cell fate and allow selection of a subset of 80 compounds (Table 1). This subset was then used for further analyses such as dose-response and time-lapse measurements. Clustering of compounds though DHM-based analysis is illustrated on Fig. 4. From the 80 compounds tested by DHM on HeLa cells, a first cluster of 10 compounds can be identified (black circle), characterized by a drop in confluency and an increase in OPD signal, compared to the control (black dot). This cluster includes for example our positive control, doxorubicin (red dot), a molecule that has already been shown to induce cell death through different cellular mechanisms, apoptosis, necrosis, or autophagy [24], or colchicine (green dot), a powerful inhibitor of microtubule polymerization through binding to tubulin [25].

The power of time-lapse experiments for determining the evolution of cell phenotypes upon drug action is reported in Fig. 5 where the OPD and confluence were monitored over time for the two test anticancer drugs (doxorubicin and colchicine). As illustrated, the action of the two drugs on HeLa cells is different over

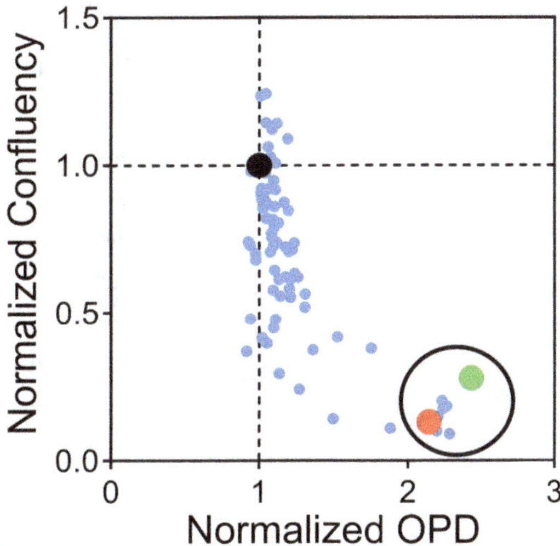

Fig. 4 Clustering cytotoxic compounds by DHI. HeLa cells were seeded in presence of 10 μM final of each of the 80 compounds from the "cancer set" and DHI was performed after 48 h of culture. Scatter plot of OPD versus Confluency, normalized by DMSO control (*black dot*) shows a clustering of some compounds displaying a lower confluency and an increased OPD signal. Doxorubicin (*red dot*) or colchicine (*green dot*) is included in this cluster

time, with a faster effect of doxorubicin, compared to a more gradual and delayed effect of colchicine, reflecting the differences in mode of action of the molecules. This representation, when used with for many drugs, allows a fast comparison of tested compounds in respect of the cell phenotypes they generated. This approach of cytotoxic assay though quantitative image analysis using DHM can be applied to cells of various origin, as we successfully tested our "cancer set" on a series of representative cancer cell lines, thus allowing screening approaches for specific compounds targeting specific cancers or cell types. It is important to highlight that these population analyses methods are complemented by the highly informative images obtained at each acquisition and allow further multidimensional analysis for adding predictive value to the compounds selected.

3.2 Cell Proliferation Assay

Cell migration and proliferation are central to a variety of functions such as wound healing, cell differentiation, embryonic development, tumor growth, and metastasis. A better understanding of the mechanism by which cells proliferate or migrate may lead to the development of novel therapeutic strategies, in particular for cancer research, where rated metastasis and tumor invasion appear as the main applications of cell migration assays [26].

Label-free DHI provides an informative and fast detection method of active compounds inhibiting cell proliferation using

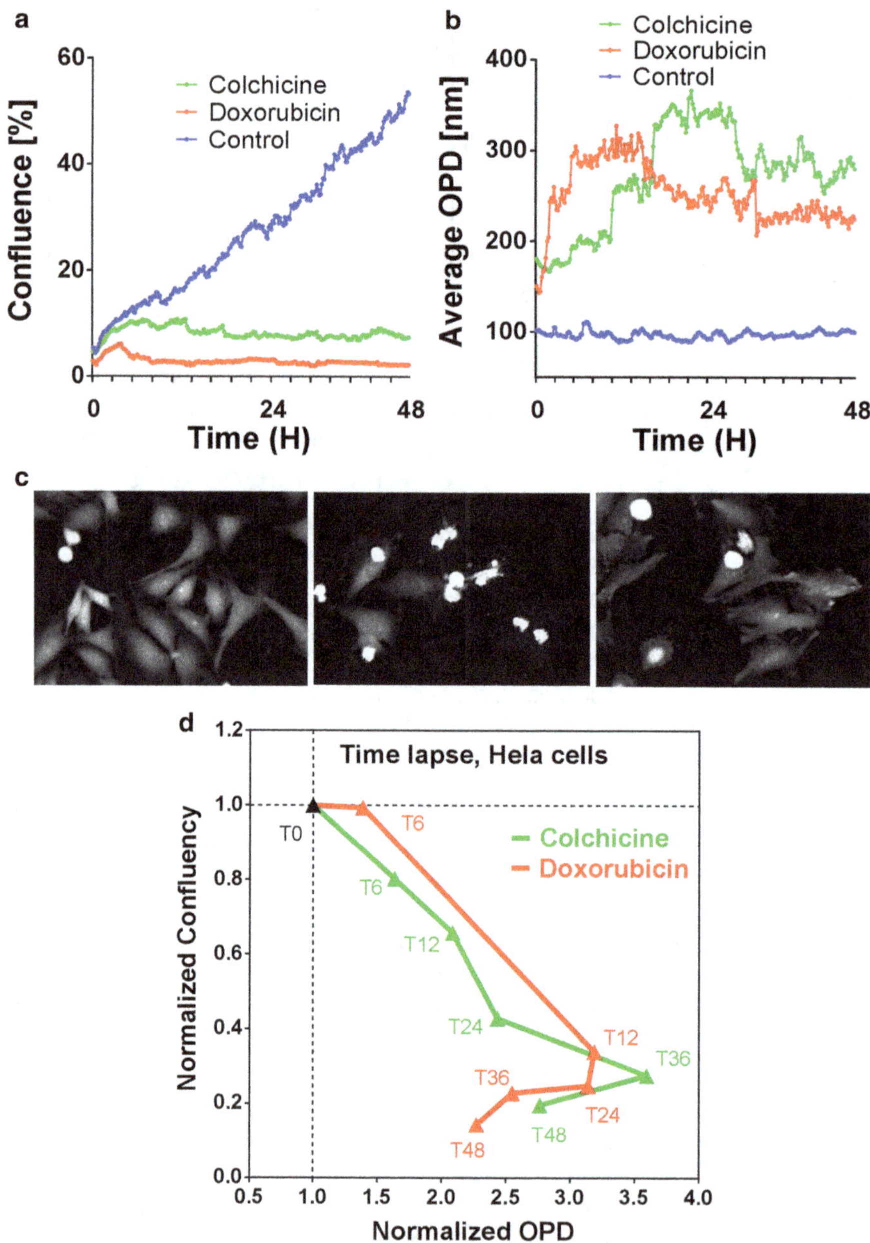

Fig. 5 Time-lapse monitoring of HeLa cells for a DHI cytotoxycity assay. HeLa cells were cultured in an environmental chamber in presence of DMSO (*blue*), 10 μM doxorubicin (*red*), or 10 μM colchicine (*green*): Quantitative phase image acquisition was performed every 15 min by DHM, over a period of 48 h. After reconstruction, raw confluency (**a**) and raw OPD (**b**) were calculated and plotted for each time point. (**c**) Example of reconstructed quantitative phase images acquired after 8 h in presence of control DMSO (*left*), doxorubicin (*middle*), and colchicine (*right*). Cells treated with colchicine, a powerful inhibitor of microtubule polymerisation through binding to tubulin, display in particular a typical morphological change. (**d**) Evolution of confluency plotted versus OPD after normalization by control condition (DMSO), over 48 h, from the T0 starting point (*black dot*) to the following representative time points (6 h, 12 h, 24 h, 36 h, and 48 h), showing a decrease of confluency and an increase of OPD over time for the treated cells (doxorubicin and colchicine), but with main differences in speed, reflecting differences in mode of action of the molecules

both time-lapse and end-point measurements. Moreover, active compounds can be categorized according to their potency through the generation of dose responses but also according to the phenotype generated. In addition, cytotoxicity measurements are obtained without further postprocessing or analysis using the average OPD information. Our methodological approach presented here allows easy and cost-effective characterization of hits for their ability to perturb cell proliferation and simultaneously to gather valuable information related to cell phenotypic changes induced by the effect of the chemical compounds.

1. Plate HeLa cells on Oris™-Pro 96-well plates (Platypus Technologies). The silicon-based stoppers provide a temporary physical barrier preventing cells adherence to the center of the well generating an annular monolayer of cells with a central cell-free area (exclusion zone) into which cell movement can occur.

2. Treat cells for 40 h with increasing concentrations of cytochalasin D. This compound is a cell permeable potent inhibitor of the polymerization and elongation of actin.

3. Acquire 25 images using a $10\times/0.22$ NA objective per well at the speed of about 2 images/s. This leads to a total of 20 min for acquiring 2,400 images of a full 96-well plate. Acquire time-points each hour for 40 h.

4. Calculate cell confluency, the readout for proliferation, for each compound at specific time points by simple thresholding of the images.

The EC_{50} value calculated from the dose–response curve generated at the 40 h end point (Fig. 6) for the cytochalasin D was in agreement with previously reported data, and reflected the cell cycle arrest in G1/S induced by cytochalasin D, through the activation of p53-dependent pathways [27]. In addition, the increase in average OPD measured by DHM at the same time as confluency reflected the global cytotoxicity of cytochalasin D, as manifested by generalized cell contraction and zeiosis [28]. Thus, high-content temporal and spatial information both have been easily generated with our label-free DHM imaging approach. This demonstrates that chemical compounds can be easily evaluated and quantified for their ability to prevent cell proliferation. By extension, DHM could therefore be used also in screening of proper migration inhibition activity using classic wound healing assays in a HCS context [29]. Moreover, the phenotypic changes of cells can be recorded in parallel for giving additional valuable information about the compounds action over time at the cell level. Our method is suitable for large-scale screening at single compound concentration and focused high-content analysis of selected molecules during hits-validation or hits-to-leads process.

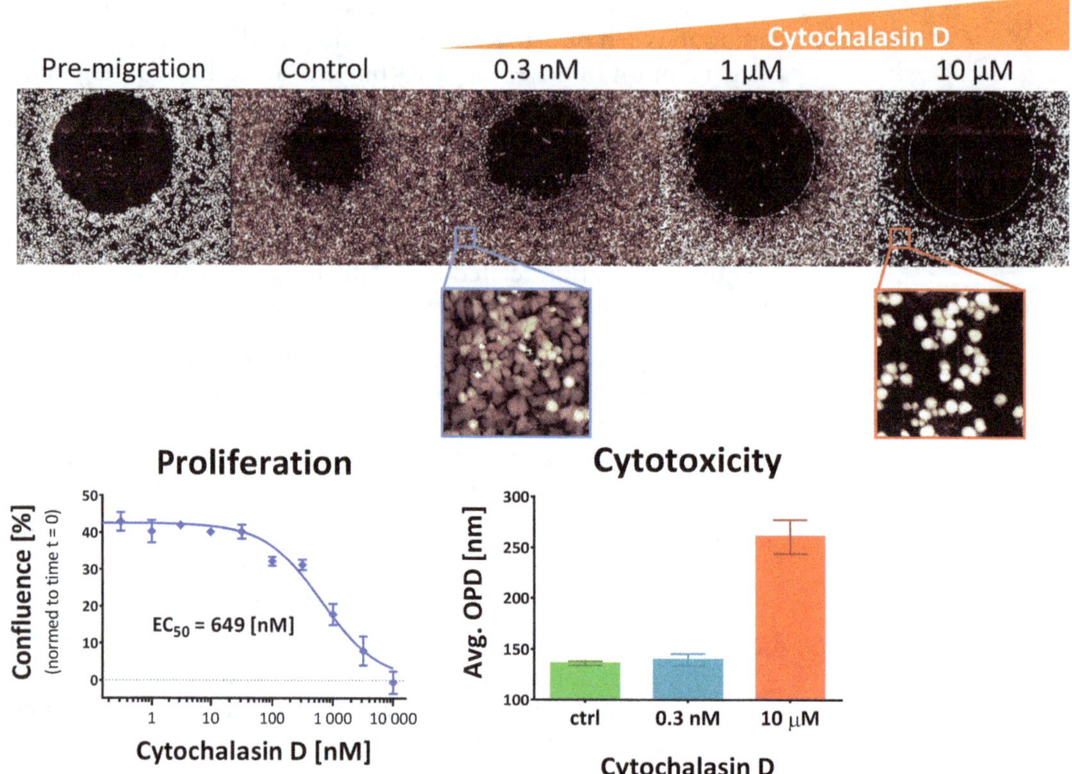

Fig. 6 Proliferation and cytotoxic dose–response curves by DHI. Parallel proliferation and cytotoxic measurements of the effect of serial dilution of cytochalasin D (inhibitor of actin polymerization) on HeLa cells over a recording period of 40 h. We observed a decreased proliferation and increased cytotoxic effect with high dose of cytochalasin D

3.3 Chloride Fluxes Related Receptors; GABA$_A$ Receptor

Gamma-aminobutyric acid (GABA) is the principal inhibitory neurotransmitter in the mammalian CNS acting via metabotropic GABA$_B$ and ionotropic GABA$_A$ receptors [28]. GABA$_A$, an ion channel member of the "cys-loop" ion channel superfamily [30], leads to an influx of chloride ions upon its activation. The modulation of GABA$_A$ as a target is a clinically proven mechanism for a range of CNS indications [31].

As for many ligand-gated ion channels, there have been limited progresses for significantly increasing the throughput of GABA$_A$ receptor screening through invasive patch clamp experiments or by using fluorescent dyes. Recently, it has been demonstrated that the noninvasive optical DHM method allowed monitoring of ion channel activity in a label-free manner.

DHM provides a quantitative determination of transmembrane chloride fluxes mediated by the activation of chloride channels associated with GABA$_A$ receptors. The signal originated from the ion-associated water fluxes following the GABA$_A$ receptor activation [14], a parameter to which the DHM is particularly sensitive [32]. Here we report the use and validation of this so-called "optical electrode" method for label-free screening of this important class of receptors.

1. Plate HEK 293 cells stably expressing various configurations of rat $GABA_A$ receptors (HEK-GABA) (Hoffmann-LaRoche, Basel, Switzerland) on previously poly-D-ornithine-coated BD-falcon imaging plates (ref. 353219) at a density of 40,000 cells/well and used at 4 DIV (at high confluency). The description of the constructs and cell culture protocols have been previously reported [14]. In the present application, the HEK-GABA cells express the $\alpha5\beta3\gamma2s$ subunits of the $GABA_A$ receptor.

2. Prepare serial-dilutions of 5 known $GABA_A$ agonists in a NaSCN assay buffer. This buffer is to maximize the chloride current upon $GABA_A$-receptor activation. The agonists are GABA, isoguvacine hydrochloride (Sigma Aldrich), muscimol (Toronto Research Chemicals), pip-4-sulfonic acid, and gaboxadol (THIP) (Santa Cruz Biotechnology). Compounds are serially diluted (0.01–100 µM, with two dilutions per log) in the NaSCN assay buffer before application.

3. Acquire a control image on the cells in culture medium just before addition of a $GABA_A$ agonist for each well.

4. Remove the culture medium in each well and replace with the NaSCN assay buffer containing the serial-dilution of the $GABA_A$ agonists.

5. Acquire images of cells 8 min after agonist treatment using DHM equipped with a 10×/0.22 NA objective. Record four images per well at the speed of about 4 min per 96-well plate.

6. Obtain average OPD values on the control and stimulated conditions.

7. Subtract control data points for each well to reduce inter-well variability.

8. Calculate EC_{50} for each of the compounds by fitted data, for instance using Prism 6 (GraphPad software, La Jolla, California) using the *log (agonist) vs. response 4 parameter* fitting option.

The measured EC_{50} values were ranked and compared to electrophysiology recordings (Fig. 7) (performed according to the protocol described in ref. [14]) using cells obtained from the same culture. The values and ranking measured by DHM and electrophysiology are in good agreement. It should be noted that it only took 30 min to generate all the data points with DHM whereas with electrophysiology 2 full working days were necessary, mostly due to the fact that electrophysiological recordings can only be performed on a single cell at a time.

The differences in efficacy between the agonists tested are due to the fact that gaboxadol and isoguvacine are partial agonists of

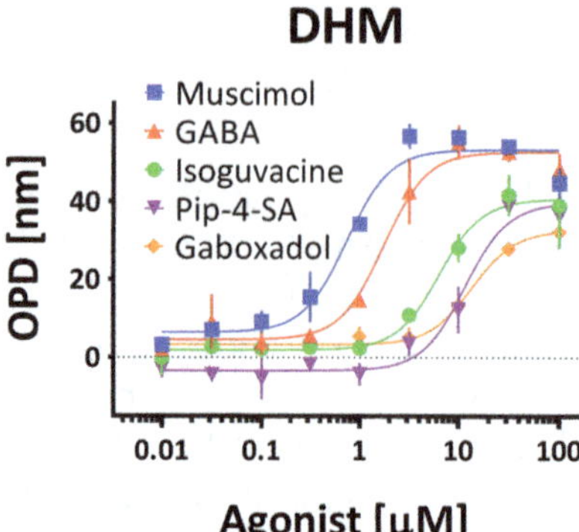

Compound	EC_{50} (µM)	
	DHM	Electrophysiology
Muscimol	0.74	1.00
GABA	1.75	1.86
Isoguvacine	6.41	9.79
Pip-4-SA	11.7	10.4
Gaboxadol	13.8	11.4

Fig. 7 EC_{50} ranking of $GABA_A$ agonists by DHI and electrophysiology. Five known specific $GABA_A$ agonists were measured using the DHM "optical electrode" and on a patch-clamp setup. EC_{50} obtained by both methods were in excellent agreement. Data are mean ± SEM

GABA-receptor [33, 34]. Differences in potency for the panel of agonists tested are expected for different subunits composition of $GABA_A$ [35, 36].

4   Conclusions and Future Prospects

Running comparative screens using different cell types would allow selecting profiled compounds according to the phenotypes generated as illustrated in the proof-of-principle exercise reported here. Moreover, the highly informative aspect of the analyzed data provide insights about the cellular phenotypes generated and possible indications about the mechanism of action of the drugs for a given cell type. This contributes to the annotation of compounds for an appropriate selection or prioritization of screening hits.

In addition to traditional phenotypic screens, cellular target-based assays can be performed by DHI as illustrated in the present work for the chloride channel $GABA_A$ receptor. Furthermore, it has been demonstrated that the activity of the therapeutically important chloride related receptor CFTR can also be monitored by DHM, opening new opportunities for the development of high-content assays for this group of receptors with expected higher throughput.

The convenient utilization of DHM for time-lapse experiments during several days for various experimental conditions represents an important advantage in terms of real time monitoring of cellular events provoked by the action of interfering compounds.

In summary, label-free quantitative DHM imaging is a technique delivering HCS data that can be scalable in throughput by the combination of easily implemented, fast, and cost-effective methodological approaches.

5 Notes

1. The acquisition speed should be fast enough to sample the response of the biological system investigated. The current maximum speed for acquiring four images per well in a 96-well plate is less than 4 min. If faster acquisitions are needed, only a few wells can be imaged (minimum acquisition speed for a single image, 400 µs). The length of the acquisition is also dictated by the experimental requirements but can last for few days, provided that cells are maintained in a controlled environment.

2. The experimental questions would define the choice of microscope objective magnification. Generally a Leica 10×/0.22 NA (Leica Microsystems GmbH, Wetzlar, Germany, ref. 11506263) offers the best compromise between sampling a large number of cells per field of view and good resolution. A 20×/0.4 could be preferred if subcellular structures (vesicles, nucleus shape, etc.) are investigated. A minimum of about 30 cells should be imaged per condition. Magnifications between 4× and 40× are commonly used. Air objectives are preferred for ease of use (longer working distance and no need for oil or water addition).

3. For instance, to discriminate dead cells after treatment with doxorubicin the training sets were defined as follows: "control" (untreated, elongated, and well-attached cells), "round" (round and intense cells—used for cells treated with doxorubicin), or segmentation error objects (Fig. 2). Other classes of objects could be created, depending on the type of cytotoxicity assay performed. For example a "vesicles" class could be used for cells treated with chloroquine, defined by less attached cells with presence of small and round vesicles [9]. This exemplifies also the types of assays that require the use of higher microscope objectives, 20× instead of 10× in the case of DHM-based assays.

Acknowledgements

This work was supported by the CTI program (grant No. 12669.1 PFLS-LS). The authors thank the staff of Lyncée Tec SA for their technical support on the DHM imaging system, Sandra Borel and Nathalie Ballanfat from the BSF-EPFL for cell preparation and culture, Dr. Pascal Jourdain for electrophysiology experiments, and Dr. Marc Chambon for fruitful discussions and pertinent comments about the manuscript.

References

1. Bickle M (2010) The beautiful cell: high-content screening in drug discovery. Anal Bioanal Chem 398(1):219–226. doi:10.1007/s00216-010-3788-3

2. McCoy JP Jr (2011) High-content screening: getting more from less. Nat Methods 8(5):390–391. doi:10.1038/nmeth.1599

3. Kell DB (2013) Finding novel pharmaceuticals in the systems biology era using multiple effective drug targets, phenotypic screening and knowledge of transporters: where drug discovery went wrong and how to fix it. FEBS J 280(23):5957–5980. doi:10.1111/febs.12268

4. Wagner M, Weber P, Bruns T, Strauss WS, Wittig R, Schneckenburger H (2010) Light dose is a limiting factor to maintain cell viability in fluorescence microscopy and single molecule detection. Int J Mol Sci 11(3):956–966. doi:10.3390/ijms11030956

5. Schneckenburger H, Weber P, Wagner M, Schickinger S, Richter V, Bruns T, Strauss WS, Wittig R (2012) Light exposure and cell viability in fluorescence microscopy. J Microsc 245(3):311–318. doi:10.1111/j.1365-2818.2011.03576.x

6. Le Harzic R, Riemann I, König K, Wüllner C, Donitzky C (2007) Influence of femtosecond laser pulse irradiation on the viability of cells at 1035, 517, and 345 nm. J Appl Phys 102(11):114701. doi:10.1063/1.2818107

7. Graves R (2011) Incorporating transmitted light modalities into high-content analysis assays. In: Mayr LM, Cooper M (eds) Label-free technologies for drug discovery. Wiley, Chichester, West Sussex, pp 101–110

8. Kuhn J, Shaffer E, Mena J, Breton B, Parent J, Rappaz B, Chambon M, Emery Y, Magistretti P, Depeursinge C, Marquet P, Turcatti G (2013) Label-free cytotoxity screening assay by digital holographic microscopy. Assay Drug Dev Technol 11(2):101–107. doi:10.1089/adt.2012.476

9. Rappaz B, Breton B, Shaffer E, Turcatti G (2014) Digital holographic microscopy: a quantitative label-free microscopy technique for phenotypic screening. Comb Chem High Throughput Screen 17(1):80–88, CCHTS-EPUB-56550

10. Marquet P, Rappaz B, Magistretti PJ, Cuche E, Emery Y, Colomb T, Depeursinge C (2005) Digital holographic microscopy: a noninvasive contrast imaging technique allowing quantitative visualization of living cells with subwavelength axial accuracy. Opt Lett 30(5):468–470. doi:10.1364/OL.30.000468

11. Moon I, Daneshpanah M, Anand A, Javidi B (2011) Cell identification computational 3-D holographic microscopy. Opt Photon News 22(6):18–23. doi:10.1364/OPN.22.6.000018

12. Rappaz B, Barbul A, Emery Y, Korenstein R, Depeursinge C, Magistretti PJ, Marquet P (2008) Comparative study of human erythrocytes by digital holographic microscopy, confocal microscopy, and impedance volume analyzer. Cytometry A 73(10):895–903. doi:10.1002/cyto.a.20605

13. Rappaz B, Cano E, Colomb T, Kuhn J, Depeursinge C, Simanis V, Magistretti PJ, Marquet P (2009) Noninvasive characterization of the fission yeast cell cycle by monitoring dry mass with digital holographic microscopy. J Biomed Opt 14(3):034049. doi:10.1117/1.3147385

14. Jourdain P, Boss D, Rappaz B, Moratal C, Hernandez MC, Depeursinge C, Magistretti PJ, Marquet P (2012) Simultaneous optical recording in multiple cells by digital holographic microscopy of chloride current associated to activation of the ligand-gated chloride channel GABA(A) receptor. PLoS One 7(12): e51041. doi:10.1371/journal.pone.0051041

15. Jourdain P, Becq F, Lengacher S, Boinot C, Magistretti PJ, Marquet P (2014) The human CFTR protein expressed in CHO cells activates aquaporin-3 in a cAMP-dependent pathway: study by digital holographic microscopy. J Cell Sci 127(Pt 3):546–556. doi:10.1242/jcs.133629

16. Colomb T, Pavillon N, Kuhn J, Cuche E, Depeursinge C, Emery Y (2010) Extended depth-of-focus by digital holographic microscopy. Opt Lett 35(11):1840–1842. doi:10.1364/OL.35.001840

17. Ferraro P, Grilli S, Alfieri D, Nicola SD, Finizio A, Pierattini G, Javidi B, Coppola G, Striano V (2005) Extended focused image in microscopy by digital Holography. Opt Express 13(18):6738–6749. doi:10.1364/OPEX.13.006738

18. Jourdain P, Pavillon N, Moratal C, Boss D, Rappaz B, Depeursinge C, Marquet P, Magistretti PJ (2011) Determination of transmembrane water fluxes in neurons elicited by glutamate ionotropic receptors and by the cotransporters KCC2 and NKCC1: a digital holographic microscopy study. J Neurosci 31(33):11846–11854, 31/33/11846

19. Pavillon N, Kuhn J, Moratal C, Jourdain P, Depeursinge C, Magistretti PJ, Marquet P (2012) Early cell death detection with digital holographic microscopy. PLoS One 7(1): e30912. doi:10.1371/journal.pone.0030912

20. Carpenter AE, Jones TR, Lamprecht MR, Clarke C, Kang IH, Friman O, Guertin DA,

Chang JH, Lindquist RA, Moffat J, Golland P, Sabatini DM (2006) Cell Profiler: image analysis software for identifying and quantifying cell phenotypes. Genome Biol 7(10):R100, gb-2006-7-10-r100

21. Jones TR, Kang IH, Wheeler DB, Lindquist RA, Papallo A, Sabatini DM, Golland P, Carpenter AE (2008) Cell profiler analyst: data exploration and analysis software for complex image-based screens. BMC Bioinformatics 9:482. doi:10.1186/1471-2105-9-482

22. Zhang J-H, Chung TDY, Oldenburg KR (1999) A simple statistical parameter for use in evaluation and validation of high throughput screening assays. J Biomol Screen 4(2):67–73. doi:10.1177/108705719900400206

23. Kozak K, Csucs G (2010) Kernelized Z' factor in multiparametric screening technology. RNA Biol 7(5):615–620. doi:10.4161/rna.7.5.13239

24. Zhang YW, Shi J, Li YJ, Wei L (2009) Cardiomyocyte death in doxorubicin-induced cardiotoxicity. Arch Immunol Ther Exp (Warsz) 57(6):435–445. doi:10.1007/s00005-009-0051-8

25. Skoufias DA, Wilson L (1992) Mechanism of inhibition of microtubule polymerization by colchicine: inhibitory potencies of unliganded colchicine and tubulin-colchicine complexes. Biochemistry 31(3):738–746

26. Friedl P, Wolf K (2003) Tumour-cell invasion and migration: diversity and escape mechanisms. Nat Rev Cancer 3(5):362–374. doi:10.1038/nrc1075

27. Hayot C, Debeir O, Van Ham P, Van Damme M, Kiss R, Decaestecker C (2006) Characterization of the activities of actin-affecting drugs on tumor cell migration. Toxicol Appl Pharmacol 211(1):30–40. doi:10.1016/j.taap.2005.06.006

28. Godman G, Woda B, Kolberg R, Berl S (1980) Redistribution of contractile and cytoskeletal components induced by cytochalasin. II. In HeLa and HEp2 cells. Eur J Cell Biol 22(2): 745–754

29. Yarrow JC, Perlman ZE, Westwood NJ, Mitchison TJ (2004) A high-throughput cell migration assay using scratch wound healing, a comparison of image-based readout methods. BMC Biotechnol 4:21. doi:10.1186/1472-6750-4-21

30. Harrington WN, Godman GC (1980) A selective inhibitor of cell proliferation from normal serum. Proc Natl Acad Sci U S A 77(1): 423–427

31. Godman G, Woda B, Kolberg R, Berl S (1980) Redistribution of contractile and cytoskeletal components induced by cytochalasin. I. In Hmf cells, a nontransformed fibroblastoid line. Eur J Cell Biol 22(2):733–744

32. Rappaz B, Marquet P, Cuche E, Emery Y, Depeursinge C, Magistretti P (2005) Measurement of the integral refractive index and dynamic cell morphometry of living cells with digital holographic microscopy. Opt Express 13(23):9361–9373. doi:10.1364/OPEX.13.009361

33. Karobath M, Lippitsch M (1979) THIP and isoguvacine are partial agonists of GABA-stimulated benzodiazepine receptor binding. Eur J Pharmacol 58(4):485–488

34. Mortensen M, Kristiansen U, Ebert B, Frolund B, Krogsgaard-Larsen P, Smart TG (2004) Activation of single heteromeric GABA(A) receptor ion channels by full and partial agonists. J Physiol 557(Pt 2):389–413. doi:10.1113/jphysiol.2003.054734

35. Mortensen M, Wafford KA, Wingrove P, Ebert B (2003) Pharmacology of GABAA receptors exhibiting different levels of spontaneous activity. Eur J Pharmacol 476(1–2):17–24. doi:10.1016/S0014-2999(03)02125-3

36. Hansen SL, Ebert B, Fjalland B, Kristiansen U (2001) Effects of GABA(A) receptor partial agonists in primary cultures of cerebellar granule neurons and cerebral cortical neurons reflect different receptor subunit compositions. Br J Pharmacol 133(4):539–549. doi:10.1038/sj.bjp.0704121

Chapter 18

Label-Free Profiling of Cell Adhesion: Determination of the Dissociation Constant for Native Cell Membrane Adhesion Receptor-Ligand Interaction

Norbert Orgovan, Beatrix Peter, Szilvia Bősze, Jeremy J. Ramsden, Bálint Szabó, and Robert Horvath

Abstract

Here we describe the protocol and workflow for a label-free cell adhesion assay utilizing the high-throughput Epic BenchTop (BT) optical biosensor. We also describe how the dissociation constant for the binding between integrins in their native cell membrane and their ligands immobilized on the planar sensor surface can be determined from the biosensor data. To achieve this, cell adhesion has to be measured on surfaces having fine-tuned ligand densities. The present protocol can be applied to determine the dissociation constant of the binding between any matrix adhesion receptor embedded in its native cell membrane and its ligand, provided that a coating molecule with appropriate functionalization is available. The effect of drugs or other chemicals on this molecular interaction and subsequent cellular adhesion can be investigated in a straightforward way.

Key words Adhesion kinetics, Adhesion tailoring, Cell adhesion, Integrin, RGD-tuning, Optical biosensor, Resonant waveguide grating

1 Introduction

Cellular adhesion is central to life. Cells usually establish an anchorage with the extracellular matrix or neighboring cells in the tissue using cell adhesion receptors embedded in the cell membrane, such as integrins [1, 2], cadherins [3], selectins [4], syndecans [5], and the immunglobulin superfamily of adhesion receptors [6]. Since nowadays many modern drugs intervene at the level of cellular adhesion [7–9], there is an ever-increasing demand for techniques that enable the effects of such drugs to be screened in a straightforward and reliable way which moreover produce highly informative (e.g., multiparameter and/or kinetic) data.

Traditional methods for measuring cellular adhesion, including phase-contrast microscopy or mechanical assays, where the adhered

Ye Fang (ed.), *Label-Free Biosensor Methods in Drug Discovery*, Methods in Pharmacology and Toxicology, DOI 10.1007/978-1-4939-2617-6_18, © Springer Science+Business Media New York 2015

cells are subjected to a fluid flow, are cumbersome and hence generally unsuitable for (1) high throughput needed in drug discovery, and (2) kinetic monitoring with high temporal resolution and high signal-to-noise ratio. In contrast, surface-sensitive label-free biosensors are inherently capable of generating good-quality kinetic data. Evanescent field-based label-free optical biosensors including optical waveguide lightmode spectroscopy (OWLS) [10–16], photonic crystal biosensors [17], grating coupling interferometry (GCI) [18–20], and resonant waveguide grating (RWG or Epic) biosensors [21, 22] are considered to be especially straightforward means to monitor cell adhesion, since they can in situ detect refractive index changes in the 100–200 nm thick layer closest to the sensor surface, where the anchorage between the cell and its substratum takes place [10, 23]. Moreover, the probing depth of these biosensors can be fine-tuned through waveguide structure design, so dynamic information from various depths can be simultaneously collected using multimode waveguides [24–26], potentially permitting the monitoring of changes inside the cell or in its nucleus triggered by surface adhesion [26].

In the present protocol we describe how the adhesion kinetics of living cells on a surface coated with integrin ligands can be characterized in detail. We use an optical biosensor, an Epic BenchTop (BT) system system (*see* **Note 1**), to monitor cell adhesion with unprecedented quality in a high-throughput way. The biosensor data recorded at various ligand densities are used to determine the dissociation constant, so the binding between the RGD ligand and its adhesion receptors embedded in their native cell membrane is characterized in a label-free and perturbation-free manner [22]. Of note, the present protocol is equally applicable for other types of ligands and adhesion receptors and can also be used to measure the effects of drugs interfering with cell adhesion.

2   Materials

2.1 Instruments and Microplates

1. Epic BenchTop system (Corning Incorporated, Corning, NY, USA) (*see* **Note 1**).

2. Corning Epic 96- or 384-well biosensor microplate (*see* **Notes 1** and **2**).

2.2 Solutions for Cell Culture

1. Complete culture medium: Dulbecco's modified Eagle's medium (DMEM) supplemented with 10 % fetal bovine serum (FBS), 4 mM L-glutamine (*see* **Note 3**), 40 μg/ml gentamycin, 0.25 μg/ml amphotericin B. Store the complete medium at 2–8 °C for short periods.

2. Washing solution: 1× phosphate-buffered saline (PBS, obtained from Sigma).

3. Cell detachment solution: 1.0 % or less trypsin-EDTA, or EDTA without trypsin, or Accutane, or Cellstripper (*see* **Note 4**).

2.3 Buffers

1. Buffer for surface coating solutions: 10 mM *N-2-hydroxyethylpiperazine*-N-2-ethane sulfonic acid (HEPES, Sigma), pH 7.4. Sterile solutions are stable under normal conditions.

2. Buffer for cell adhesion assays: Hank's balanced salt solution (HBSS, from Sigma) supplemented with 20 mM HEPES. Store at 15–30 °C.

2.4 Surface Coating Materials

1. Poly(L-lysine)-graft-poly(ethylene glycol) (PLL-*g*-PEG, from SuSoS AG, Dübendorf, Switzerland) (*see* **Note 5**).

2. PLL-*g*-PEG/PEG-GGGGYGRGDSP (PLL-*g*-PEG-RGD, from SuSoS AG, Dübendorf, Switzerland) (*see* **Note 6**).

Prepare separate stock solutions from PLL-*g*-PEG and PLL-*g*-PEG-RGD by dissolving their powders in 10 mM HEPES, pH 7.4 to a concentration of 0.5–1.0 mg/ml (*see* **Note 6**). The concentration of the two stock solutions should be set the same. Powders stored at < −20 °C remain functional for 1 year or more. Solutions sterilized by filtration through 0.22 μm pores can be stored at 4 °C for 2 weeks or at −20 °C for up to 3 months.

3 Methods

3.1 Cell Adhesion Assay on the Epic BT

1. Mix the PLL-*g*-PEG and PLL-*g*-PEG-RGD solutions in different ratios to create coating solutions with different amounts of RGD.

2. Pre-wet the biosensors with the buffer used to prepare the coating solutions (*see* **Notes 2, 7**, and **8**), place the microplate in the Epic BT instrument, and establish a baseline. Experiments should be done at least in triplicate (3 wells per treatment) with the appropriate controls (e.g., wells lacking RGD) (Fig. 1).

3. Following the stabilization of the Epic baseline signal (<5 pm/5 min, generally taking 30 min), pause the measurement, take out the plate, replace the buffer with the coating solutions, and incubate on a mini rocker shaker for 0.5 h at room temperature (*see* **Note 9**).

4. Place the plate back into the Epic BT instrument and restart the measurement to record the signal arising due to the adsorption from the coating solutions. Continue monitoring until saturation is reached (5–10 min).

5. Take the plate out of the instrument. Remove the coating solutions and rinse the wells three times with the assay buffer to remove any unabsorbed/reversibly adsorbed material from the wells, and dose the wells with fresh assay buffer.

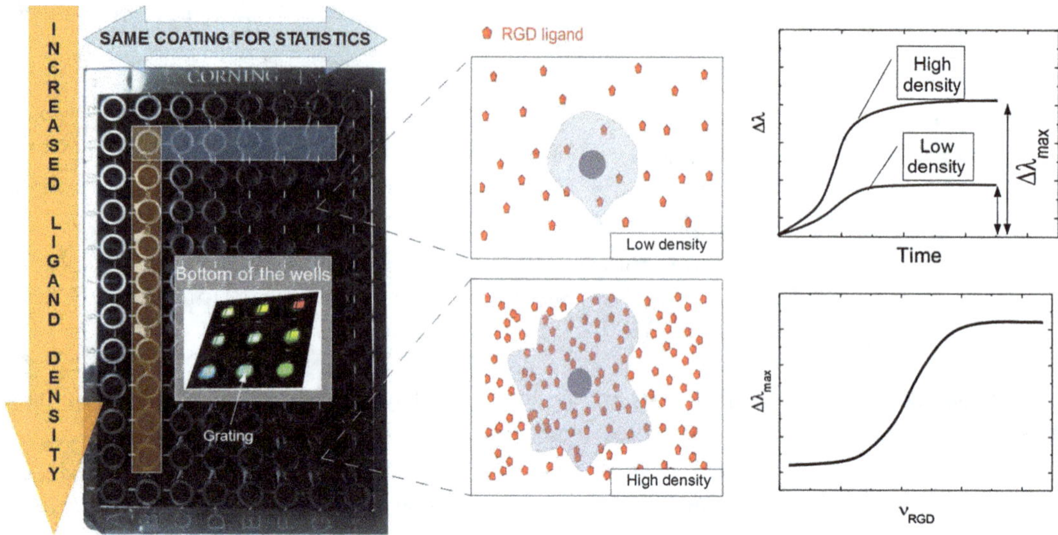

Fig. 1 Monitoring the adhesion kinetics of cells with an Epic biosensor on different ligand densities enables the dissociation constant characterizing the interaction of native cell membrane receptors and their ligands to be determined. On the *left*, a photograph of an SBS-standard 96-well Epic sensor microplate is shown. Each well contains a biosensor (a 2×2 mm nano-grating embedded in a high-refractive index waveguiding film) at its bottom; the nano-gratings are visible due to diffraction (shown for nine wells imaged from the back of the plate in the inset *lower right*). To determine the dissociation constant of the binding between adhesion ligands and their receptors embedded in their native cell membrane, the adhesion process has to be measured at different ligand densities (here: RGD densities). In the illustrating image, replicates are in the same column (shown in *blue*), and ligand densities are increased from row to row (shown in *orange*). Very low surface ligand densities fail to promote cell adhesion, while cells spread extensively on surfaces presenting a high number of ligands (compare the images in the *middle*), giving rise to a bigger biosensor signal (schematic graph in the *top right corner*). The sigmoidal spreading curves measured at different ligand densities are fitted one by one with the logistic Eq. (5) to determine the maximum biosensor signal, the rate constant of spreading, and the time of inflexion ($\Delta\lambda_{max}$, r, m, respectively). The interaction between the adhesion receptors and their ligands immobilized on the surface are considered as a monovalent binding reaction, and the data replotted as $\Delta\lambda_{max}$ against ν_{RGD} (RGD density on the surface, $[\nu_{RGD}] = \mu m^{-2}$) can be fitted with Eq. (7) describing the steady state of such a reaction (schematic graph in *bottom right corner*). Fitting yields the value of the two-dimensional dissociation constant, from which the three-dimensional dissociation constant can be easily obtained, Eq. (8)

6. Place the microplate back into the instrument and establish a new baseline for the subsequent cell spreading assay.

7. Pre-warm the culturing medium, PBS, and cell dissociation solution to 37 °C. Harvest the cells as usual (*see* **Notes 4** and **10**), then centrifuge, and resuspend them in the cell adhesion assay buffer. Prepare a cell suspension with an appropriate number of cells.

8. Pause the measurement and take out the plate.

9. Seed the cells (*see* **Note 11**), rapidly replace the plate in the instrument, and resume the measurement. Ideally, all cells

should sediment simultaneously, resulting in a uniform distribution of cells on the bottom of the wells [16].

10. Monitor cell spreading until the biosensor signals reach a steady state (generally 2–4 h) (*see* **Notes 12** and **13**).

11. Take out the plate and investigate the cells under a phase-contrast microscope.

In adhesion receptor-targeted drug discovery, the workflow of the assay is somewhat different than the adhesion assay described above (*see* **Note 14**).

3.2 Estimation of the Average Number of Ligands per Unit Area

1. Calculate the molar surface density (ρ_{RGD}) from the mixing ratio of the two copolymer solutions [22, 27]:

$$\rho_{RGD} = \frac{\Gamma}{M_{Pol}} \frac{Q}{100} \frac{N_{Lys}}{g} P, \tag{1}$$

where Γ is the mass per unit area adsorbed to the smooth surface, M_{Pol} is the molecular weight of the RGD-functionalized copolymer, Q is the volume percent of the PLL-*g*-PEG-RGD solution in the mixed solution of copolymers, $N_{Lys} = 96$ is the average number of lysine monomers in a PLL backbone, $g = 3.7$ is the grafting ratio (giving the number of Lys units per PEG side chain), and $P = 0.12$ is the fraction of RGD-functionalized PEG chains in the PLL-*g*-PEG-RGD molecules [27]. These values are for the products we actually used in our experiments but may be different for different products. M_{Pol} is estimated from the approximate molecular weights of the components of the corresponding copolymer, i.e., that of the PLL backbone $\left(M_{PLL} = 14\,\text{kDa}\right)$, the unfunctionalized PEG side chains $\left(M_{PEG} = 2.3\,\text{kDa}\right)$, the PEG side chains for functionalization $\left(M_{PEG*} = 3.4\,\text{kDa}\right)$, and the peptide $\left(M_{RGD} = 1035\,\text{Da}\right)$:

$$M_{Pol} = M_{PLL} + \frac{N_{Lys}}{g}\left\{(1-P)M_{PEG} + P\left(M_{PEG*} + M_{RGD}\right)\right\}. \tag{2}$$

This yields $M_{Pol} = 80.3\,\text{kDa}$. The mass surface density of the copolymers adsorbed to a Nb_2O_5 substratum has been reported to be $\Gamma \approx 184$ ng cm^{-2} (independently of *g* or *P*) [28].

2. Calculate the average ligand-to-ligand distance. Assuming a hexagonal distribution of ligands the following equation can be used [27]:

$$d_{RGD-RGD} = \sqrt{\frac{2}{\sqrt{3}}\frac{1}{\rho_{RGD}\cdot N_A}}, \tag{3}$$

where N_A is Avogadro's number $\left(N_A = 6.022\cdot 10^{23}\ \text{mol}^{-1}\right)$.

3. Estimate the average number of ligands per unit area as

$$\nu_{\mathrm{RGD}} = \frac{F}{\left(d_{\mathrm{RGD-RGD}}/2\right)^2 \pi}, \tag{4}$$

where $F \approx 0.9069$ is the proportion of the surface covered by non-overlapping circles of equal sizes packed in a hexagonal arrangement [22].

3.3 Calculating the Three-Dimensional (3D) Dissociation Constant from the Biosensor Data

1. Carry out background correction on the raw data by subtracting the signal from the control wells coated with pure PLL-*g*-PEG from the other signals from the RGD-coating wells.

2. Fit the logistic function to the background-corrected spreading curves measured in individual wells [11, 22]:

$$\lambda(t) = \frac{\lambda_{\max}}{1 + \exp\left(-r\left(t - m\right)\right)}, \tag{5}$$

where $\Delta\lambda_{\max}$ is the signal value at the maximum (plateau) of the spreading curve, termed *spreading constraint*, r is the *rate constant of spreading*, and m is the constant of integration, which gives the time when inflexion occurs, at which the ordinate is exactly $\Delta\lambda_{\max}/2$ [11]. We found that cell spreading data can usually be well fitted with this equation. This three-parameter equation is the simplest one that describes a sigmoidal curve, but has an inherent limitation; the sigmoid is symmetrical.

3. Calculate the mean and standard deviation of the three parameters from the replicates.

4. Plot $\Delta\lambda_{\max}$ against ν_{RGD} (Fig. 1). Consider the receptor-ligand interaction as a first-order reaction. Denoting the 2D (surface) concentrations of the unbound ligand (RGD), unbound receptor (integrin), and their bound form as L, I and B, respectively, the receptor-ligand reaction is

$$L + I \underset{k_{\mathrm{a}}}{\overset{k_{\mathrm{d}}}{\rightleftharpoons}} B. \tag{6}$$

According to the kinetic mass action law (KMAL), at steady state (equilibrium) the attachment and detachment reactions characterized by 2D (two-dimensional) rate coefficients k_{a} and k_{d}, respectively, have equal rates and

$$B_{\mathrm{eqm}} = \frac{L_0 I_0}{L_0 + {}^{2\mathrm{D}}K_{\mathrm{d}}}, \tag{7}$$

where $L_0 = L + B = \nu_{RGD}$, $I_0 = I + B$, and $^{2D}K_d = k_d / k_a$ is the two-dimensional dissociation constant. We assume that B_{eqm} is directly proportional to the optical response measured at saturation ($\Delta\lambda_{max}$). Thus, fitting Eq. (7) to the data replotted as $\Delta\lambda_{max}$ vs. ν_{RGD}, one can obtain K_d for the interaction between the RGD-specific integrins and their ligand immobilized on the surface [22].

5. Calculate the three-dimensional dissociation constant using the following relation:

$$^{3D}K_d = \frac{^{2D}K_d}{l_c},\tag{8}$$

where l_c is a characteristic length of the interacting systems, commonly referred to as the confinement length [29, 30]. We assume that l_c is the average cell-substrate separation distance: the extent of separation is the result of the combined effect of nonspecific repulsion and specific bonding forces between the cell and the underlying substrate [29]. Various techniques including internal reflection microscopy [31], surface plasmon resonance microscopy [32], and impedance-based biosensing [33] have been utilized to determine the separation distance, and the obtained average values are typically in the range of $40 - 160$ nm . Lacking more precise information, an assumption of $l_c = 100$ nm seems to be reasonable in most cases [22].

Following this procedure, we have previously determined the three-dimensional dissociation constant characterizing the interaction of the RGD motifs (of the PLL-*g*-PEG-RGD molecule) and the native RGD-specific integrins of HeLa cells [22]. The obtained value, $^{3D}K_d \approx 30$ μM, was compared to previous experimental values determined by others, and taking into account the multiple differences in both the investigated systems and the utilized techniques, it was considered to be a highly reasonable value [22].

4 Notes

1. The Epic BT system [22, 34, 35] enables high-throughput label-free detection of molecules at a solid–liquid interface. The instrument accepts 96- or 384-well *Society for Biomolecular Screening* (SBS) standard format Epic biosensor microplates. The bottom of each well of the Epic microplate is a planar optical waveguide. It is a thin layer of niobium pentoxide (which has a high refractive index, and is transparent and biocompatible) deposited on a thicker glass substratum. An optical grating, positioned in the center of each well and covering

about half the area, is embedded into the waveguide to incouple the illuminating beam. Incoupled light undergoes total internal reflections at the inner surfaces of the waveguide, and its phase is shifted upon each reflection. The extent of the acquired phase shift depends on the refractive index (RI) of the medium closest to the reflecting surface (because an exponentially decaying evanescent electromagnetic field penetrates into a ~ 150 nm thick layer of the neighboring medium where it probes the local RI [10, 12, 23]). Waveguiding occurs only at a certain illuminating wavelength, called the resonant wavelength (λ). Any process accompanied by RI variations in the ~ 150 nm thick layer over the biosensor surface (e.g., medium RI change, molecular adsorption, density change due to cellular spreading, mass redistribution inside the surface-adhered cells) alters the acquired phase shift. This detunes the resonance, but waveguiding can resume at a different illuminating wavelength $\lambda' \neq \lambda$. The primary signal output of the Epic BT system is the shift of the resonant wavelength $\left(\Delta\lambda = \lambda' - \lambda \right)$ in each well. $\Delta\lambda$ is proportional to the alteration in the effective refractive index N of the substrate-cell-medium system. At constant cell number and cell volume, N is related in a simple way to the degree of spreading [10, 13, 36].

In practice, all wells of an Epic microplate are simultaneously interrogated every 3 s by sweeping the illuminating wavelength through a range of 15,000 pm with 0.25 pm precision [34]. The guided light is outcoupled by the same grating as that used for incoupling, and the resonant wavelength distribution from the grating area within each well is imaged with a spatial resolution of ~90 μm using a complementary metal oxide semiconductor (CMOS) camera. The two-dimensional resonant wavelength map allows patterns in single wells (corresponding to areas of, e.g., aggregated spread cells, or a group of dead ones in a cellular monolayer) to be identified and permits data filtration to improve image quality.

The small footprint and tolerance to high temperatures of the Epic BT allow one to place it into a non-humidified cell culture incubator and, therefore, the environmental conditions that cells experience in vivo can be better approximated during the experiment.

2. If an experiment does not require the throughput offered by a 96- or 384-well Epic microplate, then seal the unused wells with an aluminum foil to keep them sterile until future use (specially cut foil is available from Corning).

3. L-Glutamine is unstable in solution if stored at +2 °C or higher temperatures; it has a half-life of approximately 1 month if stored in the refrigerator. Importantly, the degradation of L-glutamine leads to NH_4^+ which can be toxic for cells if accumulated. It is the best to add L-glutamine to the solution directly before use.

4. Trypsin can dramatically alter the adhesion properties of cells by cleaving adhesion receptors, including integrins [37]. Therefore, the duration of trypsinization should be minimized. It is even better to use the chelator EDTA in itself, or Accutase, or the non-enzymatic dissociation solution called Cellstripper to gently release spread cells from a surface.

5. PLL-*g*-PEG is a synthetic copolymer designed to be protein resistant and cell repellent if adsorbed to a surface [38, 39]. PLL-*g*-PEG-RGD is the RGD-functionalized counterpart of PLL-*g*-PEG. The RGD tripeptide is a minimal recognition sequence of a group of integrins [40, 41], which are the major receptors establishing the connection between cells and the neighboring extracellular matrix. Surface-adsorbed PLL-*g*-PEG-RGD is designed to specifically trigger cell adhesion [22, 28].

6. PLL-*g*-PEG and PLL-*g*-PEG-RGD in their powder form tend to acquire an electrostatic charge and become difficult to handle.

7. If possible, leave the wells around the edges of the microplate empty. Results measured in the wells closest to the edge of the microplate tend to be significantly different than those measured in wells closer to the center, a phenomenon called the edge effect. The edge effect is likely caused by several factors that are hard to identify and characterize. The most important is that edges of the plate heat or cool at a different rate than areas closer to the center of the plate, and as one result, the evaporation rate in these wells will also be different.

8. Upon filling the microplate wells, air bubbles can potentially remain near the sensor surface. Since an air bubble has a grossly different refractive index compared to the liquid medium or analyte, its presence would severely distort the biosensor experiment—therefore great care has to be taken to check whether there are bubbles near the surface of the sensors, and eliminate them if any.

9. The molecular layers created from PLL-*g*-PEG and PLL-*g*-PEG-RGD may be imperfect and molecules secreted by the cells may unspecifically adsorb to the surface at locations of small defects in the PEG brushes [22, 27]. Adsorption should be minimized as its direct contribution to the biosensor signal makes the data harder to evaluate and interpret. If significant nonspecific adsorption occurs, try creating ultradense PLL-*g*-PEG layers by incubating the coating solutions at high temperatures which diminishes the number of small defects [39]. On a surface containing PLL-*g*-PEG-RGD, secreted material might specifically bind the amino acid sequence used for functionalization. If the biosensor signal does not fully resemble a

sigmoidal spreading curve, but rather a sigmoid superposed on a hyperbolic adsorption signal, then the data set might be ambiguous and is more difficult to interpret.

10. Serum starvation of cells prior to the experiment may help to get more consistent results as the cells will be in the same cell cycle state. To achieve starvation, cells should be placed in serum-free culture medium for typically 12–24 h. Shorter generation times will require shorter incubation times.

11. Seeding numbers should be chosen in a way to minimize the number of cell-cell contacts while maximizing the number of cells in each well. We found empirically that 8,000–10,000 and 3,000–5,000 cells per well for a 96 and a 384 microplate generally gave satisfactory results.

12. The biosensor response—integrating changes in both the size of the contact area and the optical density therein (dependent on the extents of actin cytoskeleton polymerization, integrin clustering, adhesion complex formation and maturation, etc.)—is a more accurate measure of cell adhesion and spreading than those measures predominantly used in microscope image analysis (number of attached cells and average contact area) [22].

13. For many cell types, it may have greater biological relevance to carry out experiments at 37 °C rather than at ambient conditions. This can be done by placing the Epic BT into a (non-humidified) incubator. However, evaporation from the limited-volume sample wells may cause the osmolality of the medium to significantly increase which stresses the cells. To avoid this, seal the top of the wells with a special gas-permeable film (breathable sealing tape, Corning cat. no. #3345).

14. In adhesion receptor-targeted drug discovery, the workflow of the assay is somewhat different than the simple adhesion assay described in this protocol. The ideal experimental design may depend on the presumed mechanism of effect of the given drug, and different approaches often yield complementary information. For a drug that intervenes at the level of the adhesion receptors themselves or the adhesion cascade (thus targets the cell and not its environment, i.e., the ligands of the adhesion receptors), basically three strategies exist. One may (1) preincubate the cells with the effector molecule, then remove the excess material, and monitor the mid- to long time effects of the treatment; (2) add the drug to the cell suspension and directly afterwards initiate the cell spreading assay to investigate how the kinetics of the adhesion process is altered; (3) begin the treatment and the Epic measurement after the cells already obtained their characteristic well-spread morphology in the wells of the biosensor microplate.

References

1. Barczyk M, Carracedo S, Gullberg D (2010) Integrins. Cell Tissue Res 339:269–280. doi:10.1007/s00441-009-0834-6

2. García AJ (2005) Get a grip: integrins in cell-biomaterial interactions. Biomaterials 26:7525–7529. doi:10.1016/j.biomaterials.2005.05.029

3. Patel SD, Chen CP, Bahna F et al (2003) Cadherin-mediated cell–cell adhesion: sticking together as a family. Curr Opin Struct Biol 13:690–698. doi:10.1016/j.sbi.2003.10.007

4. McEver RP (2002) Selectins: lectins that initiate cell adhesion under flow. Curr Opin Cell Biol 14:581–586. doi:10.1016/S0955-0674(02)00367-8

5. Kwon M-J, Jang B, Yi JY et al (2012) Syndecans play dual roles as cell adhesion receptors and docking receptors. FEBS Lett 586:2207–2211. doi:10.1016/j.febslet.2012.05.037

6. Aricescu AR, Jones EY (2007) Immunoglobulin superfamily cell adhesion molecules: zippers and signals. Curr Opin Cell Biol 19:543–550. doi:10.1016/j.ceb.2007.09.010

7. Dunehoo AL, Anderson M, Majumdar S et al (2006) Cell adhesion molecules for targeted drug delivery. J Pharm Sci 95:1856–1872. doi:10.1002/jps.20676

8. Desgrosellier JS, Cheresh DA (2010) Integrins in cancer: biological implications and therapeutic opportunities. Nat Rev Cancer 10:9–22. doi:10.1038/nrc2748

9. Panés J, Perry M, Granger DN (1999) Leukocyte-endothelial cell adhesion: avenues for therapeutic intervention. Br J Pharmacol 126:537–550. doi:10.1038/sj.bjp.0702328

10. Ramsden JJ, Horvath R (2009) Optical biosensors for cell adhesion. J Recept Signal Transduct Res 29:211–223. doi:10.1080/10799890903064119

11. Aref A, Horvath R, Ramsden JJ (2010) Spreading kinetics for quantifying cell state during stem cell differentiation. J Biol Phys Chem 10:1–7

12. Ramsden JJ, Li SY, Heinzle E, Prenosil JE (1995) Optical method for measurement of number and shape of attached cells in real time. Cytometry 19:97–102

13. Aref A, Horvath R, McColl J, Ramsden JJ (2009) Optical monitoring of stem cell-substratum interactions. J Biomed Opt 14:010501. doi:10.1117/1.3065541

14. Fang Y (2011) Label-free biosensors for cell biology. Int J Electrochem 2011:460850. doi:10.4061/2011/460850

15. Orgovan N, Salánki R, Sándor N et al (2013) In-situ and label-free optical monitoring of the adhesion and spreading of primary monocytes isolated from human blood: dependence on serum concentration levels. Biosens Bioelectron 54:339–344. doi:10.1016/j.bios.2013.10.076

16. Orgovan N, Patko D, Hos C et al (2014) Sample handling in surface sensitive chemical and biological sensing: A practical review of basic fluidics and analyte transport. Adv Colloid Interface Sci 211C:1–16. doi:10.1016/j.cis.2014.03.011

17. Shamah SM, Cunningham BT (2011) Label-free cell-based assays using photonic crystal optical biosensors. Analyst 136:1090–1102. doi:10.1039/C0AN00899K

18. Patko D, Cottier K, Hamori A, Horvath R (2012) Single beam grating coupled interferometry: high resolution miniaturized label-free sensor for plate based parallel screening. Opt Express 20:23162–23173. doi:10.1364/OE.20.023162

19. Patko D, Gyorgy B, Nemeth A et al (2013) Label-free optical monitoring of surface adhesion of extracellular vesicles by grating coupled interferometry. Sensors Actuators B Chem 188:697–701. doi:10.1016/j.snb.2013.07.035

20. Patko D, Mártonfalvi Z, Kovacs B et al (2014) Microfluidic channels laser-cut in thin double-sided tapes: Cost-effective biocompatible fluidics in minutes from design to final integration with optical biochips. Sensors Actuators B Chem 196:352–356. doi:10.1016/j.snb.2014.01.107

21. Fang Y, Ferrie AM, Fontaine NH et al (2006) Resonant waveguide grating biosensor for living cell sensing. Biophys J 91:1925–1940. doi:10.1529/biophysj.105.077818

22. Orgovan N, Peter B, Bősze S et al (2014) Dependence of cancer cell adhesion kinetics on integrin ligand surface density measured by a high-throughput label-free resonant waveguide grating biosensor. Sci Rep 4:4034. doi:10.1038/srep04034

23. Tiefenthaler K, Lukosz W (1989) Sensitivity of grating couplers as integrated-optical chemical sensors. J Opt Soc Am B 6:209–220. doi:10.1364/JOSAB.6.000209

24. Horvath R, Lindvold LR, Larsen NB (2002) Reverse-symmetry waveguides: theory and fabrication. Appl Phys B Lasers Opt 74:383–393. doi:10.1007/s003400200823

25. Horvath R, Pedersen HC, Skivesen N et al (2005) Monitoring of living cell attachment and

spreading using reverse symmetry waveguide sensing. Appl Phys Lett 86:071101. doi:10.1063/1.1862756

26. Horvath R, Cottier K, Pedersen HC, Ramsden JJ (2008) Multidepth screening of living cells using optical waveguides. Biosens Bioelectron 24:805–810. doi:10.1016/j.bios.2008.06.059

27. Schuler M, Owen GR, Hamilton DW et al (2006) Biomimetic modification of titanium dental implant model surfaces using the RGDSP-peptide sequence: a cell morphology study. Biomaterials 27:4003–4015. doi:10.1016/j.biomaterials.2006.03.009

28. VandeVondele S, Vörös J, Hubbell JA (2003) RGD-grafted poly-L-lysine-graft-(polyethylene glycol) copolymers block non-specific protein adsorption while promoting cell adhesion. Biotechnol Bioeng 82:784–790. doi:10.1002/bit.10625

29. Bell GI, Dembo M, Bongrand P (1984) Cell adhesion. Competition between nonspecific repulsion and specific bonding. Biophys J 45:1051–1064

30. Dustin ML, Bromley SK, Davis MM, Zhu C (2001) Identification of self through two-dimensional chemistry and synapses. Annu Rev Cell Dev Biol 17:133–157. doi:10.1146/annurev.cellbio.17.1.133

31. Izzard CS, Lochner LR (1976) Cell-to-substrate contacts in living fibroblasts: an interference reflexion study with an evaluation of the technique. J Cell Sci 21:129–159

32. Giebel K-F, Bechinger C, Herminghaus S et al (1999) Imaging of cell/substrate contacts of living cells with surface plasmon resonance microscopy. Biophys J 76:509–516

33. Lo CM, Glogauer M, Rossi M, Ferrier J (1998) Cell-substrate separation: effect of applied force and temperature. Eur Biophys J 27:9–17

34. Ferrie AM, Wu Q, Fang Y (2010) Resonant waveguide grating imager for live cell sensing. Appl Phys Lett 97:223704. doi:10.1063/1.3522894

35. Orgovan N, Kovacs B, Farkas E et al (2014) Bulk and surface sensitivity of a resonant waveguide grating imager. Appl Phys Lett 104:083506. doi:10.1063/1.4866460

36. Cottier K, Horvath R (2008) Imageless microscopy of surface patterns using optical waveguides. Appl Phys B 91:319–327. doi:10.1007/s00340-008-2994-6

37. Brown MA, Wallace CS, Anamelechi CC et al (2007) The use of mild trypsinization conditions in the detachment of endothelial cells to promote subsequent endothelialization on synthetic surfaces. Biomaterials 28:3928–3935. doi:10.1016/j.biomaterials.2007.05.009

38. Kenausis GL, Vo J, Elbert DL et al (2000) Poly(L-lysine)-g-poly(ethylene glycol) layers on metal oxide surfaces: attachment mechanism and effects of polymer architecture on resistance to protein adsorption. J Phys Chem B 104:3298–3309. doi:10.1021/jp993359m

39. Ogaki R, Zoffmann Andersen O, Jensen GV et al (2012) Temperature-induced ultradense PEG polyelectrolyte surface grafting provides effective long-term bioresistance against mammalian cells, serum, and whole blood. Biomacromolecules 13:3668–3677. doi:10.1021/bm301125g

40. Ruoslahti E (1996) RGD and other recognition sequences for integrins. Annu Rev Cell Dev Biol 12:697–715

41. Hersel U, Dahmen C, Kessler H (2003) RGD modified polymers: biomaterials for stimulated cell adhesion and beyond. Biomaterials 24:4385–4415. doi:10.1016/S0142-9612(03)00343-0

Chapter 19

Label-Free Impedance-Based Monitoring of Cell Migration and Invasion

Ridha Limame and Olivier De Wever

Abstract

Cell migration and invasion involve the active translocation of cells along surfaces and through tissues and are key processes during different stages of life from early embryonic development to adulthood in both normal and pathophysiological conditions. During cancer progression towards metastatic disease, the cellular mechanisms underlying motility and invasion tend to be hijacked by cancer cells in order to disseminate throughout the body. An important mechanism driving cell motility is *chemotaxis*, the directional movement of cells along a chemical gradient.

Based on the setup of a conventional dual chamber Transwell system separated by a microporous membrane, the application of gold microelectrodes on the bottom side of the membrane enables the continuous detection and relative quantification, expressed as a Cell Index, of migrating or invading cells in real time, without interventions of fixing and staining. Nevertheless, post-fixation fluorescent or colorimetric endpoint measurements are possible and allow one to translate the dimensionless Cell Index parameter of the last measured time point into morphometric/colorimetric/fluorescence data.

Key words Cell migration, Extracellular matrix, Impedance, Invasion, Kinetic real-time, *xCELLigence*

1 Introduction

Cell migration, also referred as motility, is defined as the active movement of cells from one point to another and typically implies sequential phases of polarization, protrusion of the front end and elongation of the cell, ending with retraction of the rear end, resulting in a net translocation [1]. Invasion involves penetration of the surrounding extracellular matrix (ECM) by the moving cell, either in a destructive manner by proteolytic enzyme activity (mesenchymal invasion) or by short cycles of elongation and contraction enabling cell "gliding" between matrix fibers, similarly to the movement of the amoeba *Dictyostelium discoideum* (amoeboid invasion) [2]. Recently it was found that the limits of cell migration are determined by matrix porosity and deformation of the nucleus. With decreasing pore sizes, composed by ECM fibrils,

Ye Fang (ed.), *Label-Free Biosensor Methods in Drug Discovery*, Methods in Pharmacology and Toxicology,
DOI 10.1007/978-1-4939-2617-6_19, © Springer Science+Business Media New York 2015

nuclei, and thus cells, become physically halted and dependent on both proteolytic enzyme activity to increase the pore size and mechanocoupling of integrins with actomyosin to move forward the nucleus through the pore [3]. Processes of motility and invasion are important in driving gastrulation, neural development, and morphogenesis. During adulthood, pathophysiological processes of inflammation and wound healing are largely dependent on immune cell migration. Moreover, cancer cells are known to make use of the cellular motility machinery in their progression towards metastatic disease. An important mechanism in driving migration and invasion in these (patho)physiological processes is *chemotaxis*, the directional motility of cells along a chemical concentration gradient of soluble factors [4].

In a laboratory context, migration is modeled as motion in 2D on a flat surface, such as glass or tissue-treated plastic. Traditionally, migratory behavior is studied in vitro by assessing the gradual closure of an artificial scratch (or "wound") in a cultured cell monolayer (wound healing or scratch assay). In order to consider *chemotaxis*, Transwell assays traditionally shape the main technique of choice. Initially reported in 1962 by Stephen Boyden to study leukocyte chemotaxis [5], Transwells consist of an upper ("insert") and a lower chamber ("well"), separated by a microporous polycarbonate membrane that allows for passage of different mammalian or prokaryotic cell types depending on the applied pore size (bacteria: 0.7 µm, macrophages, leukocytes: 5 µm, epithelial/*carcinoma* cells: 8 µm). As cell movement, both in a migratory and invasive fashion, is a de facto active (energy consuming) process, these assays are designed to avoid passive fall-through of cells towards the wells. Adherent cells will initially attach to the upper side of the membrane and, when responsive to the chemical gradient, squeeze themselves through the pores and reattach to the bottom side of the membrane.

As epithelial cells are structurally confined by a highly specialized sheet-like ECM, named the basement membrane, progression of epithelial cancers or *carcinomas* implies breaching this barrier. This process is generally called local tissue invasion and is mimicked in vitro by the application of an ECM component, typically derived from the ECM of mouse sarcomas (Matrigel™), which needs to be traversed by the invading cells prior to their arrival at the bottom side of the microporous membrane.

Although applied as the gold standard method for assessing cell migration and invasion, Transwell assays are constrained by its means of detection using a fixing and staining reagent at one predetermined time point, providing only snapshot information. Real-time impedance-based monitoring of cell migration and invasion is established on the principle of conventional Transwell plates, as outlined above, and circumvents the endpoint nature of traditional experimentation. A meshwork of gold microelectrodes covering the bottom side of the microporous membrane, connected with a detection system, is able to sense any presence of cells arriving from the upper side, based on impedance changes. In general, the background electrode impedance is initially measured in a cell-free environment containing medium only and is reflected as a baseline Cell Index (CI). Cell addition in the upper chamber and the gradual arrival and settlement of cells on the electrodes at the bottom side will result in changes of impedance, proportional to the number of cells. This allows continuous monitoring ("real-time") of the process without intervention and yields time-dependent (dynamic) information, typically displayed in a CI as a function of time graph.

Our experience and the experiments described in this chapter are limited to the *xCELLigence* Real-Time Cell Analysis (RTCA) DP device (ACEA Biosciences). However, other similar systems have become commercially available and share the principle of impedance-based, label-free detection of cell behavior in real time.

Both proliferation and motion can be followed in real time and, therefore, compound effects on these processes may be studied in complementary experiments. For example, cytotoxic or cytostatic actions of a molecule on certain cell types can be defined by exposing the cells of interest to different concentrations and live monitoring of the response. After identification of the compound dosage leading to a 50 % reduction of proliferation ("IC_{50}"), additional effects of the molecule on cell migration or invasion as separate cellular functionalities can be addressed by selectively applying a nontoxic dose and assessing putative inhibitory effects on cell motility. Such an approach was applied in our lab to uncover anti-invasive activities of the SRC non-receptor tyrosine kinase-inhibiting small molecule compound M475275 on the triple negative breast cancer cell line MDA-MB-231. Exposure of these cells to a low dose, defined as nontoxic based on a previously defined IC_{50} (not shown), a blocking effect on invasion could be found when compared to vehicle control-treated cells (Fig. 1).

In this chapter, we will describe wet-lab benchwork procedures, potential pitfalls, and workarounds, associated with real-time cell migration and invasion assessments.

2 Materials

2.1 Equipments and Software

1. *xCELLigence* RTCA (Acea Biosciences, San Diego, CA, USA) (*see* **Note 1**).

2. Humidified CO_2-incubator.

3. Hemocytometer for manual cell counting or an automatic cell counter (electronic pipet or chamber-based).

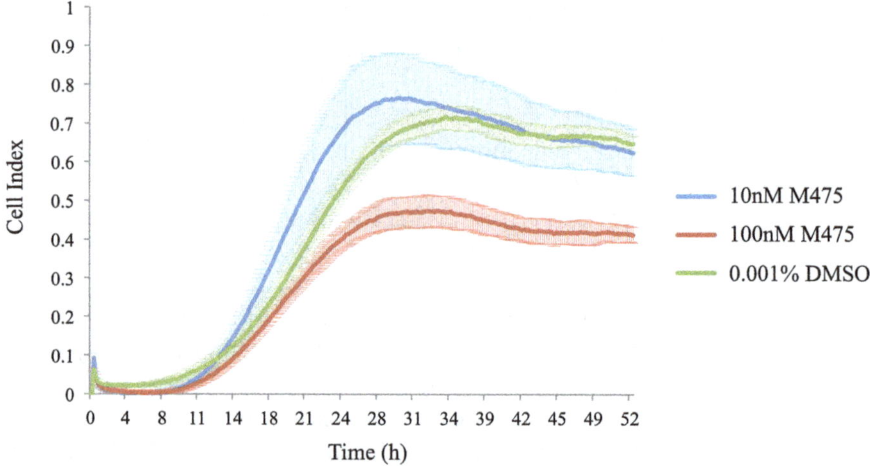

Fig. 1 Real-time measurement of Matrigel invasion by MDA-MB-231 cells on the *xCELLigence* RTCA DP device. Cells were seeded on Matrigel (5 % v/v in SF medium), exposed to the indicated concentrations of the small molecule SRC-inhibitor M475275, and allowed to invade during 50 h. Data presents mean ± s.d. of four replicates

2.2 Cell Culture Reagents and Devices

1. Growth medium containing fetal bovine serum (FBS) and/or growth additives/chemoattractants.

2. Medium without FBS (serum-free, SF) or containing 0.5–2 % FBS or bovine serum albumin (BSA), depending on the needs of the cells of interest.

3. Trypsin/EDTA or TrypLE™ EXPRESS (Life Technologies) (*see* **Note 2**).

4. Trypan Blue (0.4 % solution, Life Technologies).

5. Cell Invasion and Migration (CIM) plate-16, hereafter referred as "CIM16" (ACEA Biosciences) (*see* **Note 3**).

6. Metal plate holder (ACEA Biosciences). This serves to carry CIM-plate 16 while handling.

7. Calibrated pipettes and associated sterile tips: <100 µL, <1,000 µL, <5 mL.

8. Sterile tubes: <15 mL, <50 mL.

9. Matrigel® Basement Membrane Matrix growth factor reduced (Corning Incorporated) (*see* **Notes 4–6**).

10. Methanol 20 % (v/v) + crystal violet 0.5 % (w/v) (*see* **Notes 7 and 8**).

3   Methods

3.1 Impedance-Based Cell Migration Assay

This section describes a general protocol to use the *xCelligence* RTCA DP in combination with a modified Transwell plate (CIM-16) to measure single cell migration. This protocol includes multiple essential steps, including media and chemoattractant preparation, impedance device setup and equilibration, cell preparation, real-time impedance measurement before and after cell addition, and optional confirmation by endpoint staining.

1. Warm media and chemoattractants to 37 °C for 30 min.

2. Open both the upper chamber (UC) and the lower chamber (LC) of a CIM16 plate only within a laminar flow hood. For orientation purposes, mark both parts with a blue dot on the upper left corner, as well as the corresponding engraved masks on the plate holder fitting the LCs. All wells are surrounded by a thin silicon ring on the upper side.

3. Place the lower chamber onto the plate holder.

4. Add 160 µL of the appropriate chemoattractants in the lower chamber wells. Avoid air bubble formation and remove any air from the well contents before proceeding. When finished, menisci should be visible on all wells.

5. Turn the plate holder with the LC 90° (horizontally) by picking it up. *Do not slide.*

6. Remove the UC from the package and place it onto the LC with the blue dot corresponding to the one on the LC. As the bottom side of the UC is covered with gold microelectrodes, the UC should not be put directly on the flow hood bench, but on the hard plastic provided in the package if not immediately topped on the LC. Press the UC thoroughly and evenly onto the LC until two click sounds are heard. The UC is now sealed on the LC by the silicon rings and should not be removed until after the end of the assay. Air bubble entrapment between the chemoattractant surface in the LC and the electrodes will result in a drastic rise of CI values and should be avoided.

7. Turn the plate holder back to the original position on the flow hood bench (vertically) by picking it up. *Do not slide.*

8. Add 50 µL (minimal 30 µL) pre-warmed SF media to the UC inserts, hereby critically aiming to cover the entire membrane surface for hydration.

9. In order to maintain local hydration during the assay, fill all interspaces between the UC inserts with sterile PBS, dH_2O, or SF media. We mostly use the same SF media as applied in the inserts, since it would minimize interference when accidentally spilled in the inserts.

10. Place the plastic lid on top of the CIM16 plate, covering the insert openings.

11. Lock the completed CIM16 plate into the xCELLigence device in the incubator and leave it for 1 h to equilibrate at 37 °C.

12. After equilibration, perform an initial measurement step on the CIM16 plate in the device, establishing the background signal of cell-free medium.

13. Unlock the CIM16 plate from the device and transfer it back to the flow hood using the metal plate holder.

14. Add all cell suspensions to the respective inserts (100 µL SF medium per insert, totalling the volume in the inserts to 150 µL) according to the experimental design and cover the insert openings using the plastic lid (*see* **Note 9**).

15. Leave the CIM16 plate on the plate holder for 30 min at room temperature in the flow hood. During this step, cells gradually drop down and attach to the membranes.

16. After 30 min at room temperature, lock the CIM16 plate back into the device and start the experiment.

17. After completion of impedance measurement, remove media carefully from the inserts without touching the membranes.

18. Unlock the CIM-16 UC and LC by pressing the parallel lids on the LC inward, and place the UC inverted or tilted on the bench. Avoid any contact with the bottom side of the UC before fixing.

19. Remove media from the LC wells and replace with 160 µL crystal violet (0.5 %)/methanol (20 %) per well.

20. Press the UC onto the LC, such that the membranes make contact with the well contents.

21. Keep the CIM-16 plate at RT for 5 min so cells are fixed and stained simultaneously.

22. Separate UC and LC of the CIM-16 plate, discard the LC, and rinse the UC in a beaker containing dH$_2$O.

23. Remove the cells residing at the upper side of the membranes carefully using a cotton swab. Make sure not to press through the membranes. Optional: the UC may be rinsed again in dH$_2$O in order to remove all remaining debris.

24. Place the UC inverted (bottom side of the membranes facing upward) in darkness overnight.

25. Next to crystal violet, DAPI nuclear staining, or fluorescent probes to reveal the F-actin cytoskeleton (phalloidin), proliferation markers such as Ki67 can be visualized on the cell material.

26. Fixation can also be avoided by performing 3-(4,5-dimethylthiazol-2-yl)-2,5-diphenyltetrazolium bromide reduction (MTT) or sulforhodamine B (SRB) staining (*see* **Note 10** for **steps 17–26**).

3.2 Impedance-Based Cell Invasion Assay

This section describes a general protocol to use the *xCelligence* RTCA DP system in combination with a Matrigel-coated modified Transwell plate (CIM-16) to measure the invasion of single cells through a Matrigel-coated microporous plate. The steps to initiate cell invasion experiments are almost identical to those of the migration experiments described above, with the typical difference of adding an ECM barrier on top of the microporous membrane, prior to all other actions.

1. Dilute the ice-thawed Matrigel with ice-cold SF medium to the desired concentration, roughly ranging from 1/10 to 1/40, and keep vials consistently on ice (*see* **Note 11**).

2. Place the UC on the plate holder and add 50 µL of the Matrigel to each of four inserts. Do not touch the membrane and avoid air bubble formation within the added Matrigel, by stopping at the first arrest and not pressing through to the second pipet stop. If (an) air bubble(s) become(s) apparent at sight, these can be removed by careful aspiration using a 100 µL tip.

3. Immediately remove 30 µL of the Matrigel solution from each insert carefully without touching the membrane, leaving 20 µL of Matrigel per insert. This approach provides the highest reliability to obtain homogeneous gels.

4. Allow the complete gelation of Matrigel. It is of importance to consider a minimal incubation time of 4 h at 37 °C in order to have the Matrigel properly solidified.

5. After Matrigel gelation, repeat **steps 3–26** in Section 3.1 to perform baseline measurement, cell addition, cell invasion measurement, and endpoint staining confirmation.

---

4 Results and Discussion

4.1 Migration

The reduced detection limit of the *xCelligence* impedance-based system requires meticulous culturing, detaching, and counting of cells prior to the assay. Since small differences in cell seeding may be detected, it is of importance to carefully prepare cell suspensions and to properly pipet technical replicates, in order to avoid "funnel-shaped" escalation of standard deviation values (as reported in [6]). As a general rule, it should be avoided to dispense from proportionally large volumes, e.g., dispensing volumes of 100 µL per insert from a 5 or 10 mL cell suspension will often result in technical variability (Table 1). Similarly, cell suspensions should be properly resuspended to obtain a homogeneous mixture of cells before addition to inserts. Table 1 refers to some common issues that may be encountered, together with possible solutions.

Table 1
Q/A of commonly occurring symptoms during assays

Symptom	Problem	Solution
Cells with known migratory capability do not yield an appropriate CI signal	Cells are seeded in clusters	Prepare a homogeneous suspension of single cells (avoid cell clumps and clusters
	Number of cells seeded is too small	Apply more cells per insert
Variability of CI patterns between technical replicate wells	Signal differs highly between replicate wells resulting in large SD values	Prepare a homogeneous suspension of single cells (avoid cell clumps and clusters)
		Dispense cells from a small volume ($N+1$, where N = number of wells)
CI < 0 over majority or entire duration of experiment	Inhomogeneous gelification of Matrigel layers	Handle Matrigel consequently on ice
	Matrigel density too high	Apply Matrigel in higher degrees of dilution
	Number of cells seeded is too small	Apply more cells per insert
Sudden increase of CI occurring in multiple wells at different times (Fig. 4)	Not all silicon rings are tightly attached to the bottom side of the UC, resulting in entrapment of air between electrodes and medium	Thoroughly and evenly press UC onto LC until two click sounds are heard. To ensure adequate sealing, press UC onto LC at all sides around the plate

As applicable for any other functional assay, cell culturing routines should be standardized in order to increase the biological reproducibility. This implies consequent subculturing and avoiding cell lines to grow to complete (100 %) confluency. In general, experiments are initiated from cell cultures that have reached 70–80 % confluency and it is recommended to apply this strategy consequently throughout the assessment of biological replicates from a certain cell type, as results may vary when cells are derived from different degrees of confluency (Fig. 2).

Each cell type or cell line is characterized by its proper genomic and functional characteristics. However, variability may exist between different clones of a particular cell line. Next to confirmation of cell line identity by short tandem repeat profiling [7, 8], initial experiments should be carried out to obtain information on basic proliferative and migratory/invasive behavior of the cells of interest, before proceeding with addressing biological hypotheses. This can be approached by performing a serial cell dilution experiment to identify the optimal cell seeding number (Fig. 3). In addition, a combination of migration and Matrigel invasion using different dilutions can be applied on one cell line in a single plate.

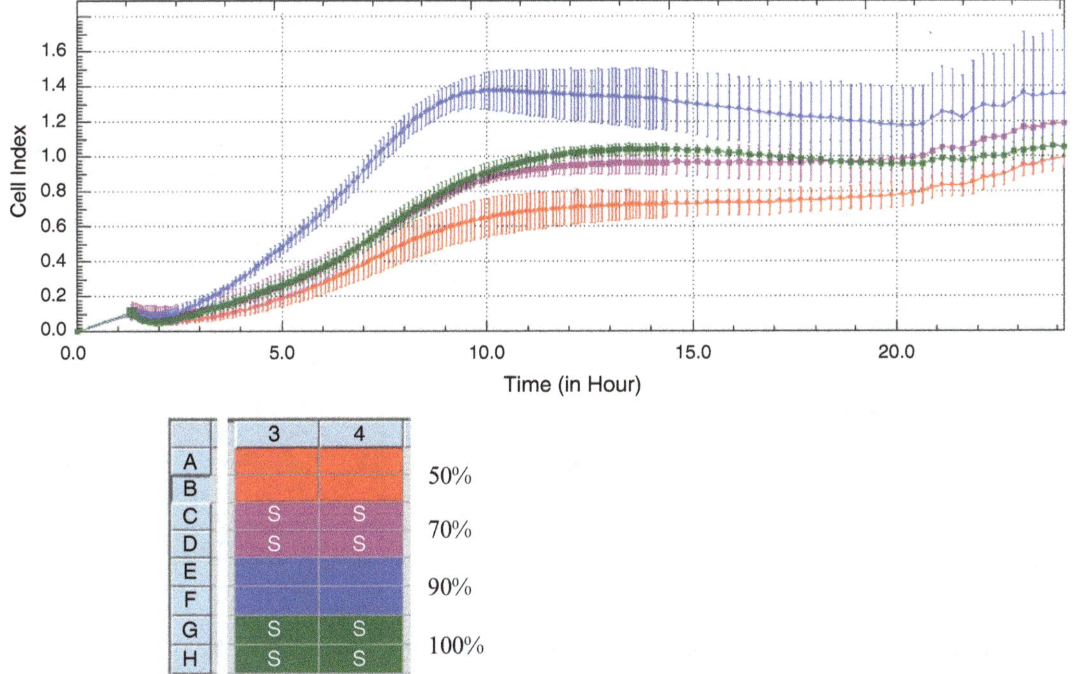

Fig. 2 Dynamic migration patterns of MDA-MB-231 breast cancer cells as measured in tetraplicates in real time and displayed by the *xCELLigence* RTCA DP system. Cells were initially seeded in different dilutions, grown to different degrees of flask confluency (50, 70, 90, and 100 %), and deprived of FBS 24 h prior to the assay. Full growth medium containing 10 % FBS was used as chemoattractant; cells were seeded in SF medium. Well distribution and color key for the graphs is shown

4.2 Invasion

There are several important factors for achieving high-quality cell invasion using the label-free technique. First, the application of Matrigel is a major source of variability, both in classic Transwells and real-time impedance-based measurement of invasion. Matrigel is highly sensitive to gelification at temperatures >4 °C, which may result in heterogeneous gel formation and interfere with reproducibility. To obtain gels as uniform as possible, one shall always work on ice and use pre-cooled and ice-cold materials when handling the Matrigel. One shall thaw Matrigel aliquots on ice and mix with ice-cold SF medium. By preference, pre-cooled pipet tips (–20 °C) should be used, if possible on an insulating cold block. For invasion assays, both the metal plate holder and the UC are to be pre-cooled (–20 °C) overnight.

Second, air bubbles can introduce significant issues for real-time label-free measurements. One shall avoid air bubble entrapment in gels and, if occurring, air bubbles should be carefully removed using a tip <100 or <10 μL.

Third, the mechanical stability and integrity of Matrigel is also important. One shall not proceed with adding media to gelifying upper chambers of the CIM16 plates before 4 h of incubation at

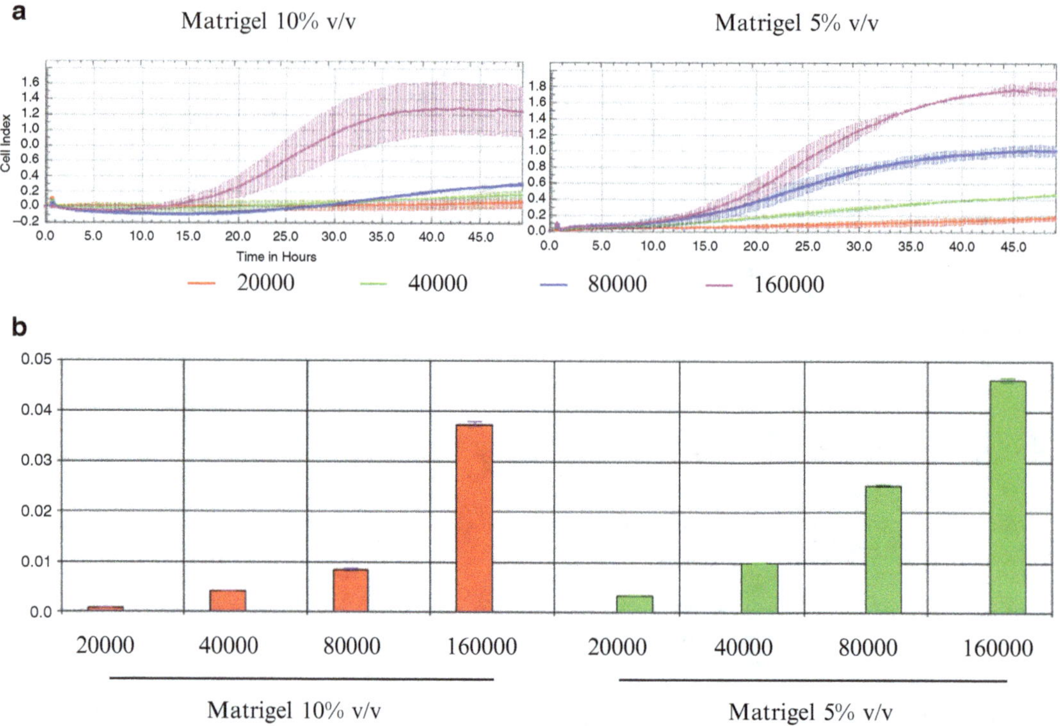

Fig. 3 (a) Real-time monitoring of invasion of a dilution series of MDA-MB-231 breast cancer cells through two Matrigel concentrations (10 % and 5 % v/v in SF medium). *Color bars* indicate seeded cell numbers. (b) Slope calculation of the real-time patterns to quantitate invasion. Slopes have been calculated over the entire duration of the experiment. Timeframes considered for slope calculation can be selected as appropriate. Data presents mean ± s.d. of two replicates

37 °C, since incomplete gelation of Matrigel may compromise the assay results. Furthermore, due to the manual application, Matrigel becomes an extra variable in the experiment and may result in increased variability between technical replicates. An initiating experiment may comprise two different cell lines with generally known and highly differing degrees of invasiveness, e.g., MDA-MB-231 and MCF-7 being highly and weakly invasive breast cancer cell lines, respectively. Visualizing the differential behavior between such extremes can add to the experience of performing these experiments.

It is recommended to test several Matrigel dilutions in order to assess the invasive response of a given cell line. In our report [6], we identified a correlation between Matrigel invasion on conventional Transwells and *xCELLigence* RTCA, based on surface area and cell seeding density using the same liquid volume of Matrigel (20 μL). Roughly, applying a 2.3-fold increase on the Matrigel dilution in Transwell inserts yielded similar dynamics of invasion on MDA-MB-231 cells on the *xCELLigence* RTCA. This might be useful to calculate a potential correlate on *xCELLigence*, if in-house knowledge exists for certain cell lines on Transwell setups.

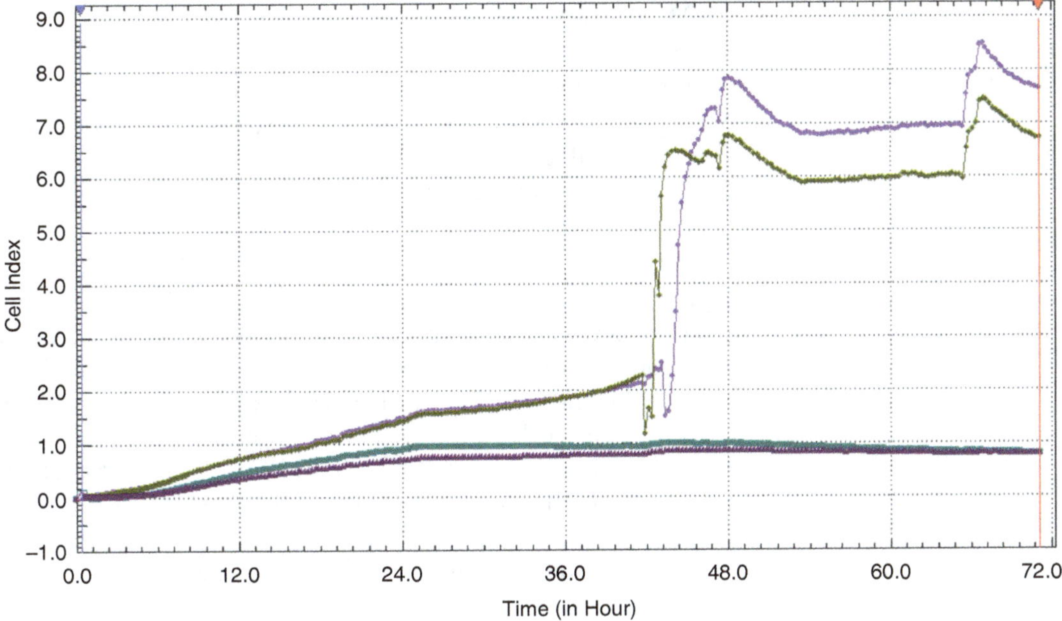

Fig. 4 Example of aberrant real-time invasion profiles, caused by inadequate sealing of the CIM16-plate

5   Notes

1. It is strongly advised to have the detection platform (*xCELLigence* RTCA or other) placed in a dedicated incubator, if possible with careful monitoring of humidity (>95 %). In order to maintain humidity, incubator doors should remain closed during the entire progress of an experiment. Changes in humidity, as caused by frequent opening and closing, may result in accelerated evaporation of the media, increasing concentrations of cell metabolites, well dry-out and aberrant detection signal patterns (Fig. 4). Ideally, an incubator equipped with an access port for cable transfer should be used.

2. As *in vitro* transmembrane cell migration and invasion experiments focus on single cell movement, care should be taken to prepare a suspension of single cells by avoiding clusters. This requires more intensive exposure to Trypsin/EDTA and resuspension within the Trypsin/EDTA solution, with the possibility of increasing cell stress and death in the detached population. Viability testing of the cell population prior to seeding is therefore essential.

3. The CIM16 is a 16-well dual chamber plate, with the upper chamber (containing the inserts) and the lower chamber (containing the wells). UCs and LCs are separately packed in sterile conditions.

4. ECM is critical for cell invasion studies. Except for ECM, all other necessary materials are similar for both migration and invasion assays.

5. Matrigel is the most commonly used extracellular matrix substitute, available in several different forms, including a regular (Matrigel® Basement Membrane Matrix), a high concentration (HC), and a growth factor-reduced (GFR) formulation, the latter of which is often used for in vitro purposes.

6. Upon arrival, the ECM component shall be distributed into small volume aliquots, depending on the lab-specific usage (50–200 μL). Matrigel gelifies quickly and spontaneously at room temperature. To avoid partial gelification during handling, always work on ice (4 °C) and essentially use pre-cooled tips and microtubes (stored at –20 °C). Do not repeatedly freeze/thaw the Matrigel. Long-term (3–6 months) store Matrigel aliquots at –20 °C and thaw on ice. For in vitro assays, Matrigel is diluted in the SF variant of the growth medium of the cells of interest. When diluting the Matrigel, always use ice-cold SF medium (4 °C) and keep vials on ice.

7. This is to perform endpoint staining. It is estimated that ~2.5 mL crystal violet solution for staining one CIM-16 plate is needed. Crystal violet staining is a frequently used light microscopic method of staining. This endpoint staining is performed after impedance measurement and cells are fixed.

8. Caution: methanol is highly toxic and crystal violet is a strong and unremovable dye. Precautions should be taken to protect clothes and bench. Use protective gloves.

9. Cells are prepared by detaching cells cultured in standard vessels (T25/T75 flasks, petri dishes, or well plates), followed by resuspension in SF medium. The cell preparation is initiated during the incubation time of the CIM16 plate. Caution: if animal trypsin is used as detachment agent, FBS-containing medium needs to be used to block enzymatic activity. After cell counting and viability assessment, the appropriate number of cells can be transferred to a fresh tube, centrifuged ($100 \times g$, 3 min) and resuspended in SF medium, followed by another two to three rounds of centrifugation ($100 \times g$, 3 min) to remove FBS remnants. When preparing cell suspensions, it is advised to include the dead volume associated with pipetting by adding an extra imaginary insert to the calculation of suspensions.

10. **Steps 17–26** describe an endpoint staining protocol. The total procedure takes about 15 min, and is optional. Although essentially not required, fixing and staining of CIM-16 insert membranes may be useful to obtain a visual correlation with the actual CI endpoint at the end of the experiment, hereby

providing an additional confirmation of the results measured in real time. This can easily be achieved by performing a staining protocol resembling that of classic Transwells.

11. All handlings involving Matrigel should be carried out in 4 °C conditions. Therefore, pipet tips, (micro)tubes, CIM16 plate, and plate holder should be stored at–20 °C overnight before starting the experiment.

References

1. Lauffenburger DA, Horwitz AF (1996) Cell migration: a physically integrated molecular process. Cell 84:359–369
2. Friedl P, Wolf K (2003) Tumour-cell invasion and migration: diversity and escape mechanisms. Nat Rev Cancer 3:362–374. doi:10.1038/nrc1075
3. Wolf K, Te Lindert M, Krause M, Alexander S, Te Riet J, Willis AL, Hoffman RM, Figdor CG, Weiss SJ, Friedl P (2013) Physical limits of cell migration: control by ECM space and nuclear deformation and tuning by proteolysis and traction force. J Cell Biol 201:1069–1084. doi:10.1083/jcb.201210152
4. Roussos ET, Condeelis JS, Patsialou A (2011) Chemotaxis in cancer. Nat Rev Cancer 11:573–587. doi:10.1038/nrc3078
5. Boyden S (1962) The chemotactic effect of mixtures of antibody and antigen on polymorphonuclear leucocytes. J Exp Med 115:453–466
6. Limame R, Wouters A, Pauwels B, Fransen E, Peeters M, Lardon F, de Wever O, Pauwels P (2012) Comparative analysis of dynamic cell viability, migration and invasion assessments by novel real-time technology and classic endpoint assays. PLoS One 7:e46536. doi:10.1371/journal.pone.0046536
7. Masters JR, Thomson JA, Daly-Burns B, Reid YA, Dirks WG, Packer P, Toji LH, Ohno T, Tanabe H, Arlett CF, Kelland LR, Harrison M, Virmani A, Ward TH, Ayres KL, Debenham PG (2001) Short tandem repeat profiling provides an international reference standard for human cell lines. Proc Natl Acad Sci U S A 98:8012–8017. doi:10.1073/pnas.121616198
8. Romano P, Manniello A, Aresu O, Armento M, Cesaro M, Parodi B (2009) Cell line data base: structure and recent improvements towards molecular authentication of human cell lines. Nucleic Acids Res 37:D925–D932. doi:10.1093/nar/gkn730

Infrared Surface Plasmon Spectroscopy Decodes Early Processes in Epithelial Host Cells upon Enteropathogenic *Escherichia coli* Infection

Victor Yashunsky and Benjamin Aroeti

Abstract

Enteropathogenic *Escherichia coli* (EPEC) is a generally noninvasive bacterial pathogen that causes diarrhea in humans. This microbe infects mainly the enterocytes of the small intestine. In this chapter we describe newly developed method, infrared surface plasmon resonance (IR-SPR) spectroscopy, for sensing pathogen infection of living cells. The IR-SPR method enables real-time and label-free monitoring of EPEC infection through highly sensitive measurement of the refractive index and height of the host epithelial cell monolayer. Our findings indicate the great potential of the IR-SPR tool to study the dynamics of host-pathogen interactions with high spatiotemporal sensitivity.

Key words EPEC, Epithelial host cells, Surface plasmon resonance, Infrared, Spectroscopy

1 Introduction

Enteropathogenic *Escherichia coli* (EPEC) infection is a major cause of infant diarrhea in the developing world [1]. EPEC bacterium colonizes on the apical surface of the small intestine's epithelial cells, where it forms characteristic attaching and effacing (A/E) lesions (Fig. 1). EPEC utilizes a type-III secretion system (T3SS) to introduce bacterial effector proteins into its host epithelial cells. Several effectors have been implicated in brush border remodeling and the induction of the A/E effects, which significantly contribute to EPEC pathogenesis (reviewed in [2]). These include effectors that promote local effacement of microvilli, intimate bacterial attachment to the host, and induce F-actin-rich protrusions beneath the adhering bacteria, often termed actin-rich pedestals [3].

Type-III-secreted virulent effectors can also disrupt the integrity of the epithelial cell monolayer. For instance, previous studies have reported that several effectors (e.g., EspG, EspF, Map, and NleA) are involved in disrupting the epithelial tight

Ye Fang (ed.), *Label-Free Biosensor Methods in Drug Discovery*, Methods in Pharmacology and Toxicology,
DOI 10.1007/978-1-4939-2617-6_20, © Springer Science+Business Media New York 2015

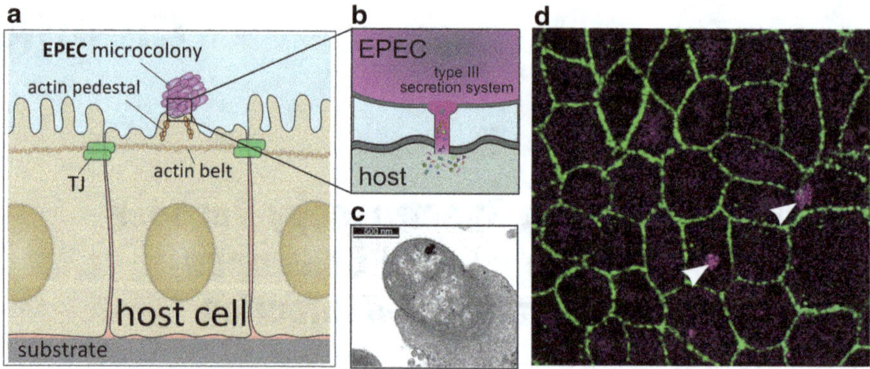

Fig. 1 Schematic representation of the EPEC infection effects on the epithelial host cell architecture. (**a**) Columnar epithelial cells maintain close intercellular contacts via junctional complexes (e.g., tight junctions (TJ), adherence junctions, gap junctions, and desmosomes). Tight junctions and adherence junctions linked to actin fibers and interconnect individual cells into a continuous and rigid epithelial cell sheet. Upon infection, EPEC microcolony attached to the apical cell surface of host epithelial cells injects a series of protein effectors into the host cells via T3SS (panel **b**), which remodels the TJs and the actin cytoskeleton. (**c**) Electron micrograph of bacterium attached to actin-rich pedestal. Finally, EPEC infection results in failure of the epithelial barrier function. (**d**) Confocal image of live MDCK cells immersed in sulforhodamine B (SRB)-labeled medium that visualizes the borders between cells (*green*) and EPEC microcolonies (*purple*)

junctions' (TJs) structure and barrier functions [4–9], when other intercellular junctions, such as desmosomes, remain unperturbed [10, 11]. Focal adhesions are affected by EPEC infection in a T3SS-dependent manner, although the specific effectors that mediate these effects have not yet been identified [12]. A conceivable hypothesis is that the effects that EPEC infection has on intercellular junctions, focal adhesions, and the cytoskeleton impact the overall epithelial host cell architecture, and thus the integrity and organization of the epithelial cell tissue. However, despite the importance of these effects, little research has been conducted to investigate them.

Existing epithelial barrier function assays, such as transepithelial resistance or small molecule permeability, provide ambiguous information regarding structural changes in host cell structure [13–15]. It is worth noting that in some cases host cell structure can be also significantly altered without losing their barrier function. For example, infection with EPEC mutant (EspM) may lead to bulging or even extrusion of the host cells, whereas epithelial monolayer maintains a normal barrier function [16].

We have recently developed infrared surface plasmon resonance (IR-SPR) spectroscopy as a novel biophysical tool for studying living cells [17–19]. Using the IR-SPR system we developed a variety of methods and measurement techniques to study structural properties of epithelial cells [20–23]. In this chapter we describe the utilization of IR-SPR for measurement of host-pathogen interactions in real time and in a label-free manner.

Specifically, we focus on detection of early effects of EPEC infection to the epithelial host cell structure. Our IR-SPR measurements reveal that EPEC infection reduces the host cell's refractive index and shortens its height, enabling screening of pathogen impact on epithelium host.

2 IR-SPR Biosensor Theory

The term surface plasmon resonance (SPR) is commonly used to describe collective oscillations in the electron density at the surface of a metal and dielectric medium stimulated by incident light. First experimental work was reported in 1968, when Otto [24] and Kretschmann and Raether [25] independently reported the optical excitation of surface plasmons. Application of SPR-based sensors to biomolecular interaction monitoring was first demonstrated in 1983 by Lundstrom [26]. Since then, SPR has found its way into practical applications in sensitive detectors, capable of detecting sub-monomolecular coverage without use of labels [27–31].

The vast majority of today's commercial SPR biosensors operating in visible wavelength range provide highly quantitative measurement of molecular interactions [29]. Extension of the SPR methodology to the near- and mid-infrared wavelength range introduces a new prospect for biosensing applications [32]: (I) Infrared (IR) surface plasmons penetrate much deeper and are more appropriate for studying cells [33–35]. In particular, the penetration depth of mid-IR surface plasmon can be extended up to several microns, which allows probing a significant portion of living cells [17]. (II) Infrared spectral region contains "fingerprints" of the most common molecular vibrations and thus can provide information on a molecular composition and coordination, which are crucial for bimolecular analysis [36, 37]. (III) Since conductive losses in the infrared range are lower than those in the visible range, the IR-SPR can be more sensitive than its visible range counterparts. These special properties open possibilities for development of new applications for surface plasmon methodology, such as whole cell biosensing, as we describe in this chapter.

2.1 IR-SPR Working Principle

Our IR-SPR system employs Kretschmann configuration [38] for excitation of surface plasmon. Namely, p-polarized (TM-mode), collimated light beam undergoes total internal reflection at a ZnS prism/ thin gold-film/cell interface (analyte), *see* Fig. 2a. Due to dispersion, the resonance occurs when the real part of SP wavevector $k'_{SP} = k_0 \mathrm{Re}\left[\sqrt{\varepsilon_m \varepsilon_d (\varepsilon_m + \varepsilon_d)}\right]$ equals to the parallel component of the light wavevector, namely, $k_x = k_0 n_p \sin\theta$. Here, ε_m and $\varepsilon_d = (n_d + i\kappa_d)^2$ dielectric constants of metal and analyte, n_p is prism refractive, k_0 is light wavevector (ω/c), and θ is incident angle (Fig. 2a). IR-SPR operates at a fixed angle in wavelength interrogation mode allowing

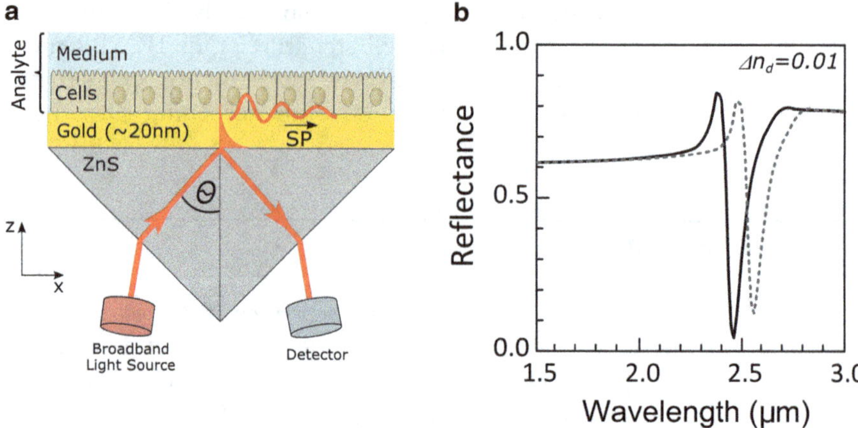

Fig. 2 Optical excitation of SP using prism coupling. (**a**) Scheme of experimental setup for SP excitation based on Kretschmann geometry (*unscaled*). SP resonance is observed as a sharp shadow in the reflected light at an angle θ. Note that SP excitation angle is beyond the critical angle; hence the refractive index of the prism has to be higher than that of the dielectric layer $n_d < n_{prism}$. (**b**) Numerical simulation based on Fresnel equations for tri-layer structure (ZnS/18 nm Au/water). (**b**) SP resonance appears as reflectance deep for wavelength interrogation. *Black solid line* spectrum corresponds to pure water dielectric and *dashed gray* spectrum simulates ~5 % sugar solution with slightly higher refractive index ($\Delta n_d = 0.01$)

measurement of the analyte refractive index (Fig. 2b) based on the following approximated expression [27, 30]

$$n_{\rm d}\left(\lambda\right) = \varepsilon_{\rm d}^{1/2}\left(\lambda_{\rm sp}\right) = n_{\rm prism}\sin\theta\left[\varepsilon_{\rm m} \big/ \left(\varepsilon_{\rm m} - n_{\rm prism}^2 \sin^2\theta\right)\right]^{1/2} \quad (1)$$

The reflectivity at the SP (R) can be approximated by the following Lorentzian [38, 39]:

$$R = \left|r_{\rm mp}\right|^2\left(1 - \frac{4k_{\rm sp}''\Gamma_{\rm rad}}{\left(k_x - k_{\rm sp}'\right)^2 + \left(k_{\rm sp}'' + \Gamma_{\rm rad}\right)^2}\right) \quad (2)$$

where $r_{\rm mp}$ is the Fresnel reflection coefficient at the metal-prism interface and $\Gamma_{\rm rad}$ is the radiation loss resulting from the finite thickness of the metal film. At resonance the reflectivity achieves its minimal value,

$$R_{\rm min} = \left|r_{\rm mp}\frac{k_{\rm sp}'' - \Gamma_{\rm rad}}{k_{\rm sp}'' + \Gamma_{\rm rad}}\right|^2 \quad (3)$$

which is determined by the imaginary part of the SP wavevector, $k''_{\rm sp}$. Hence, SPR depth ($R_{\rm min}$) follows the losses in the analyte, which as we show later correlates with cell-substrate attachment morphology [21].

2.2 IR-SPR in Aqueous Media

The majority of the biosensing applications take place in aqueous media. Thus, SPR-based biosensor design has to consider specific aspects related to optical properties of the aqueous environment, especially in the infrared wavelength range where water exhibits nontrivial dielectric properties. These properties reflect on the key properties for SPR measurement and analysis. Two key characteristics of SPR biosensor are penetration (probing) depth δ_z and propagation length L_x.

Figure 3a, b shows the real and the imaginary components of the complex refractive index of water in the wavelength range of 1–4 µm. The SP wave is affected by changes in the refractive index of the analyte in vicinity of the Au film. The thickness of this layer, namely, the penetration depth into the analyte layer, is $\delta_z = 1/2k_z$. The penetration depth strongly depends on wavelength, in particular, the penetration depth of the SP at the Au/water interface grows from $\delta_z = 0.3$ µm at $\lambda \sim 1$ µm to $\delta_z = 5$ µm at $\lambda \sim 4$ µm (Fig. 3c).

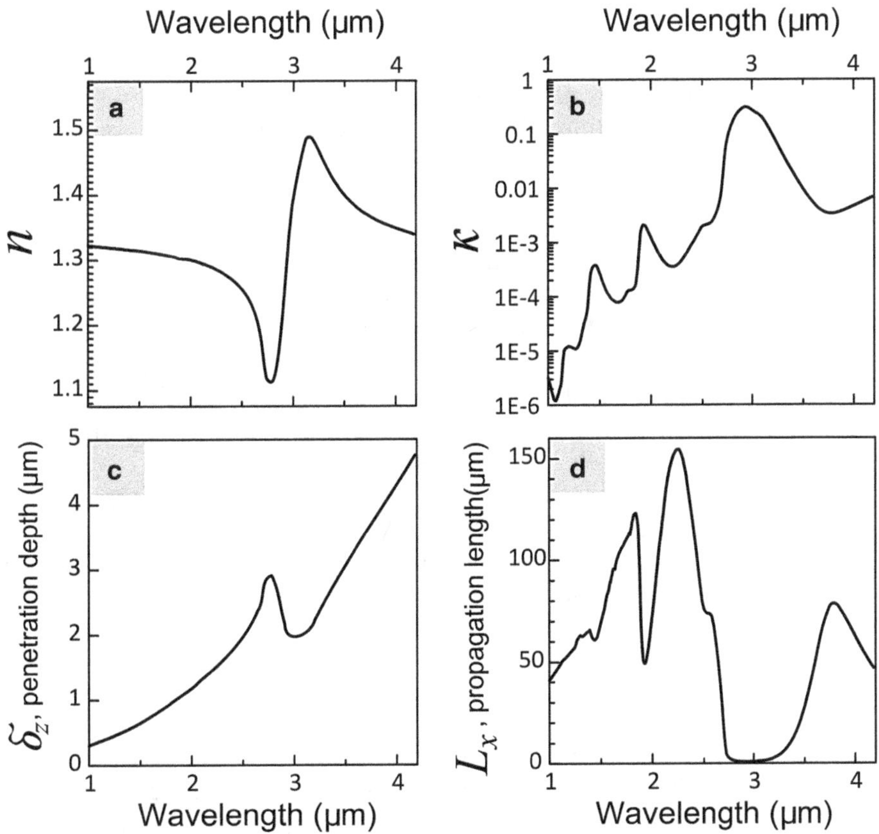

Fig. 3 Optical constants and characteristic lengths of water associated with IR-SPR biosensing. (**a, b**) The real and the imaginary parts of the complex refractive index of water in near- and mid-infrared wavelength range. (**a**) The real part of water refractive index n. (**b**) The imaginary parts of water refractive index κ. Data adopted from [36]. (**c, d**) The penetration depth and propagation length of surface plasmon in water dielectric. (**c**) The SP penetration depth, δ_z in z-direction. (**d**) The SP propagation length, L_x in x-direction

For any practical use, penetration depth can be estimated based on the following equation [38, 39]:

$$\delta_z = \mathrm{Im}\left[\frac{\lambda_{\min}}{4\pi n_{\mathrm{d}}}\left(\mid \varepsilon_{\mathrm{m}} \mid -n_{\mathrm{d}}^2\right)^{1/2}\right] \qquad (4)$$

Since SP is a damped propagating wave, its lateral resolution in the direction of propagation defined by the characteristic propagation length L_x along the Au/water interface. Water absorption in infrared wavelength range has major impact on the SP propagation length. Figure 3d shows the dependence of the SP propagation length on the light wavelength at the ZnS/Au/water interface. The following approximated equation predicts the lateral resolution of our SPR biosensor [17]:

$$L_x = \frac{\lambda_{\min}}{4\pi}\left(\frac{\varepsilon'_{\mathrm{m}} + \varepsilon'_{\mathrm{d}}}{\varepsilon'_{\mathrm{m}}\varepsilon'_{\mathrm{d}}}\right)^{3/2} \bigg/ \left(\frac{\varepsilon''_{\mathrm{m}}}{\varepsilon'^2_{\mathrm{m}}} + \frac{\varepsilon''_{\mathrm{d}}}{\varepsilon'^2_{\mathrm{d}}}\right) \qquad (5)$$

Propagation length along the cell layer can be adjusted by fine tuning of the SPR wavelength, which determines by the incident angle, from a few μm to 150 μm (~10 cells). This parameter should be carefully chosen to enable sensitive monitoring of changes in cell morphology [17].

2.3 Analysis of Epithelial Cell Monolayer with IR-SPR

Cultured cells immersed in aqueous culture medium that enables their viability. Main component in cell volume is cytosol or cytoplasm, which occupies about 70 % of cell volume and contains around 80 % water. Thus, real part of refractive index (n) of cells exceeds that of the culture medium due to presence of approximately 30 % of organic substances. Additionally, intracellular organelles add scattering losses and increase the imaginary part (κ) of the cell refractive index for the shorter wavelengths ($\lambda < 2$ μm). In the mid-infrared range ($\lambda > 2$ μm) energy loss is dominated by water absorption.

For inhomogeneous media such as cells, the effective refractive index sensed by the SP wave is a weighted average in z-direction,

$$\sqrt{\varepsilon_{\mathrm{d}}} = n_{\mathrm{d}} + \mathrm{i}\kappa_{\mathrm{d}} = \frac{1}{\delta_z}\int\limits_{z=0}^{z=\infty}\left[n(z) + \mathrm{i}\kappa(z)\right]\exp(-z/\delta_z)\,dz \qquad (6)$$

The real part of refractive index n_{d} yields the total biomass inside the SP field while the imaginary part of the refractive index κ_{d} provides information on the cell morphology.

2.4 IR Waveguide Modes Excitation in Epithelial Cell Monolayers

From a "physicist's point of view," a ~10 μm-thick cell monolayer tightly attached to flat substrate and bathed with growth medium, together forming a dielectric tri-layer structure with progressively decreasing refractive indices, $n_{\mathrm{substrate}} > n_{\mathrm{cell}} > n_{\mathrm{medium}}$ (Fig. 4a, lower panel).

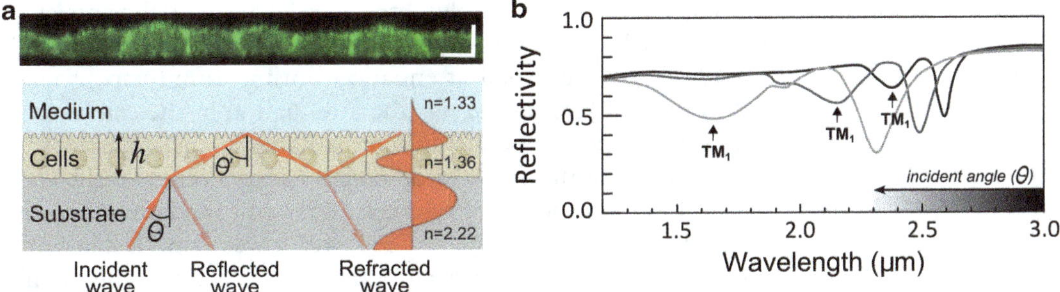

Fig. 4 Excitation of IR waveguide modes in MDCK epithelial cell monolayer. (**a**) Schematic representation of intracellular leaky waveguide mode propagation in a living cell monolayer. *Upper panel* shows cross section of epithelial MDCK cell monolayer stably expressing LifeAct-GFP and imaged by confocal microscopy. Scale bars: 10 μm. *Lower panel* illustrates the mechanism of the waveguide mode excitation in a living cell monolayer. An electromagnetic wave penetrates at an incident angle θ from the high-refractive-index substrate ($n = 2.22@\lambda = 2$ μm) into a cell monolayer having a lower refractive index ($n_{cell} = 1.36@\lambda = 2$ μm). Because n_{medium} is lower than n_{cell} ($\Delta n = 0.33@\lambda = 2$ μm), the wave undergoes total internal reflection at the cell-medium interface. The wave then impinges on the cell-substrate interface where it is partially reflected (*solid red arrow*) and refracted (*pale red arrow*). Excitation of the radiative (leaky) waveguide mode occurs when the reflected and refracted waves at the substrate-cell interface interfere destructively, confining the energy within the cell layer. (**b**) Waveguide modes (TM₁) in infrared reflectance spectrum from four-layer assembly (ZnS/18 nm Au/MDCK monolayer/medium). Waveguide modes appear as shallow reflectivity dip on the spectrum. Different incident angles θ produce waveguide modes at different wavelength

When the angle of incidence at the cell-medium interface exceeds the critical angle ($\sim78°$) at the cell-medium interface, the cell monolayer can support leaky waveguide modes also known as radiative modes. The waveguide resonance occurs when the total phase shift for the round-trip propagation is an integral multiple of 2π. Namely, $2\varphi + \phi_{cm} + \phi_{cs} = 2m\pi$, where $\varphi = n_{cell}k_0 h\cos\theta$ is the phase shift on wave propagation through the cell layer, and ϕ_{cs}, ϕ_{cm} are phase shifts on reflection from the cell-medium and cell-substrate interfaces, respectively. Here, $k_0 = 2\pi/\lambda$ is the incident wavevector and h is the cell layer thickness. For p-polarized incident light these relations yield a set of resonant wavelengths corresponding to TM₁, TM₂,... modes [40],

$$\lambda_{TM} = \frac{4\pi n_{cell} h \cos\theta}{2\pi m - \phi_{sc} - \phi_{cm}} \qquad (7)$$

where $m = 1,2,...$ The resonant wavelengths can be tuned by varying the angle θ.

The reflectivity from the tri-layer assembly is given by the Airy formula [40]

$$R = \left| \frac{r_{sc} + r_{cm}e^{2(i\phi - \alpha)}}{1 + r_{sc}r_{cm}e^{2(i\phi - \alpha)}} \right|^2 \qquad (8)$$

where r_{sc} and r_{cm} are complex Fresnel reflection coefficients at the substrate-cell and cell-medium interfaces, correspondingly; $\alpha = \mu_{cel}lh/\cos\theta$ is the total attenuation during round-trip propagation in the cell layer and μ_{cell} is the attenuation in the cell layer per unit length. At certain wavelengths/angles the reflectivity R achieves its minimum due to destructive interference of the waves reflected from the substrate-cell and cell-medium interfaces (reflected and refracted waves; Fig. 4a, lower panel). This minimum corresponds to the waveguide mode excitation. The minimal reflectivity (R) is determined by the wave attenuation, α. Apart from the intracellular absorption and scattering, there can be dynamic losses associated with the incomplete cell-cell attachment. This allows exploiting the magnitude of the waveguide resonance as an indicator of dynamic changes in the cell-cell connectivity and cell monolayer integrity [22].

The reflection from the cell-substrate interface can be significantly improved by introducing a thin conducting layer on top of the substrate. This has some effect on the resonant wavelength λ_{TM}, since the phase shift at the cell-substrate interface becomes $\phi_{cs} \approx \pi$ (Eq. 7).

2.5 Estimation of the Refractive Index and Average Cell Height

IR-SPR measurements provide infrared reflectivity spectra from the cell-prism assembly at a given incident angle. Surface plasmon and waveguide resonant wavenumbers can be extracted from these spectra. In principle, this information is enough to estimate the effective refractive index of the analyte (cell monolayer, Eq. 6) and the analyte thickness (cell height, Eq. 7). However, we used a more rigorous procedure, by fitting each spectrum with Fresnel equations for reflection from the four-layer assembly: a ZnS prism, a 20 nm Au layer, a cell monolayer, and the aqueous medium using MATLAB software. The MATLAB codes are freely available at http://irspr.blogspot.co.il. The optical constants (i.e., n and κ) of ZnS, Au, and water, which represented the extracellular medium, adopted from "Handbook of optical constants of solids" [41] and from independent IR-SPR measurements [36]. Our fitting procedure involves only one fitting parameter for each optical resonance (i.e., SPR and TM_1 resonance), the effective refractive index for SPR of the cell monolayer and cell height for TM_1 resonance [36, 42].

3 Materials

3.1 Cell Line and Cell Culture Media

1. Madin-Darby canine kidney type II (originally obtained from Prof. Keith Mostov, UCSF, USA).

2. Minimal Essential Medium (MEM, Biological Industries, Beit Haemek, Israel).

3. Fetal calf serum (FCS, Biological Industries, Beit Haemek, Israel).

4. Trypsin-EDTA solution (Trypsin, trypsin/EDTA 1:2,000 in Puck's saline A; Biological Industries, Beit Haemek, Israel).

5. Routine MDCK cell culture medium (MEM): MEM supplemented with 5 % (vol/vol) FCS, 2 mM glutamine, 1 % (vol/vol) antibiotics.

6. MDCK cell culture medium for IR-SPR experiments (MEM-Hepes): MEM supplemented with 5 % (vol/vol) FCS and 1 % (vol/vol) antibiotics and 20 mM Hepes (pH 7.4).

3.2 Reagents and Equipment for Cell Culture

1. HEPES buffer: 1 M HEPES, pH 7.3 (Biological Industries, Beit Haemek, Israel).

2. Hank's Balanced Salt Solution (HBSS): 1× with calcium and magnesium and phenol red (Biological Industries, Beit Haemek, Israel).

3. Tissue culture antibiotics solution: Penicillin-Streptomycin and Amphotericin B Solution (Biological Industries, Beit Haemek, Israel).

4. LB bacterial medium: Bacto Tryptone and Bacto Yeast Extract (Difco Laboratories, Becton, Dickinson and Company; Sparks, MD, USA) and NaCl (Bio-Lab ltd., Jerusalem, Israel).

5. LB-Agar: LB medium supplemented with Bacto-Agar (Difco Laboratories, Becton, Dickinson and Company; Sparks, MD, USA).

6. Ampicillin, Sodium Salt (CALBIOCHEM, San Diego, CA, USA).

7. Kanamycin Sulfate (CALBIOCHEM, San Diego, CA, USA).

8. Streptomycin Sulfate (Biological Industries, Beit Haemek, Israel).

9. 10 cm culture dish (Thermo Fisher Scientific Nunc A/S, Roskilde, Denmark).

3.3 IR-SPR System

1. FTIR (Equinox 55, Bruker Optik, Ettlingen, Germany).

2. MCT (Liquid Nitrogen cooled HgCdTe Infrared detector, InfraRed Associates, Stuart, FL, USA).

3. ZnS prism (ISP Optics, Irvington, NY, USA).

4. IR polarizer (Specac, Orpington, UK).

5. Off-axis parabolic mirrors (Ø25.4 mm/50.8 mm, Au coating, Edmund Optics, Barrington, NJ, USA).

6. Flat mirror (Ø25mm, Au coating, Edmund Optics, Barrington, NJ, USA).

7. Syringe pump (BASi MD-1000, Bioanalytical Systems, West Lafayette, IN, USA).

8. CMOS camera (Lw 575; Lumenera, Ottawa, Ontario, Canada).

9. Continuous zoom objective (12× zoom, Navitar, Wharton, NJ, USA).

3.4 Software for Data Acquisition and Analysis

1. MATLAB (MATLAB 7.10, The MathWorks, Natick, MA, USA).

2. OPUS (OPUS NT 6.5, Bruker Optik, Ettlingen, Germany).

3. ImageJ (ImageJ 1.48p, W. Rasband, National Institutes of Health, Bethesda, MD, USA).

4 Methods

4.1 Bacterial Strains and Activation for Cell Infection

The bacterial strains used in this study included E2348/69 (EPEC-*wt*) [43], E2348/69 escV::miniTn5kan (EPEC-*escV*) [44]. To prepare the bacteria for host cell infection, a single colony of Enteropathogenic *E. coli* (EPEC) was picked from a Luria-Bertani (LB) agar plate and placed into a bacterial tube containing 3 ml LB media supplemented with the appropriate antibiotic solution (100 µg/ml ampicillin or 50 µg/ml kanamycin, respectively). Bacteria were cultured overnight at 37 °C without shaking. The type-III secretion system (T3SS) of EPEC was preactivated by diluting the overnight bacterial culture (1:50) in MEM followed by 3 h incubation in a humidified atmosphere of 5 % CO_2 at 37 °C without shaking [45]. Infection of MDCK cell monolayers was performed with preactivated bacteria in the range of 5–10 MOI (multiplicity of infection).

4.2 MDCK Cell Culture

Madin-Darby canine kidney (MDCK) epithelial cell monolayer is a common host system for bacteria infection studies [46, 47]. For IR-SPR experiments, MDCK cells were routinely cultured in minimal essential medium (MEM), supplemented with 5 % (vol/vol) fetal calf serum (FCS) and 1 % (vol/vol) antibiotics. Cells were maintained in a humidified incubator at 37 °C and a 5 % CO_2 atmosphere for 3–5 days to reach full confluence (Fig. 5a) [21]. Next, MDCK cells were cultured on IR-SPR chip (i.e., Au-coated ZnS prism) as follows: cells were detached from the dish by trypsinization and suspended in 10 ml of MEM Hanks' salts (cell density of ~10^6 cells/ml) (Fig. 5b). Half ml of the MEM medium with suspended cells was immediately seeded on top of the IR-SPR chip mounted on a home-made polycarbonate holder (Fig. 5c). The cell suspension completely covered the Au chip surface, providing homogeneous distribution of cells. Cells were allowed adhering to the substrate for 2 h inside CO_2 incubator (5 % CO_2,

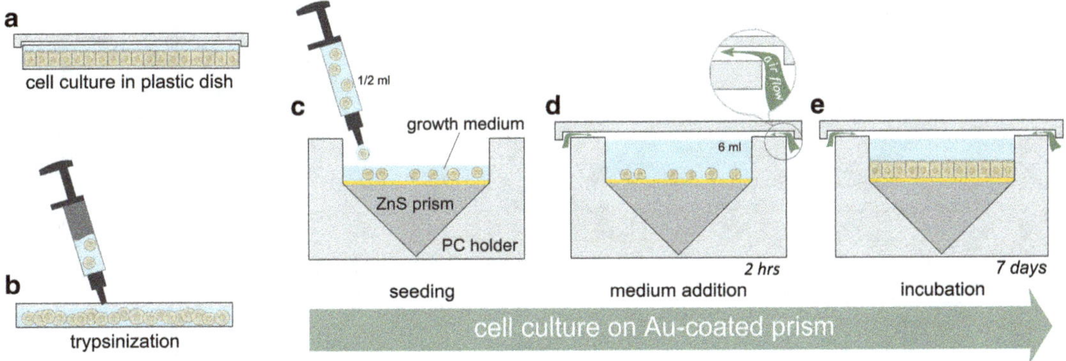

Fig. 5 MDCK cell culture on IR-SPR chips. (**a**) Routine culture of MDCK cells in plastic dish to full confluence. (**b**) Detachment of cells from dish by trypsinization. (**c**) Initial seeding of ½ ml of cell suspension on top of the gold-coated base of IR-SPR chip inside special prism holder. (**d**) Addition of 6 ml of the cell growth medium after 2 h incubation in CO_2 incubator. (**e**) Further incubation of cells in the CO_2 incubator until a fully confluent and polarized epithelial cell monolayer is formed

37 °C, 90 % humidity). Thereafter, 6 mls of MEM were gently added (Fig. 5d), and the chip was placed in a CO_2 incubator for another 7 days until a confluent and polarized cell monolayer was formed on top of the Au-surface (Fig. 5e). On fourth day, cells were washed twice with PBS and 6 ml of fresh MEM medium added. At the 7th day the chip with cells was inserted into pre-heated flow chamber (37 °C) installed into the IR-SPR setup. To avoid changes in pH in the flow chamber, cells were continuously perfused with MEM medium supplemented with 20 mM Hepes (pH 7.4). To retain stable pH in 2 ml flow chamber, the flow rate of the medium set in the range between 0.5 and 5 µl/min.

4.3 IR-SPR System

The IR-SPR experimental setup is shown in Fig. 6a. It includes a right-angle ZnS prism (20×40 mm^2 base) with a 20-nm-thick gold coating attached to a 2 ml flow chamber filled with MEM-Hepes medium. The temperature of the flow chamber was stabilized at 37 ± 0.1 °C with Peltier-based homemade temperature controller. The flow rate was controlled via a motorized syringe pump equipped with a variable speed controller. The prism-flow cell assembly was mounted on the vertical translation stage. The infrared SP was excited in Kretschmann's geometry with a Fourier-Transform Infrared (FTIR) spectrometer as a broadband infrared source with spectral range 1–5 µm (2,000–10,000 cm^{-1}). The infrared beam was collimated by two off-axis parabolic mirrors (*M1 and M2*) polarized and reflected from the prism, and then focused by another off-axis parabolic mirror (*M3*) onto a liquid-nitrogen-cooled MCT (HgCdTe) detector.

The IR-SPR system equipped with complementary optical imaging module (Fig. 6b). This allowed performing simultaneous optical time-lapsed imaging of the cells cultured on the Au-coated

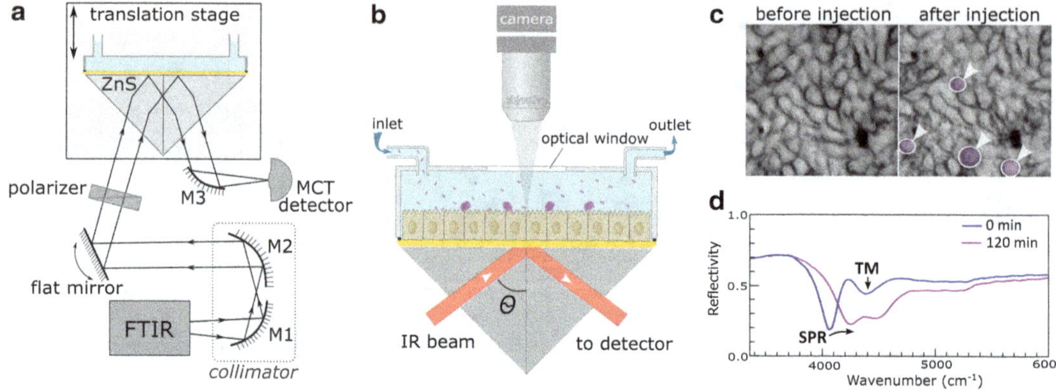

Fig. 6 IR-SPR experimental system. (**a**) Optical configuration for SPR excitation in infrared based on Kretschmann geometry. (**b**) Flow chamber with installed IR-SPR chip (Au-coated prism) equipped with upright optical imaging module. (**c**) Images of MDCK cell monolayer cultured in the flow chamber before (0 min) and after 120 min of bacteria injection. Cell-attached acterial microcolonies are indicated with arrowheads. (**d**) IR-SPR spectra before and after bacteria injection show SP and waveguide resonances at different experimental times

prism surface (Fig. 6c). The images were taken in the reflection mode through a 0.5 mm thick optical window by a CMOS camera connected to the high magnification continuous zoom objective using a halogen lamp supplemented with upright co-axial illumination. The optical imaging was synchronized with the FTIR scans. Figure 6c shows an example of two optical images with corresponding FTIR spectra (Fig. 6d).

5   IR-SPR Measurement of EPEC Infection

EPEC infection was achieved by exposing the IR-SPR chip cultured with polarized MDCK cell monolayer to preactivated EPEC bacteria in the flow chamber. Initially, infrared reflectivity spectra at an oblique incidence was recorded for about an hour before bacteria introduction to ensure stable IR-SPR spectrum (Fig. 7a, b). Then, bacteria-containing medium was introduced in to the flow chamber through the inlet and this injection phase lasted for 30 min with flow rate of 50 μl/min (started at $t = 0$ min) to rich the desired 5–10 MOI (Fig. 7c). Thereafter, bacteria injection was stopped and replaced by slower MEM-Hepes medium flow (0.5 μl/min) for the rest of the experiment. Figure 7a, b shows the time evolution of the entire infrared reflectivity spectrum upon host cell-bacteria interaction as 2D heat map. The entire measurement lasted for at least 200 min. At the end of each experiment, cells were removed from the Au substrate by introducing Trypsin/EDTA solution into the flow chamber for 30 min and additional IR-SPR spectrum was obtained. This step was not necessary for the estimation of relative changes, although it allowed calculating the absolute refractive index and cell height values [23].

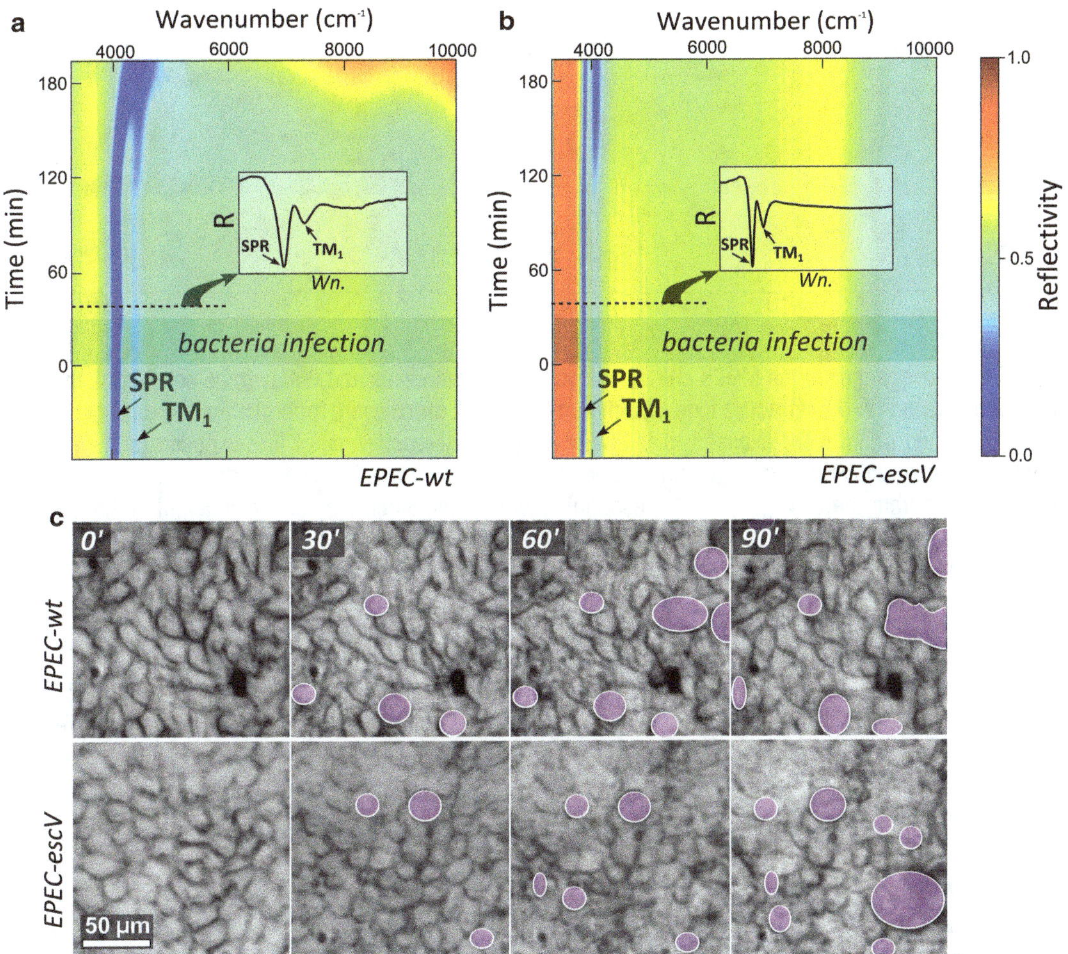

Fig. 7 Monitoring EPEC infection by the IR-SPR system. (**a, b**) Time evolution of infrared reflectivity spectrum upon EPEC infection. EPEC-*wt* and EPEC-*escV* injection lasted for 30 min (*t*= 0–30 min highlighted by a *darkened box*). The entire measurement lasted ~200 min. The *insets* show single spectrum 40 min after beginning of bacteria injection. SPR and TM₁ resonance appear as reflectivity minima or as blue valleys on the color heat map. (**c**) Representative images of cells and bacteria show the accumulation of EPEC-*wt* and EPEC-*escV* microcolonies (in purple) on the host MDCK cell monolayer. Images were taken simultaneously with the IR-SPR measurements. Adapted from Yashunsky V et al. (2013) PLoS One 8(10):e78431, doi:10.1371/journal.pone. 0078431 [21]

Analysis of the IR-SPR spectra enabled quantitative measurement of the EPEC infection induced effect, *see* Fig. 7a, b respectively. Time dependence of SPR and waveguide (TM1) resonance wavenumbers disclosed different and independent information about the host MDCK cell monolayer structure. The change in SPR wavenumber was translated to change in refractive index at basolateral region of cells, namely, the change in the water content, as it is previously explained in Section 2.3. The TM₁ resonance was used to determine the absolute height of intact cell

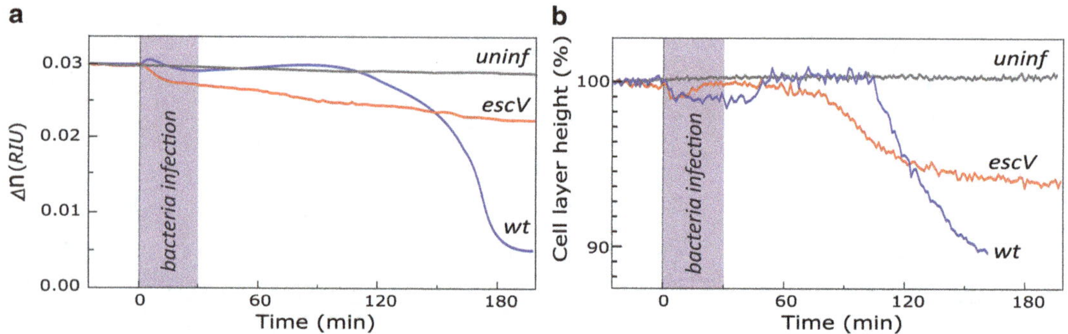

Fig. 8 Temporal changes in the MDCK cell monolayer refractive indices and the average cell height. (a) Time-dependent changes in the refractive index. Confluent MDCK cell monolayers formed after 6–7 days of culturing on an Au-coated prism were exposed to EPEC-*wt* (*blue*), EPEC-*escV* (*red*), or just exposed to bacteria-free growth medium–uninfected (*gray*). (b) Time-dependent changes in the TM$_1$ waveguide mode. The cell height was calculated from the waveguide (TM$_1$) resonant wavenumber. Since the initial cell height in these experiments varied between 8.1 and 9.2 µm, we compare the relative cell height normalized to its initial value (i.e., cell height at $t=0$ is 100 %). Adapted from Yashunsky V et al. (2013) PLoS One 8(10):e78431, doi:10.1371/journal.pone.0078431 [21]

monolayer with very high precision (*see* Section 2.4) [22]. Typical height of the 7 days old MDCK cells prior to bacterial infection varied between 8.1 and 9.2 µm. Thus, to compare different experiments the relative change in cell height was normalized to initial cell height (Fig. 8b).

5.1 Measurement of Cell Refractive Index upon EPEC Infection

Prior to infection, the infrared reflectivity dip corresponding to the SPR (4,080 cm^{-1}, Fig. 7a inset) remained unchanged for 60 min ($t<0$ min). In the case of EPEC-wt infection, after ~180 min of the SPR shifts toward 4,700 cm^{-1} (Fig. 7a). Such strong shift toward shorter wavelength (blueshift) clearly indicates about an increase of the water volume in the basolateral region of host cell monolayer. Indeed, this interpretation was confirmed by live confocal microscopy, which revealed enlarged basolateral intercellular gaps and intensive generation of macrovesicles at basolateral cell region [20].

For quantitative analysis of the effect the temporal dynamics of SPR wavenumber translated into the change of the effective refractive index $\Delta n = n_{\text{cell}} - n_{\text{medium}}$. Figure 8a shows typical temporal dynamics of Δn during bacterial infection with EPEC-wt. Throughout the injection stage, when medium containing activated EPEC-wt bacteria was introduced into the flow chamber ($t=0$–30 min), Δn gradually decreased from 0.030 to 0.029. During the subsequent 60 min, Δn returned to its initial value of 0.030 ($t=90$ min, Fig. 8a). Thereafter, the Δn value dropped sharply and irreversibly for about 80 min, and reached a refractive index value of $\Delta n = 0.004$ (Fig. 8a), which slightly exceeds that of a stripped-off prism (i.e., a prism without cells) with plain growth medium. Cell infection at a lower MOI resulted in a slower rate and delayed the drop in Δn, respectively, indicating that the timing of the Δn drop is dependent on the host cell infection intensity.

5.2 Measurement of Host Cell Layer Height upon EPEC Infection

The satellite minor reflectivity dip at a shorter wavelength ($4{,}400$ cm^{-1}, Fig. 7a) corresponds to the TM_1 resonance (*see* Fig. 7a, b). Before introducing the bacteria into the flow chamber (i.e., at $t < 0$ min), according to our numerical fitting model (*see* **Section 7, Notes**), the TM_1 resonance value corresponds to average cell height of 9.01 ± 0.05 μm. Upon infection with EPEC-wt, the cell height decreased by 1.5 % (0.14 μm) for 35 min ($t = 10$–45 min), and then rapidly recovered to its original value, and remained unchanged for 50 min ($t = 50$–100 min). Starting $t = 100$ min, the cell height dropped down by 10 % (1 μm) over a time span of 60 min ($t = 100$–160 min; Fig. 8b). After that time ($t > 160$ min), the TM_1-waveguide resonance was completely smeared. This indicates a severe impairment of the cell monolayer integrity. These data suggest that an average cell height is a very sensitive indicator of early effects that the bacteria have on host cell monolayer structure.

5.3 Selective Detection of EPEC Pathogens

The ability of EPEC bacteria to translocate its effector proteins into the host cells is considered to be critical for EPEC pathogenesis [6]. To deliver virulent effector proteins into its host, EPEC utilizes a type-III secretion system (T3SS). T3SS is essential for the ability of EPEC to infect successfully its host cells [48]. To test the specificity of IR-SPR measurement in sensing EPEC infection of epithelial hosts MDCK cell monolayers were either infected with the T3SS-defective EPEC-*escV* or remained uninfected and just exposed to plain growth medium containing small amounts of LB, equivalent to those introduced when cells are exposed to bacteria. Figure 8a, b compares the dynamics of cell refractive index and cell height as they exposed to different bacterial strains; EPEC-*wt*, EPEC-*escV*, or uninfected cells.

Figure 8a shows that the refractive index of uninfected cells remained essentially unaffected over the entire experimental time (over 180 min and up to 3 days, *not shown*). In all experiments in which cells were exposed to bacteria, a small transient variation of the cell refractive index was observed upon injection. We attribute this to the effects produced upon injection of bacteria-containing medium. Infection with EPEC-*escV* resulted in a gradual decrease in the cell refractive index ($\Delta n_{escV} = 0.022$, over 180 min). Nonetheless, the reduction in Δn values was much smaller than what was observed after 180 min for EPEC-wt infected cells ($\Delta n_{wt} = 0.004$).

Figure 8b shows that for uninfected cells, the average cell monolayer height remains nearly constant over time. A minor drop in the average cell monolayer height (1.5 %) was observed immediately upon bacteria injection into the flow chamber. Similar to SPR or Δn fluctuation, we attribute this transient variation in cell height to the mere injection of bacteria-containing medium. In the case of EPEC-*escV* and EPEC-*wt* infected cells, the average cell height recovered after 40 min and 60 min, respectively, and remained unchanged for an additional 60 min. Then EPEC-*escV* infected cells exhibited a much slower and smaller reduction of the cell height (6 %) compared to EPEC-*wt* infected cells, whose cell height decreased by 10 % in the course of 60 min. Moreover, the experiments with EPEC-*wt* infected cells always showed that the waveguide mode disappeared approximately 160 min after bacteria injection, whereas in case EPEC-*escV* infection, the waveguide mode was still detectable up to 4 h postinfection (*not shown*).

Together these data show that translocated type-III-secreted effectors decisively contribute to early fluctuations and subsequent reduction in the refractive index and cell height reduction of EPEC infected cells. Thereby, these parameters may serve to identify pathogenic and nonpathogenic bacterial strains by a simple procedure and in a relatively short time.

6   Summary and Future Prospects

Label-free cellular biosensors have found applications in a variety of cellular processes, such as cell adhesion, toxicity, receptor signaling, and viral infection [28, 31, 49]. In this chapter we introduced a novel method of IR-SPR for real-time monitoring of structural changes in epithelial host cell layers and its implication in detecting EPEC infection. Similar to other label-free methods, IR-SPR measures integrated and phenotypic responses at whole cell level. However, IR-SPR exhibits several unique advantages. These include simultaneous and independent dynamic measurements of cell-substrate interaction, intercellular intactness, and height and uniformity of the epithelial monolayer.

We foresee that IR-SPR capabilities will be further developed and used as a powerful tool for sensing diverse processes of host cell-pathogen interactions and as a rapid and highly sensitive method for screening various effects that pathogenic bacteria induce on their hosts.

7   Notes

1. For IR-SPR calibration, each IR-SPR experiment started by the following calibration steps. Flat mirror angle, translational stage, and focusing mirror (M3) adjusted to produce incident angle (θ_{ext}) of 22.5 ± 0.5° (Fig. 6a, b). The polarizer set to obtain *s*-polarized spectrum and single measurement of *s*-polarized

spectrum performed, afterwards the polarized rotated by 90° to obtain p-polarized reflectivity spectrum. The s-polarized reflectivity spectrum (R_s) used further for normalization of the p-polarized reflectivity spectra (R_p) to eliminate undesired spectral contribution (e.g., light source, optical components, and environment), Reflectivity $= R_p(t)/R_s$. The spectra were collected using an FTIR spectrometer operated with OPUS software (Bruker Optik). The measurements were performed at 8 cm^{-1} spectral resolution and represented an average over eight scans, which lasted for 25 s with a repetition rate of 70 s.

Acknowledgments

VY deeply thanks Dan Davidov (HUJI) and Michael Golosovsky (HUJI) for their scientific guidance. We also thank Leorah Kharilker (HUJI), Efrat Zlotkin-Rivkin (HUJI), and Vladislav Lirtsman (HUJI) for helping with experiments; Ilan Rosenshine (HUJI) and Michael Donnenberg (UMD) for providing EPEC strains. BA acknowledges the support from the Start-Up grant Tack A from Yissum, the Israel Science Foundation (ISF), funded by the Israel Academy of Sciences (Grants 1167/08 and 1483/13), and a grant from the Israel Cancer Association.

Glossary

EPEC	Enteropathogenic *Escherichia coli*
IR	Infrared
Lx	Surface plasmon propagation length
MDCK	Madin-Darby canine kidney
SP	Surface plasmon
SPR	Surface plasmon resonance
T3SS	Type-III secretion system
TJ	Tight junction
TM	Transverse magnetic
δz	Surface plasmon penetration depth

References

1. Ochoa TJ, Contreras CA (2011) Enteropathogenic Escherichia coli infection in children. Curr Opin Infect Dis 24(5):478–483. doi:10.1097/QCO.0b013e32834a8b8b

2. Frankel G, Phillips AD (2008) Attaching effacing Escherichia coli and paradigms of Tir-triggered actin polymerization: getting off the pedestal. Cell Microbiol 10(3):549–556. doi:10.1111/j.1462-5822.2007.01103.x

3. Croxen MA, Finlay BB (2010) Molecular mechanisms of Escherichia coli pathogenicity. Nat Rev Microbiol 8(1):26–38. doi:10.1038/nrmicro2265

4. Aroeti B, Friedman G, Zlotkin-Rivkin E, Donnenberg M (2012) Retraction of enteropathogenic E. coli type IV pili promotes efficient host cell colonization, effector translocation and tight junction disruption.

Gut Microbes 3(3):267–271. doi:10.4161/gmic.19814

5. Bhavsar AP, Guttman JA, Finlay BB (2007) Manipulation of host-cell pathways by bacterial pathogens. Nature 449(7164):827–834. doi:10.1038/nature06247

6. Goosney DL, Gruenheid S, Finlay BB (2000) Gut feelings: enteropathogenic E. coli (EPEC) interactions with the host. Annu Rev Cell Dev Biol 16:173–189. doi:10.1146/annurev.cellbio.16.1.173

7. Shifflett DE, Clayburgh DR, Koutsouris A, Turner JR, Hecht GA (2005) Enteropathogenic E. coli disrupts tight junction barrier function and structure in vivo. Lab Invest 85(10):1308–1324. doi:10.1038/labinvest.3700330

8. Vallance BA, Finlay BB (2000) Exploitation of host cells by enteropathogenic Escherichia coli. Proc Natl Acad Sci U S A 97(16):8799–8806. doi:10.1073/pnas.97.16.8799

9. Weflen AW, Alto NM, Hecht GA (2009) Tight junctions and enteropathogenic E. coli. Ann N Y Acad Sci 1165:169–174. doi:10.1111/j.1749-6632.2012.06563.x

10. Guttman JA, Kazemi P, Lin AE, Vogl AW, Finlay BB (2007) Desmosomes are unaltered during infections by attaching and effacing pathogens. Anat Rec (Hoboken) 290(2):199–205

11. Ivanov AI, Parkos CA, Nusrat A (2010) Cytoskeletal regulation of epithelial barrier function during inflammation. Am J Pathol 177(2):512–524. doi:10.2353/ajpath.2010.100168

12. Shifrin Y, Kirschner J, Geiger B, Rosenshine I (2002) Enteropathogenic Escherichia coli induces modification of the focal adhesions of infected host cells. Cell Microbiol 4(4):235–243. doi:10.1046/j.1462-5822.2002.00188.x

13. Balda MS, Whitney JA, Flores C, González S, Cereijido M, Matter K (1996) Functional dissociation of paracellular permeability and transepithelial electrical resistance and disruption of the apical-basolateral intramembrane diffusion barrier by expression of a mutant tight junction membrane protein. J Cell Biol 134(4):1031–1049

14. Blikslager AT, Moeser AJ, Gookin JL, Jones SL, Odle J (2007) Restoration of barrier function in injured intestinal mucosa. Physiol Rev 87(2):545–564. doi:10.1152/physrev.00012.2006

15. Gookin JL, Galanko JA, Blikslager AT, Argenzio RA (2003) PG-mediated closure of paracellular pathway and not restitution is the primary determinant of barrier recovery in acutely injured porcine ileum. Am J Physiol Gastrointest Liver Physiol 285(5):G967–G979. doi:10.1152/ajpgi.00532.2002

16. Simovitch M, Sason H, Cohen S, Zahavi EE, Melamed-Book N, Weiss A, Aroeti B, Rosenshine I (2010) EspM inhibits pedestal formation by enterohaemorrhagic Escherichia coli and enteropathogenic E. coli and disrupts the architecture of a polarized epithelial monolayer. Cell Microbiol 12(4):489–505. doi:10.1111/j.1462-5822.2009.01410.x

17. Golosovsky M, Lirtsman V, Yashunsky V, Davidov D, Aroeti B (2009) Midinfrared surface-plasmon resonance: a novel biophysical tool for studying living cells. J Appl Phys 105(10):1020–1021. doi:10.1063/1.3116143

18. Yashunsky V, Lirtsman V, Zilbershtein A, Bein A, Schwartz B, Aroeti B, Golosovsky M, Davidov D (2012) Surface plasmon-based infrared spectroscopy for cell biosensing. J Biomed Opt 17(8):081409. doi:10.1117/1.JBO.17.8.081409

19. Ziblat R, Lirtsman V, Davidov D, Aroeti B (2006) Infrared surface plasmon resonance: a novel tool for real time sensing of variations in living cells. Biophys J 90(7):2592–2599. doi:10.1529/biophysj.105.072090

20. Yashunsky V, Kharilker L, Zlotkin-Rivkin E, Rund D, Melamed-Book N, Zahavi EE, Perlson E, Mercone S, Golosovsky M, Davidov D, Aroeti B (2013) Real-time sensing of enteropathogenic E. coli-induced effects on epithelial host cell height, cell-substrate interactions, and endocytic processes by infrared surface plasmon spectroscopy. PLoS One 8(10):e78431. doi:10.1371/journal.pone.0078431

21. Yashunsky V, Lirtsman V, Golosovsky M, Davidov D, Aroeti B (2010) Real-time monitoring of epithelial cell-cell and cell-substrate interactions by infrared surface plasmon spectroscopy. Biophys J 99(12):4028–4036. doi:10.1016/j.bpj.2010.10.017

22. Yashunsky V, Marciano T, Lirtsman V, Golosovsky M, Davidov D, Aroeti B (2012) Real-time sensing of cell morphology by infrared waveguide spectroscopy. PLoS One 7(10):e48454. doi:10.1371/journal.pone.0048454

23. Zilbershtein A, Bein A, Lirtsman V, Schwartz B, Golosovsky M, Davidov D (2014) Surface plasmon resonance-based infrared biosensor for cell studies with simultaneous control. J Biomed Opt 19(11):111608. doi:10.1117/1.JBO.19.11.111608

24. Otto A (1968) Excitation of nonradiative surface plasma waves in silver by the method of frustrated total reflection. Zeitschrift fur Physik 216:398–410

25. Kretschmann E, Raether H (1968) Radiative decay of non radiative surface plasmons excited by light(Surface plasma waves excitation

by light and decay into photons applied to nonradiative modes). Zeitschrift Fuer Naturforschung, Teil A 23:2135

26. Liedberg B, Nylander C, Lunström I (1983) Surface plasmon resonance for gas detection and biosensing. Sensor Actuator 4:299–304

27. Knoll W (1998) Interfaces and thin films as seen by bound electromagnetic waves. Annu Rev Phys Chem 49:569–638

28. Cooper MA (2002) Optical biosensors in drug discovery. Nat Rev Drug Discov 1(7):515–528. doi:10.1038/nrd838

29. Homola J (2003) Present and future of surface plasmon resonance biosensors. Anal Bioanal Chem 377(3):528–539. doi:10.1007/s00216-003-2101-0

30. Homola J, Yee SS, Gauglitz G (1999) Surface plasmon resonance sensors: review. Sensor Actuator B Chem 54(1–2):3–15

31. Fang Y (2011) The development of label-free cellular assays for drug discovery. Expert Opin Drug Discov 6(12):1285–1298. doi:10.1517/17460441.2012.642360

32. Stanley R (2012) Plasmonics in the mid-infrared. Nat Photon 6(7):409–411. doi:10.1038/nphoton.2012.161

33. Peterson AW, Halter M, Tona A, Bhadriraju K, Plant AL (2009) Surface plasmon resonance imaging of cells and surface-associated fibronectin. BMC Cell Biol 10:1–17. doi:10.1186/1471-2121-10-16

34. Chabot V, Cuerrier CM, Escher E, Aimez V, Grandbois M, Charette PG (2009) Biosensing based on surface plasmon resonance and living cells. Biosens Bioelectron 24(6):1667–1673. doi:10.1016/j.bios.2008.08.025

35. Yanase Y, Suzuki H, Tsutsui T, Hiragun T, Kameyoshi Y, Hide M (2007) The SPR signal in living cells reflects changes other than the area of adhesion and the formation of cell constructions. Biosens Bioelectron 22(6):1081–1086. doi:10.1016/j.bios.2006.03.011

36. Zilbershtein A, Golosovsky M, Lirtsman V, Aroeti B, Davidov D (2012) Quantitative surface plasmon spectroscopy: determination of the infrared optical constants of living cells. Vib Spectros 61:43–49. doi:10.1016/j.vibspec.2012.01.019

37. Coe JV, Rodriguez KR, Teeters-Kennedy S, Cilwa K, Heer J, Tian H, Williams SM (2007) Metal films with arrays of tiny holes: spectroscopy with infrared plasmonic scaffolding. J Phys Chem C 111(47):17459–17472. doi:10.1021/jp072909a

38. Raether H (1988) Surface-plasmons on smooth and rough surfaces and on gratings. Springer Tr Mod Phys 111:1–133

39. Johansen K, Arwin H, Lundstrom I, Liedberg B (2000) Imaging surface plasmon resonance sensor based on multiple wavelengths: sensitivity considerations. Rev Sci Instrum 71(9):3530–3538

40. Born M, Wolf E (1999) Principles of optics: electromagnetic theory of propagation, interference and diffraction of light, 7th edn. Cambridge University Press, Cambridge, UK

41. Palik ED (1984) Handbook of optical-constants. J Opt Soc Am A Opt Image Sci Vis 1(12):1297–1297

42. Yashunsky V, Zilbershtein A, Lirtsman V, Marciano T, Aroeti B, Golosovsky M, Davidov D (2012) Infrared surface plasmon spectroscopy and biosensing. Proc. SPIE 8234, Plasmonics in Biology and Medicine IX, 823419; doi:10.1117/12.907255

43. Levine MM, Bergquist EJ, Nalin DR, Waterman DH, Hornick RB, Young CR, Sotman S (1978) Escherichia coli strains that cause diarrhoea but do not produce heat-labile or heat-stable enterotoxins and are non-invasive. Lancet 1(8074):1119–1122

44. Nadler C, Shifrin Y, Nov S, Kobi S, Rosenshine I (2006) Characterization of enteropathogenic Escherichia coli mutants that fail to disrupt host cell spreading and attachment to substratum. Infect Immun 74(2):839–849. doi:10.1128/IAI. 74.2.839-849.2006

45. Rosenshine I, Ruschkowski S, Finlay BB (1996) Expression of attaching/effacing activity by enteropathogenic Escherichia coli depends on growth phase, temperature, and protein synthesis upon contact with epithelial cells. Infect Immun 64(3):966–973

46. Gassama-Diagne A, Yu W, ter Beest M, Martin-Belmonte F, Kierbel A, Engel J, Mostov K (2006) Phosphatidylinositol-3,4,5-trisphosphate regulates the formation of the basolateral plasma membrane in epithelial cells. Nat Cell Biol 8(9):963–970. doi:10.1038/ncb1461

47. Sason H, Milgrom M, Weiss AM, Melamed-Book N, Balla T, Grinstein S, Backert S, Rosenshine I, Aroeti B (2009) Enteropathogenic Escherichia coli subverts phosphatidylinositol 4, 5-bisphosphate and phosphatidylinositol 3,4,5-trisphosphate upon epithelial cell infection. Mol Biol Cell 20(1):544–555. doi:10.1091/mbc. E08-05-0516

48. Coburn B, Sekirov I, Finlay BB (2007) Type III secretion systems and disease. Clin Microbiol Rev 20(4):535–549. doi:10.1128/CMR. 00013-07

49. Xi B, Yu N, Wang X, Xu X, Abassi YA (2008) The application of cell-based label-free technology in drug discovery. Biotechnol J 3(4):484–495. doi:10.1002/biot.200800020

Chapter 21

Surface Plasmon Resonance for Clinical Diagnosis of Type I Allergy

Yuhki Yanase and Michihiro Hide

Abstract

Noninvasive real-time evaluation of living cell conditions and functions is increasingly sought after in life science. Surface plasmon resonance (SPR) sensors can sensitively detect refractive index changes on the surface of a sensor chip without any labeling in a real-time manner. In this chapter, we first review the principle of SPR sensors and the applications of SPR sensors for detection of living cell reactions. We then introduce the technique to isolate and fix basophils on an SPR sensor chip. Finally, we describe the method to visualize individual basophil activation by means of SPR imaging (SPRI) sensor and the potential of basophil activation test by SPRI for clinical diagnosis of type I allergy.

Key words Basophils, Clinical diagnosis of allergy, Mast cells, Surface plasmon resonance, SPR imaging

1 SPR Sensors

SPR sensors can detect the binding of molecules in the detection volume (evanescent field, within 500 nm on the gold surface) on a sensor chip coated with gold film (50 nm) in real time without any labeling. As shown in Fig. 1, when p-polarized light through a P-polarizer is reflected at the interface between glass and gold film at various incident angles for total reflection, the reflected light is strongly attenuated at a specific incident angle. This phenomenon, called SPR, is due to the resonance between plasmon wave derived from gold film and the evanescent wave derived from reflected light. The specific angle, called resonance angle (RA), is correlated with refractive index (RI) in a detection area on the surface of SPR sensor chip. Thus, SPR sensors can detect the RI changes in a detection area without any labeling of the substances involved in interaction by detecting the change of RA [1–3]. Figure 2 shows the typical shape of an RA change during the course of an experiment of antigen–antibody interaction. When SPR sensor chip with antibody that can capture antigen is exposed to antigens, RA increases

Ye Fang (ed.), *Label-Free Biosensor Methods in Drug Discovery*, Methods in Pharmacology and Toxicology, DOI 10.1007/978-1-4939-2617-6_21, © Springer Science+Business Media New York 2015

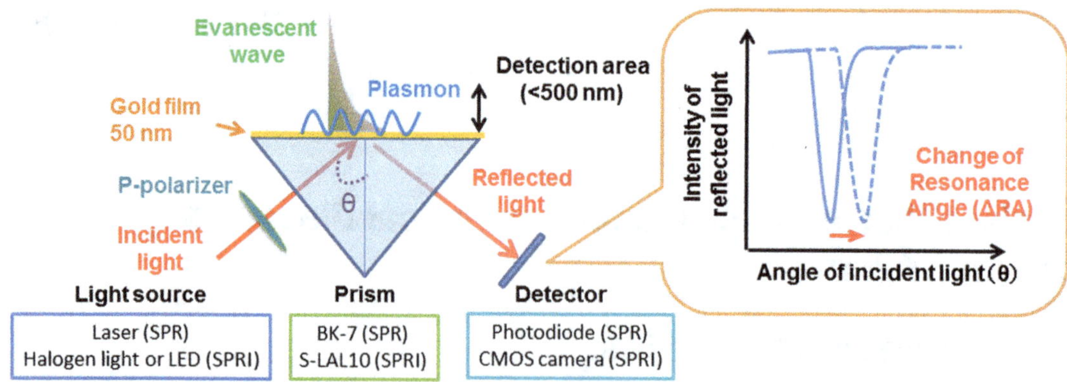

Fig. 1 Principle of SPR sensor. The SPR sensor can detect changes of RI in a detection area as a change of RA (ΔRA)

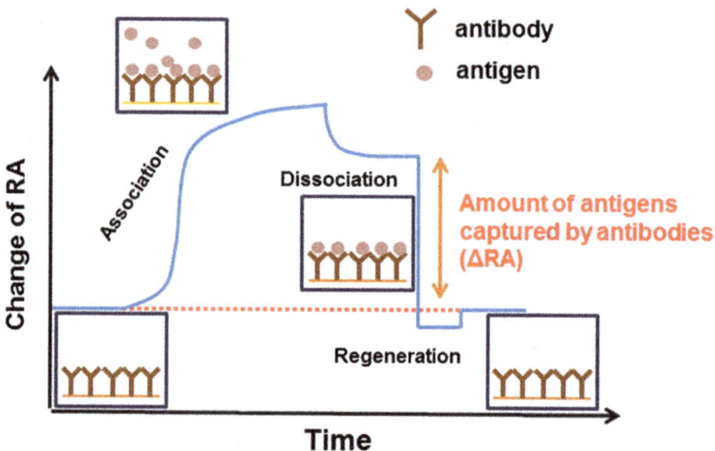

Fig. 2 Principle of detection of antigen–antibody interactions by SPR sensor. Adapted from [24]

due to the binding of antigens to antibodies (association step). RA slightly decreases, in accordance with the removal of antigens that did not bind to the antibodies in the washing process (dissociation step). The amount of antigen bound to the antibodies is calculated from ΔRA. The sensor chip with antigens captured by antibodies is regenerated by removing antigens with sodium hydroxide (regeneration step). Thus, SPR sensors can detect the interaction of molecules on a sensor chip.

2 SPR for Living Cells

During the past two decades, SPR sensors have become widely used for non-label detection of molecules interactions. In 2002, we first reported that SPR sensors not only detect binding and dissociation of biochemical substances but also reflect changes of RI in response to the activation of living mast cells. Consequentially, activation of various cells, including keratinocytes, basophils, and B lymphocytes on a sensor chip, were successfully analyzed without any labeling, suggesting the potential of SPR as a new diagnostic method for allergy and immunology [4–8]. Figure 3 shows SPR signal (real-time RI changes) in RBL-2H3 mast cells treated with IgE antibodies followed by DNP-HSA antigens. In mast cells, the binding of antigen to IgE bound to the high-affinity IgE receptor (FcεRI) on the cell surface cross-links FcεRI, results in the release of preformed and newly synthesized mediators such as histamine and arachidonic acid metabolites, and causes anaphylactic symptoms [9, 10]. When RBL-2H3 mast cells are exposed to IgE antibodies, the cells are sensitized, but not activated, with IgE which binds to FcεRI on the cells. Therefore, RI in RBL-2H3 cells does not increase. Consequentially, RI rapidly increases and gradually decreases in 40 min, when RBL-2H3 cells sensitized with IgE antibodies are stimulated with antigen (DNP-HSA) (Fig. 3). This result suggests that SPR sensors detect cell activation in response to stimuli, rather than by the simple binding of extracellular molecules to cell surface.

We have also demonstrated that reactions detected by SPR sensors are not limited to changes of the area of cell adhesion and subcellular structures of living cells which may be observed using an ordinary light microscopy. In mast cells, the activation of protein kinases Syk, Lat, Gads, and protein kinase C β (PKCβ) are indispensable for the antigen-induced RI increase of mast cells detected by SPR biosensors [11]. Moreover, we demonstrated that epidermal growth factor (EGF) induced RI changes via the

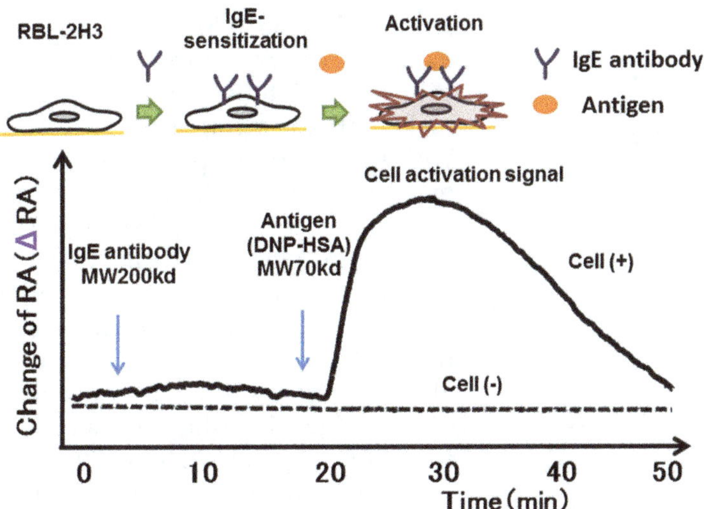

Fig. 3 SPR signals obtained by bindings of anti-DNP IgE antibody and DNP-HSA (antigen) to RBL-2H3 cells. Adapted from [24]

phosphorylation of EGFR, and suggested that the SPR biosensor could be applied to the real-time detection and diagnosis of malignant tumors [12]. Furthermore, we have developed a relatively small, simple, and portable system, using an optical fiber to detect the activation of small numbers of living cells attached to the fiber chip in a real-time manner [8]. Recently, relations between RI and cell functions have also been reported by other groups. Chabot et al. reported that SPR sensors may determine real-time adhesion and morphological changes in cells following activations by various agents [13]. An SPR sensor based on Fourier Transform infrared spectrometer operating in the near infrared wavelength range, FTIR-SPR, could also monitor changes in cell occupancy and membrane biochemical composition such as cholesterol [14, 15]. Lee et al. reported that an SPR sensor combined with olfactory receptor-expressing cells could represent a new olfactory biosensor system for the selective quantitative detection of volatile compounds [16]. A technique to detect the reaction of cancer cells against an anticancer drug with SPR sensor is reported by Kosaihira et al. [17, 18].

3   SPR Imaging (SPRI): Visualization of Individual Living Cells Activation

Conventional SPR sensors detect an average RI change in the presence of thousands of cells in an area of the sensor chip and could offer only a small number of sensing channels (<10). Consequently, it was difficult to construct an array system for cell activation, and reactions of target cells might have been readily overlooked when they were in a mixture of different cell types. Moreover, they could not reveal intracellular distribution of RI, which is important to understand the mechanism of RI changes upon cell activation. A recently developed SPR imaging (SPRI) system determines a spatial RI distribution at the SPR-active surface by measuring the distribution of light intensity which proportionally reflects RI on the surface of sensor chip in an image captured by a camera [19–21]. We therefore developed an SPRI sensor for living cell analysis in order to visualize RI changes in individual basophils [22–24]. Figure 4 shows the principal of visualization of individual cell activation. The expected resonance curve of assay buffer, cells before stimulation, and cells after stimulation are shown in (a), (b), and (c) respectively. The sensor chip is exposed to the incident light at the angle of 56°, achieving the maximum resonance of surface plasmon with assay buffer in the absence of cells. In the presence of cells whose RI is higher than buffer, the resonance angle shifts to a higher degree, resulting in the increase of reflected light intensity at the cell adherent area. When cells are stimulated, the resonance angle shifts further to the level that varies according to the stimulus and intensity of reflected light at the cell area increases.

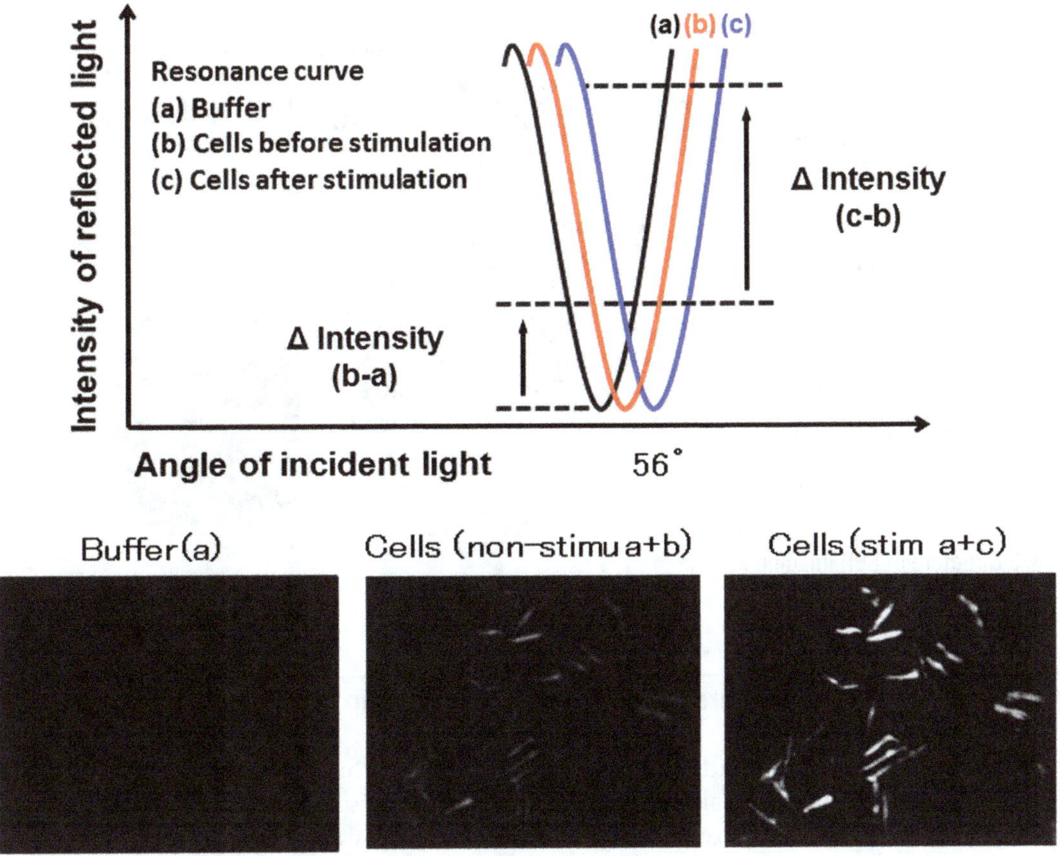

Fig. 4 Principle of visualization of individual cell reactions by SPRI. Adapted from [24]

The SPRI sensor we developed consists of a light source (Tungsten halogen light or LED (640 nm), Ocean Optics Inc, FL), P-polarizer (Sigma Koki Co., Ltd., Tokyo, Japan), prism (S-LAL10, RI = 1.72), thermostat (MiSUMi, Tokyo, Japan), Objective lens (×0.5, ×2, ×4, Edmund Optics Japan, Tokyo, Japan), and CMOS camera (ARTRAY, Tokyo, Japan). The sensor chips (S-LAL10, 20 mm × 20 mm × 1 mm, RI = 1.72) were coated with gold thin film (1 nm Cr layer and 49 nm gold layer) by means of vapor deposition (Osaka Vacuum Industrial Co., Ltd., Osaka, Japan). For collimate LED light, achromatic lens (Sigma Koki Co., Ltd) was used. Flow chamber was composed of cover glass, PEEK tubes, and silicone rubber (20 mm × 20 mm × 5 mm) of which the center was cut out as a flow space. Obtained images and changes of light intensity of individual cells were analyzed with Image-Pro (Media Cybernetics, Bethesda, MD) (Fig. 5). Visualization of RI changes in living cells by means of SPRI sensors has been summarized in several reviews [25, 26].

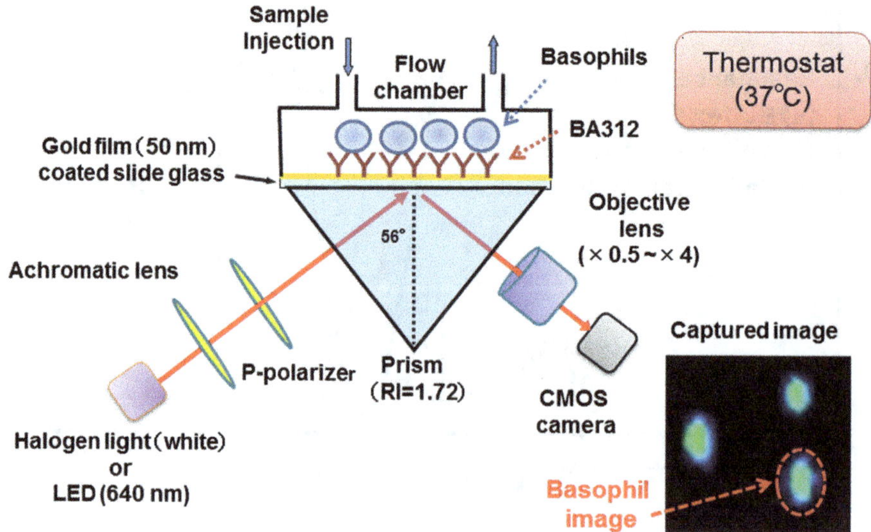

Fig. 5 Structure of SPR imaging sensor

4   Attachment of Nonadherent Cells to SPR Sensor Chip

For adherent type of cells, cell attachment can be achieved through typical cell culture. However, for suspension type of cells (i.e., nonadherent cells), it is necessary to attach them to the SPR sensor surface via specific bio-binding or nonselective electrostatic binding approach. With certain modifications the following protocols can be used to anchor other suspension cells, besides basophils.

4.1 Attachment of Basophils to Antibodies-Coated Sensor Chip

1. Clean SPR sensor chips by sonication in acetone for 5 min followed by rinsing with ethanol.

2. Immerse the chips in 1 mM dinitrophenol (DSP) solution in dimethyl sulfoxide (DMSO) for 1 h, followed by rinsing three times with water. This is to form the layer of DSP which binds to primary amines of proteins, such as antibody.

3. Apply and incubate the DSP-treated sensor chip with a solution of anti-basophilic antibody (BA312 kindly provided by Shionogi Pharmaceutical, Co., Ltd., Osaka, Japan) for 10 min at room temperature [27].

4. Rinse the surface with water once.

5. Apply and incubate with 50 µl of basophil suspension in Hepes buffer (0.03 % HSA, 0.8 % NaCl, 0.02 % KCl, 0.52 mM Na_2PO_4, 10 mM HEPES, 0.1 % Glucose, 2 mM $CaCl_2$, 1 mM $MgCl_2$, pH 7.4) for 15 min.

6. Rinse the sensor chip having basophils with buffer and then measure using SPR or SPRI.

4.2 Attachment of Floating Cells Coated with Aminoalkanethiol

1. Clean SPR sensor chips by sonication in acetone for 5 min followed by rinsing with ethanol.

2. Immerse the chips with 1 mM 8-aminooctanethiol in ethanol for 1 h, and rinse with ethanol for three times. This is to form a layer of 8-aminoalkanethiol.

3. Incubate cells suspended in appropriate buffer with the sensor chip for 20 min.

4. Rinse the chips having cells with buffer and then measure by SPR or SPRI.

4.3 Droplet method (A Method to Fix Floating Cells on Optical Fiber SPR)

1. Suspend cells in appropriate buffer at a concentration of 1×10^6 cells/ml.

2. Fill a furrowed plate with the cell suspension and turn the plate so as to make an elongated droplet containing living cells at room temperature (Fig. 6).

3. Immerse a gold-coated fiber tip into the bottom of a droplet for 15 min.

4. Quickly locate the sensor part into a flow cell and perfuse with appropriate buffer (Fig. 6) [8].

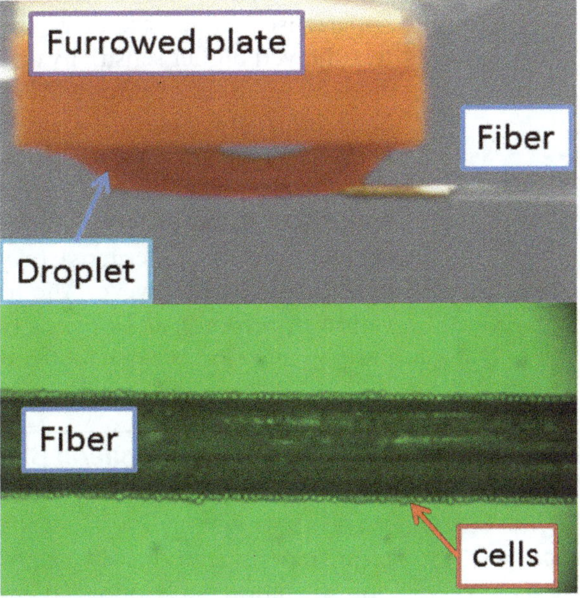

Fig. 6 Cells were fixed on a sensor tip surface by means of the "droplet method" and observed under a phase contrast microscope. Adapted from [8]

5 Diagnosis of Type I Allergy

The identification of antigens that provoke mast cell activation is crucial to avoid anaphylactic shock and the aggravation of atopic diseases, such as atopic dermatitis, allergic rhinitis, food allergy, and asthma. The detection of antigen-specific IgE in serum implies hypersensitivity against the antigen. Thus, a variety of immunological methods such as ImmunoCAP™, Ala-STAT™, and AD-VIA Centaur™ have been developed to detect antigen-specific IgE and utilized in clinical practice [28]. However, there are often substantial discrepancies between the dates of serological tests and clinical symptoms [28]. In vivo tests, such as skin test and antigen challenge test, are more reliable in reflecting clinical conditions. However, these tests may be painful and could potentially evoke anaphylactic shock when a patient is extremely sensitive to a particular antigen [29]. Moreover, the intradermal injection of an antigen may sensitize subjects who are not sensitized to the antigen. Both mast cells and basophils, which are sensitized with the same repertoire of IgE in individual subjects, release various substances, including histamine, arachidonic acid metabolites, and cytokines in response to the antigen. They also express several molecules on their surface, such as CD203c and CD69. Therefore, the in vitro histamine release test and cell surface analysis by flow cytometry for basophils of peripheral blood are sensitive and safe and give reliable information regarding antigen that causes type I hypersensitivity. Griese et al. reported that the histamine release test showed higher sensitivity and specificity than skin test or serum analysis, such as ImmunoCAP™, based on the comparison with bronchoprovocation of extrinsic asthmatic children [30]. Moreover, the basophil activation test based on CD203c upregulation has been validated as a reliable tool for the diagnosis of IgE-mediated allergies [31]. Thus, detection of basophils' reaction against antigens (allergens) may be a useful indicator of type I hypersensitivity. However, the technique to detect basophils' activation in response to antigens (allergens) with a small amount of peripheral blood is expected to be developed for clinical practice.

6 Isolation of Human Basophils from Peripheral Blood by Means of Magnetic Activated Cell Sorting (MACS)

6.1 Isolation of Human Basophils by Means of Magnetic Activated Cell Sorting (MACS)

Human peripheral blood basophils can be isolated from fresh heparinized blood of donors using Ficoll-Paque Plus (Amersham Pharmacia Biotech, Piscataway, NJ) density gradient separation followed by magnetic depletion of non-basophils (MACS basophil isolation kit II (Miltenyi Biotec GmbH, Bergisch Gladbach, Germany). An Easy sep™ human basophil enrichment kit (STEMCELL Technologies Inc., Vancouver, Canada) is also available for human basophil isolation from PBMC. Isolated basophils can be suspended in Hepes buffer for SPR or SPRI measurements.

6.2 Isolation of Human Basophils Using Magnetic Particles Containing Microfluidic Chip

In order to isolate human basophils from a small amount of peripheral blood, magnetic particles containing a microfluidic chip have been developed [32]. The separation chip consists of glass slide (RI = 1.72) and patterned PDMS containing magnetic particles (100–500 nm). The chip can trap magnetic bead-labeled non-basophils in a flow channel and collect non-labeled basophils at an outlet port. SPR detection areas (gold film-coated areas) can be mounted on the outlet port of separation chip. Thus, the chip with SPR sensing areas enables us to isolate basophils from a small amount of blood and detect their activation in response to stimuli by SPRI in single procedure.

6.3 Detection of Basophil Population by Flow Cytometry

Human basophils are CD123- and CD203c-double positive leukocytes constituting around 2 % of PBMCs. The purity of basophils before and after isolation can be detected by flow cytometer (such as Attune Acoustic Focusing Cytometer, Life technologies). The cells are generally incubated with phycoerythrin (PE)-labeled anti-CD123 antibody and APC-labeled anti-CD203c antibody (BD Biosciences, Franklin Lakes, NJ) for 30 min protected from light on ice, and then washed with PBS twice before analysis. The stained cells can be analyzed by FACSCalibur® (BD Biosciences). More than 90 % of basophils are collected using the isolation kit.

7 Method of Basophil Activation Test by SPRI

1. Place the sensor chip, to which human basophils are attached, on a prism with matching fluid (RI = 1.72).

2. Place the flow cell on a sensor chip and wash cells with suitable buffer such as Hepes buffer for human basophils.

3. Expose cells to an inhibitor for suitable time followed by stimulation.

4. Stimulate cells with an antigen in the flow chamber by injection with a manual syringe at 37 °C.

5. Take images of reflected light intensity every 10 s using CMOS camera.

6. Surround the area of individual cells by AOI (Area of interest) with Image-Pro.

7. Plot the light intensity of individual cells, from which the intensity of the area without cells is subtracted as background at each time points, versus time with Image-Pro.

Figure 7 shows the distribution of RI at indicated time points with or without anti-IgE antibody, which activates all basophils

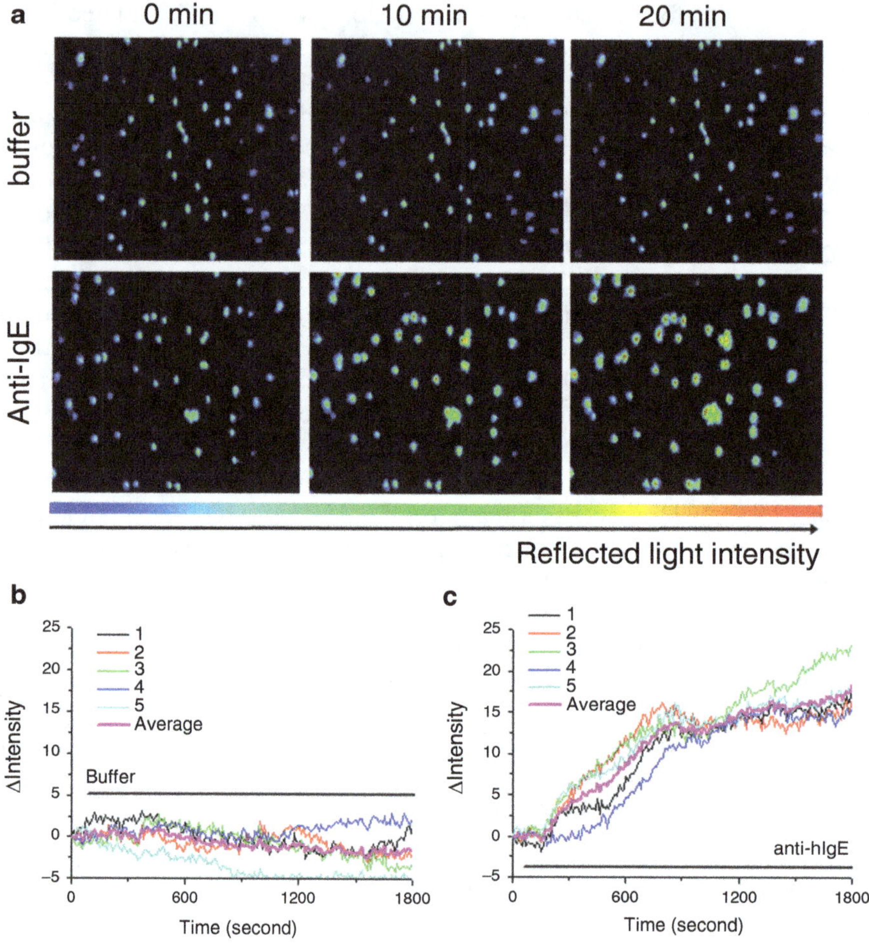

Fig. 7 RI changes in individual basophils with or without stimulation detected by SPRI. Adapted from [23]

isolated from peripheral blood, with false color. In the absence of anti-IgE antibody, RI in basophils were not changed (upper panels), but clearly increased in response to anti-IgE antibody (lower panels). The change of reflected light intensity in five randomly selected cells and their average (pink line) are plotted in Fig. 7a, b. The sensor can detect the different reaction of a basophil in response to several kinds of antigen: mite antigen, cedar pollen antigen, or sweat antigen. Thus, SPRI sensor can identify the specific antigen that causes allergic reaction in a patient by detecting reactions of basophils in response to antigens [23, 24].

8 Future Prospects

The SPRI sensor can visualize the activation of human basophils in response to specific antigens at single cell level. Further studies to establish the technique to isolate and arrange cells rapidly from patient blood, and to stimulate them with different antigens should enable us to utilize SPRI sensor as a rapid high-throughput screening system for clinical diagnosis of type I allergy with a single drop of patient's blood. Moreover, a screening assay with thousands of candidate molecules which inhibit basophil activation might enable us to find an effective medication for basophils and mast cells-related allergic diseases.

Acknowledgments

We wish to thank the Analysis Center of Life Science, Hiroshima University, for the use of their facilities. This work was supported in part by Cooperative Link of Unique Science and Technology for Economy Revitalization (CLUSTER) from Hiroshima Prefectural Institute of Industrial Science and Technology, Japan, Innovation Plaza Hiroshima of JST (Japan Science and Technology Corporation), Takeda Science Foundation, Grant-in-Aid for Scientific Research and Program for Promotion of Basic and Applied Researches for Innovation in Bio-oriented Industry, Science and technology research promotion program for agriculture, forestry, fisheries and food industry.

Glossary

CD	Cluster of differentiation
DMSO	Dimethyl sulfoxide
DNP	Dinitrophenol
DSP	Dithiobis(succinimidyl propionate)
HSA	Human serum albumin
MACS	Magnetic activated cell sorting
PBMC	Peripheral blood mononuclear cell
PDMS	Polydimethylsiloxane
RA	Resonance angle
RBL-2H3	Rat basophilic leukemia-2H3
RI	Refractive index
SPR	Surface plasmon resonance
SPRI	Surface plasmon resonance imaging

References

1. Homola J (2003) Present and future of surface plasmon resonance biosensors. Anal Bioanal Chem 377:528–539. doi:10.1007/s00216-003-2101-0

2. Szabo A, Stolz L, Granzow R (1995) Surface plasmon resonance and its use in biomolecular interaction analysis (BIA). Curr Opin Struct Biol 5:699–705

3. Mariani S, Minunni M (2014) Surface plasmon resonance applications in clinical analysis. Anal Bioanal Chem 406:2303–2323. doi:10.1007/s00216-014-7647-5

4. Hide M, Tsutsui T, Sato H, Nishimura T, Morimoto K, Yamamoto S, Yoshizato K (2002) Real-time analysis of ligand-induced cell surface and intracellular reactions of living mast

cells using a surface plasmon resonance-based biosensor. Anal Biochem 302:28–37. doi:10.1006/abio.2001.5535

5. Yanase Y, Suzuki H, Tsutsui T, Hiragun T, Kameyoshi Y, Hide M (2007) The SPR signal in living cells reflects changes other than the area of adhesion and the formation of cell constructions. Biosens Bioelectron 22:1081–1086. doi:10.1016/j.bios.2006.03.011

6. Yanase Y, Suzuki H, Tsutsui T, Uechi I, Hiragun T, Mihara S, Hide M (2007) Living cell positioning on the surface of gold film for SPR analysis. Biosens Bioelectron 23:562–567. doi:10.1016/j.bios.2007.07.005

7. Suzuki H, Yanase Y, Tsutsui T, Ishii K, Hiragun T, Hide M (2008) Applying surface plasmon resonance to monitor the IgE-mediated activation of human basophils. Allergol Int 57:347–358. doi:10.2332/allergolint.O-07-506

8. Yanase Y, Araki A, Suzuki H, Tsutsui T, Kimura T, Okamoto K, Nakatani T, Hiragun T, Hide M (2010) Development of an optical fiber SPR sensor for living cell activation. Biosens Bioelectron 25:1244–1247. doi:10.1016/j.bios.2009.09.042

9. Yanase Y, Carvou N, Frohman MA, Cockcroft S (2009) Reversible bleb formation in mast cells stimulated with antigen is Ca2+–calmodulin -dependent and bleb size is regulated by ARF6. Biochem J 425:179–193. doi:10.1042/BJ20091122

10. Yanase Y, Hide I, Mihara S, Shirai Y, Saito N, Nakata Y, Hide M, Sakai N (2011) A critical role of conventional protein kinase C in morphological changes of rodent mast cells. Immunol Cell Biol 89:149–159. doi:10.1038/icb.2010.67

11. Tanaka M, Hiragun T, Tsutsui T, Yanase Y, Suzuki H, Hide M (2008) Surface plasmon resonance-biosensor detects the downstream events of active PKCβ in antigen-stimulated mast cells. Biosens Bioelectron 23:1652–1658. doi:10.1016/j.bios.2008.01.025

12. Hiragun T, Yanase Y, Kose K, Kawaguchi T, Uchida K, Tanaka S, Hide M (2012) Surface plasmon resonance-biosensor detects the diversity of responses against epidermal growth factor in various carcinoma cell lines. Biosens Bioelectron 32:202–207. doi:10.1016/j.bios.2011.12.004

13. Chabot V, Cuerrier CM, Escher E, Aimez V, Grandbois M, Charette PG (2009) Biosensing based on surface plasmon resonance and living cells. Biosens Bioelectron 24:1667–1673. doi:10.1016/j.bios.2008.08.025

14. Yashunsky V, Shimron S, Lirtsman V, Weiss AM, Melamed-Book N, Golosovsky M, Davidov D, Aroeti B (2009) Real-time monitoring of transferrin-induced endocytic vesicle formation by mid-infrared surface plasmon resonance. Biophys J 97:1003–1012. doi:10.1016/j.bpj.2009.05.052

15. Ziblat R, Lirtsman V, Davidov D, Aroeti B (2006) Infrared surface plasmon resonance: a novel tool for real time sensing of variations in living cells. Biophys J 90:2592–2599. doi:10.1529/biophysj.105.072090

16. Lee SH, Ko HJ, Park TH (2009) Real-time monitoring of odorant-induced cellular reactions using surface plasmon resonance. Biosens Bioelectron 25:55–60. doi:10.1016/j.bios.2009.06.007

17. Kosaihira A, Ona T (2008) Rapid and quantitative method for evaluating the personal therapeutic potential of cancer drugs. Anal Bioanal Chem 391:1889–1897. doi:10.1007/s00216-008-2152-3

18. Nishijima H, Kosaihira A, Shibata J, Ona T (2010) Development of signaling echo method for cell-based quantitative efficacy evaluation of anti-cancer drugs in apoptosis without drug presence using high-precision surface plasmon resonance sensing. Anal Sci 26:529–534. doi:10.2116/analsci.26.529

19. Homola J, Vaisocherová H, Dostálek J, Piliarik M (2005) Multi-analyte surface plasmon resonance biosensing. Methods 37:26–36. doi:10.1016/j.ymeth.2005.05.003

20. Piliarik M, Vaisocherová H, Homola J (2005) A new surface plasmon resonance sensor for high-throughput screening applications. Biosens Bioelectron 20:2104–2110. doi:10.1016/j.bios.2004.09.025

21. Kodoyianni V (2011) Label-free analysis of biomolecular interactions using SPR imaging. Biotechniques 50:32–40

22. Yanase Y, Hiragun T, Kaneko S, Gould H, Greaves M, Hide M (2010) Detection of refractive index changes in individual cells by means of surface plasmon resonance imaging. Biosens Bioelectron 26:674–681. doi:10.1016/j.bios.2010.06.065

23. Yanase Y, Hiragun T, Yanase T, Kawaguchi T, Ishii K, Hide M (2012) Evaluation of peripheral blood basophil activation by means of surface plasmon resonance imaging. Biosens Bioelectron 32:62–68. doi:10.1016/j.bios.2011.11.023

24. Yanase Y, Hiragun T, Yanase T, Kawaguchi T, Ishii K, Hide M (2013) Application of SPR imaging sensor for detection of individual living cell reactions and clinical diagnosis of type I allergy. Allergol Int 62:163–169. doi:10.2332/allergolint.12-RA-0505

25. Yanase Y, Hiragun T, Ishii K, Kawaguchi T, Yanase Y, Kawai M, Sakamoto K, Hide M (2014) Surface plasmon resonance for cell-based clinical diagnosis. Sensors 14:4948–4959. doi:10.3390/s140304948

26. Méjard R, Griesser HJ, Thierry B (2014) Optical biosensing for label-free cellular studies. Trends Anal Chem 53:178–186

27. Nishi H, Nishimura S, Higashiura M, Ikeya N, Ohta H, Tsuji T, Nishimura M, Ohnishi S, Higashi H (2000) A new method for histamine release from purified peripheral blood basophils using monoclonal antibody-coated magnetic beads. J Immunol Methods 240:39–46

28. Plebani M (2003) Clinical value and measurement of specific IgE. Clin Biochem 36:453–469. doi:10.1016/S0009-9120(03)00037-7

29. Codreanu F, Morisset M, Cordebar V, Kanny G, Moneret-Vautrin DA (2006) Risk of allergy to food proteins in topical medicinal agents and cosmetics. Eur Ann Allergy Clin Immunol 38:126–130

30. Griese M, Kusenbach G, Reinhardt D (1990) Histamine release test in comparison to standard tests in diagnosis of childhood allergic asthma. Ann Allergy 65:46–51

31. Sturm EM, Kranzelbinder B, Heinemann A, Groselj-Strele A, Aberer W, Sturm GJ (2010) CD203c-based basophil activation test in allergy diagnosis: characteristics and differences to CD63 upregulation. Cytometry B Clin Cytom 78:308–318. doi:10.1002/cyto.b.20526

32. Sakamoto K, Yanase Y, Hide M, Miyake R (2013) The effective micro-isolation column for allergic diagnostic chip. In: Abstracts of the Seventh International Conference on Molecular Electronics and Bioelectronics, Fukuoka, Japan, 17–19 March 2013

A

Antibody

C

Calorimetry

Ye Fang (ed.), *Label-Free Biosensor Methods in Drug Discovery*, Methods in Pharmacology and Toxicology,
DOI 10.1007/978-1-4939-2617-6, © Springer Science+Business Media New York 2015

GPSR Compliance
The European Union's (EU) General Product Safety Regulation (GPSR) is a set
of rules that requires consumer products to be safe and our obligations to
ensure this.

If you have any concerns about our products, you can contact us on

ProductSafety@springernature.com

In case Publisher is established outside the EU, the EU authorized
representative is:

Springer Nature Customer Service Center GmbH
Europaplatz 3
69115 Heidelberg, Germany